OXFORD MEDICAL PUBLICATIONS

Alcohol and Public Policy: Evidence and Issues

Alcohol and Public Policy: Evidence and Issues

Edited by

HAROLD D. HOLDER

Director and Senior Scientist, Prevention Research Center, Berkeley, California, USA

and

GRIFFITH EDWARDS

Professor of Addiction Behaviour, Addiction Research Unit, National Addiction Centre, Institute of Psychiatry, University of London, UK

Oxford New York Toronto Tokyo

OXFORD UNIVERSITY PRESS

1995

Oxford University Press, Walton Street, Oxford OX2 6DP
Oxford New York
Athens Auckland Bangkok Bombay
Calcutta Cape Town Dar es Salaam Delhi
Florence Hong Kong Istanbul Karachi
Kuala Lumpur Madras Madrid Melbourne
Mexico City Nairobi Paris Singapore
Taipei Tokyo Toronto
and associated companies in
Berlin Ibadan

Oxford is a trade mark of Oxford University Press

Published in the United States
by Oxford University Press Inc., New York

A catalogue record for this book is available from the British Library

Library of Congress Cataloging in Publication Data
Alcohol and public policy: evidence and issues/edited by Harold D. Holder and Griffith Edwards.
p. cm.—(Oxford medical publications)
Includes bibliographical references and indexes.
1. Alcoholism—Government policy. 2. Drinking of alcoholic beverages—Social aspects. I. Holder, Harold D. II. Griffith, Edwards. III. Series.
HV5081.A33 1995 362.29'2'0973—dc20 95-12019
ISBN 0 19 262635 3

Typeset by Cotswold Typesetting Ltd, Gloucester
Printed in Great Britain on acid-free paper by
Bookcraft (Bath) Ltd, Midsomer Norton, Avon

Contents

Contributors

Peter Anderson, Alcohol Action Plan, WHO, Regional Office for Europe, Copenhagen, Denmark

Thomas F. Babor, Alcohol Research Center, University of Connecticut, USA

Sally Casswell, Alcohol and Public Health Research Unit, Runanga, Wananga, Hauora me te Paekaka, University of Auckland, New Zealand

Griffith Edwards, Addiction Research Unit, National Addiction Centre, Institute of Psychiatry, University of London, UK

Roberta G. Ferrence, Addiction Research Foundation, Toronto, Ontario, Canada

Christine Godfrey, Centre for Health Economics, University of York, UK

Harold D. Holder, Prevention Research Centre, Berkeley, California, USA

Paul H. H. M. Lemmens, University of Limburg, Maastricht, The Netherlands

Alan Maynard, Centre for Health Economics, University of York, UK

Lorraine T. Midanik, University of California at Berkeley, California, and Affiliate Senior Scientist, Alcohol Research Group, Berkeley, California, USA

Esa Österberg, Social Research Institute of Alcohol Studies, Helsinki, Finland

Anders Romelsjö, Karolinska Institute, Department of International Health and Social Medicine, Sundbyberg, Sweden

Jussi Simpura, Social Research Institute of Alcohol Studies, Helsinki, Finland

Acknowledgements

We as editors are grateful to all those colleagues within the Alcohol and Public Policies Project who have shared in the deliberations which have led to the production of this book. APPP's current membership includes Peter Anderson (WHO, Europe), Thomas F. Babor (USA), Sally Casswell (New Zealand), Griffith Edwards (UK), Roberta Ferrence (Canada), Norman Giesbrecht (Canada), Christine Godfrey (UK), Harold D. Holder (USA), Paul Lemmens (the Netherlands), Klaus Mäkelä (Finland), Lorraine T. Midanik (USA), Thor Norström (Sweden), Esa Österberg (Finland), Anders Romelsjö (Sweden), Robin Room (USA), Jussi Simpura (Finland), Ole-Jørgen Skog (Norway). We also owe particular gratitude to WHO (Europe) and to Cees Goos who, as a WHO staff member, has given APPP close support throughout its work.

The central administrative and office support for this project and for the preparation of the previous book has been provided with unstinted devotion by Patricia Davis (National Addiction Centre, London). We are also grateful for the skilled secretarial support for this volume which has been provided by Barbara Wereda and Anita C. Martin (Prevention Research Center, Berkeley).

Introduction

Research as the basis for rational policies on alcohol consumption

Harold D. Holder
Prevention Research Centre, Berkeley, California, USA

Griffith Edwards
National Addiction Centre, University of London, UK

The provenance of this book

In November 1991, a group of 17 scientists from nine different countries began working together within a national collaborative network designated the Alcohol and Public Policy Project (APPP). The aim is to provide a critical and dispassionate analysis of research which can inform alcohol policy decisions. While committed to scholarship, the purpose has been to make science speak to practical issues. Where doubts or ambiguities exist or where there are significant gaps in the available evidence, these have been identified and stated.

The first report to emanate from APPP was published in 1994 under the title *Alcohol policy and the public good* (Edwards *et al.* 1994). That book is a substantial distillate of the relevant research evidence and explores how that evidence could inform and empower policy choices to reduce alcohol problems.

The present volume represents the second published output from APPP. Here we analyse the scientific underpinning to a range of policy considerations in more detail than was possible within the confines of the first book. We see this volume as standing in its own right, but at the same time as complementary to the earlier publication. We hope that these two books, singly and together, will be of value as establishing an evidential basis for alcohol policy-making not previously available.

Public policy and alcohol: the broad perspective

The reasons why policy-makers are increasingly willing to give salience to alcohol as a policy issue relates to a growing awareness of the diversity, pervasiveness, and cost of the problems being caused by the use of this drug throughout the world. Alcohol can cause large or small problems; acute or chronic disorders; problems at the physical, psychological, or social level. There are many intersectoral connections, and alcohol policies are, for instance, of concern not only to health and welfare agencies, but to education, housing, family, public transport agencies, and the courts. Alcohol is a prime cause of road traffic, work, and domestic accidents.

Public policy has historically been used as a tool to reduce problems involving alcohol. Governments in most industrialized societies have outlawed or limited private production of alcohol and thus have made alcohol a legal product that must either be supervised by government or actually produced and distributed by government. Alcohol products are probably the most regulated legal commodity in most industrialized countries today.

Historically, governmental regulation was meant to protect the individual and the family from the risks of heavy drinking. These risks were seen as drunkenness resulting in violence, abandonment, unemployment or reduced worker productivity, and early death or illness. The control of alcohol was paternalistic, that is, 'saving a person (and his or her family) from themselves'. Thus, early public policies concerning alcohol were directed at reducing harm to the individual.

Underlying contemporary public policy about alcohol is a much broader view of alcohol-involved problems. Alcohol problems are now described by most countries and the World Health Organization (WHO) as public health concerns. One of the earliest discussions of alcohol problems as public health issues was presented by Bruun and his colleagues in 1975. This book, written by alcohol researchers from Finland, Sweden, Canada, the United Kingdom, and the United States, established a perspective on alcohol problems that went far beyond a view of the problems as limited to a few, unfortunate, dependent individuals. It examined the relationship between per capita consumption of alcohol in different countries and alcohol problems such as liver cirrhosis, accidents, and some cancers. The authors found a clear, positive relationship. They showed that, as per capita consumption rose, alcohol problems increased. Thus, average consumption of alcohol in a country was an important indicator of the overall level of alcohol problems. As a result, one of the major recommendations made by the authors was that alcohol control measures should be viewed as a public health issue. Control measures are those that affect the availability (physical access) and price (economic access) of alcohol as a means to reduce consumption and thereby reduce problems.

Bruun and his associates also outlined an extensive range of public health and public policy approaches which they believed had the potential to reduce alcohol problems. These included raising the price of alcohol, raising the minimum age to purchase and use alcohol, training servers of alcohol to work with their customers, limiting hours and days of sale, and restricting the number and types of alcohol outlets. They found that alcohol availability was controlled in some fashion in most countries of the world, even though the measures varied widely, as did drinking patterns and customs. At the time that the book was published, the scientific basis for the policy alternatives they described was promising, rather than definitive.

Since 1975, scientific investigation of public policy alternatives has been extensive. Twenty years later, the accumulated research in support of public policy as an effective tool to reduce alcohol problems is substantial. As Edwards *et al.* (1994) concluded, the major principles of Bruun and his colleagues have been confirmed: that is, regulation and restriction of alcohol availability can be effective as public policy. Since Bruun, a number of new public policy alternatives have been identified and studied. Most of them have been shown to be effective in reducing alcohol-related problems.

Decision-makers can now make better informed public policy choices because they have more evidence available to them than ever before. A recent issue of *Addiction* (1993) summarized the use of scientific evidence in the formation of alcohol policy.

Some of the more important potential connections between research and policy issues in the alcohol arena can be summarized thus:

- Alcohol problems are highly correlated with per capita consumption. This relationship appears to hold over time and across space.
- Decreases in per capita consumption produce reductions in alcohol problems, whether those decreases result from purposeful action—for example, from an alcohol tax increase—or from a non-public policy action, for example, a strike by alcohol workers.
- The greatest amount of evidence concerning public policy has been accumulated on the price-sensitivity of alcohol sales. This suggests that the demand for alcohol, as for other products, is responsive to changes in price and that as price increases, demand declines, and vice versa.
- Heavy drinkers have been shown to be affected by policy measures including price and availability. Contrary to popular view, such drinkers also respond to alcohol regulation.
- The range of potential public policies to reduce alcohol-involved problems is broad. A large number of possibilities have been proposed and scientifically examined.

Cultural diversity

Alcohol control policies reflect the differences across countries in citizens' values concerning alcohol and in the forms and extent of governmental regulation, which is in general viewed as in tune with public sentiment. What is acceptable in one country will not be acceptable in another. For example, prohibition in Saudi Arabia contrasts with an open alcohol production and distribution system in France and Italy. The rich diversity of country values is thus reflected in the wide range of policy alternatives that have been employed. In countries that have historically used government to control the production, distribution, and retail sale of alcohol, public policy has often been formulated to reduce the physical and economic access to alcohol by all citizens. This approach is frequently characterized by restrictions on advertising and promotion.

On the other hand, in countries that traditionally value low-cost and widely available alcohol, public policy may be formulated to encourage treatment and education. In countries with a tradition of private, unregulated alcohol production and sale, no effective controls may exist on alcohol availability at all. In other words, public policy concerning alcohol is as diverse as the cultural differences between and within individual countries.

This book contains a review of the scientific evidence that can be used as a basis for formulating alcohol policy, whatever the cultural preferences of an individual country. Informed policy based on good research and a recognition of local values will have the greatest probability of reducing alcohol problems over the long term.

Overview of the book

The book is organized in three sections. Part I, entitled 'Alcohol use and associated risk of harm', is a review of international drinking patterns and risks for alcohol problems at both the individual and aggregate levels. The chapter by Jussi Simpura (Finland) reviews the patterns of per capita alcohol consumption across a number of countries for which data are available. He also discusses the changes in these patterns over time. The chapter by Paul Lemmens (the Netherlands) discusses the risk of alcohol-involved problems at the individual as well as the societal level and how problems can be related to per capita consumption. Lorraine Midanik discusses the relationship between self-reported alcohol consumption and social problems. The chapter by Peter Anderson (WHO, Denmark) reviews the research evidence concerning the relationship of alcohol consumption and physical problems. Anders Romelsjö (Sweden) summarizes the research evidence concerning the relationship between alcohol consumption and a range of important issues, including accidents, violence, suicide, work performance, and inter-generational effects.

Part II, entitled 'Strategies with potential to reduce harm', summarizes scientific evidence concerning the efficacy of public policy alternatives designed to reduce alcohol problems. The first chapter in this section is by Esa Österberg (Finland) and reviews econometric research concerning the price elasticity or responsiveness of alcohol to price changes. It brings together price and income research from a number of countries. The second chapter in this section is by Thomas Babor (United States) and discusses how individually directed interventions, including alcoholism treatment, workplace programmes, and voluntary self-help groups, can contribute to society-wide efforts to reduce problems. Sally Casswell (New Zealand) discusses the important role of communications and community mobilization in effective alcohol policy. Included in this chapter is a review of research evidence concerning advertising restrictions and the use of warning labels concerning alcohol.

Part III, entitled 'Public policy and difficult choices', addresses two important issues of public policy: the role of moderate drinking in public policy considerations and the essential relationship of cost to effectiveness for prevention strategies. The first chapter here is by Roberta Ferrence (Canada). She discusses the policy issues that are involved in appropriately evaluating and using research findings suggesting that alcohol may be a protective factor against heart disease. The last chapter is by Christine Godfrey and Alan Maynard (United Kingdom). As economists, these authors outline the importance of cost and effectiveness considerations in evaluating alternative prevention strategies as a part of public policy deliberations. They provide a framework for the application of such principles to public policy and alcohol.

Balance and dispassion

APPP has throughout its deliberations sought to retain an open-mindedness and a respect for the objective evidence. The ethic of the operation has thus been that of a workshop of scientists who, in questing for the truth, owe loyalty to no special interest group. The project has no affiliation with the liquor industry or with temperance organizations. We believe that the chapters of this book will help to stake out the rational middle ground. APPP, as we have emphasized, seeks to serve rational discourse and support decision-making informed by science.

References

Bruun, K. *et al.* (1975). *Alcohol control policies in public health perspective*, Vol. 25. Finnish Foundation for Alcohol Studies, Helsinki.

Edwards, G., Anderson, P., and Babor, F. (eds) (1994). *Alcohol policy and the public good*. Oxford University Press.

Klingemann, H. K.-H., Holder, H. D., and Gutzwiller, F. (eds) (1993). Alcohol-related accidents and injuries. *Addiction*, **88**(7), Special Issue.

Part I

Alcohol use and associated risk of harm

1. Trends in alcohol consumption and drinking patterns: lessons from world-wide development

Jussi Simpura

Introduction

The purpose of this chapter is to provide an overview of changes in aggregate alcohol consumption in a world-wide perspective. In addition to levels of consumption, the issue of beverage preferences will be discussed, particularly for Western industrialized countries. The available data on drinking patterns will be used to illustrate how changes in aggregate alcohol consumption may be related to changes in personal consumption. Finally, various models to explain consumption trends will be briefly discussed.

A number of earlier works have dealt extensively with the problems of analysing international trends in alcohol consumption. In the 1970s, a thorough compilation of production and consumption statistics was produced, covering 1950–72 (FFAS 1977). This compilation was closely connected to, and extensively used in the so-called 'Purple book' on alcohol policies in the public health perspective (Bruun *et al.* 1975, in particular, chapters 4 and 5). Already at that time, the standard annual source of alcohol consumption statistics was a publication by the Dutch Distillers' Association (DDA), published in 1992 under the title *World drink trends*. Much of the material below comes from this source. Another important handbook is the report *Alcoholic beverages, taxation and control policies* by the Brewers' Association of Canada. The latest edition of that report is BAC (1992). In addition to consumption data, the Canadian report contains information on consequences of drinking, prices, and taxation, control policy measures, and also on patterns of drinking, although in a summary fashion.

A few recent reviews contain updated information and analysis of consumption trends (Moser 1992; Vanston 1991). The papers by Smart (1989, 1991) are a source on alcohol consumption in developing countries. Recently, specific analyses of the development of alcohol consumption in the European wine countries have become available: Pyörälä (1990) on all Mediterranean wine countries; Sulkunen (1989) on France; Rossi (1992) on Italy.

Some other earlier studies have provided analyses on the nature and determinants of changes in alcohol consumption. This was a central issue in a comparative study on alcohol control experiences in seven countries in the post-war era (the International Study on Alcohol Control Experiences (ISACE) study; Mäkelä *et al.* 1981; Single *et al.* 1981). An important related work is the study by Sulkunen (1983), which discusses the modernization of life styles and the consequent homogenization of alcohol consumption levels and beverage preferences. In addition, he presents the important hypothesis that successive generations play a decisive role in changes in drinking habits. Finally, econometric approaches have also been used in comparative analyses of alcohol consumption trends (Salomaa 1990; Godfrey 1989).

What are the most common hypotheses for explaining trends in alcohol consumption? In earlier studies, the idea of *long waves* of alcohol consumption has frequently been discussed (Mäkelä *et al.* 1981; Room 1991). The experience from the ISACE study gave rise to the idea that 'in a number of industrialized countries there appeared to be a regular pattern of rises and falls, to some extent linked across societies and not explainable simply in terms of economic cycles' (Room 1991). Some writers have declared that the post-war trend of growth in alcohol consumption may be over, in the industrialized countries at least (Smart 1991). An inflection point in the aggregate alcohol consumption may be found in the 1970s or 1980s for many countries. Another important issue is the idea of *homogenization* of alcohol consumption and beverage preferences. Briefly, it has appeared that in the industrialized world, differences between countries in the level of consumption tended to decrease in the post-war era; at the same time, the traditionally dominant beverage types were losing ground in favour of others. A third and related hypothesis makes a distinction between *substitution and addition* (Mäkelä *et al.* 1981) as models of changes in drinking patterns. Substitution means that new patterns substitute for old ones, whereas addition refers to changes where old patterns remain intact while new patterns are added to the existing ones. In earlier research, many of the changes in the post-war period of growth in consumption could be fitted to the addition model.

Evidently, these hypotheses cannot be discussed on the basis of consumption data alone. One has to consider the patterns of consumption, or drinking habits, to understand the underlying mechanisms of consumption change. Material from drinking habit surveys will be used below to illustrate what may have happened behind the curves. This type of material is mainly available from industrialized countries only. Issues concerning the developing countries will be considered on the basis of special studies of a completely different nature.

One emerging trend should be mentioned separately: since the 1970s, the growing importance of non-alcohol or low-alcohol beverages, both in economic terms and in the cultural context has developed. Indeed, competition between beverages is becoming increasingly visible, and the scope of research should be extended beyond the traditional domain of alcohol studies. Already, the share of non-alcohol beer is approaching 10 per cent of the total volume of beer consumption in the Netherlands (*Nachrichten für Aussenhandel* 1992). In Italy and in other Mediterranean wine countries, mineral water is gaining propularity at the table (Rossi 1992). Cultural changes, health concerns among the consumers, and the extended commercialization of food and beverage consumption, make it increasingly difficult to consider changes of alcohol consumption from the narrow premises of alcohol research only.

Understandably, a large number of alternative or parallel explanations have been presented of changes in aggregate alcohol consumption. The three major approaches focus on cultural changes, economic factors, and changes in alcohol control policies. These and some other explanations will be discussed at the end of this chapter after considering the evidence on consumption trends and drinking patterns.

Trends of aggregate alcohol consumption: global uniformity or regional diversity?

The conventional wisdom on trends in aggregate alcohol consumption mainly concerns the Western industrialized nations only. As has been shown in many studies (Mäkelä *et al.* 1981; Sulkunen 1983; Single *et al.* 1981), Western countries experienced an almost uniform growth in consumption in the post-war era until the mid 1970s. Since then, there is less agreement on how to characterize these trends. To illustrate the multitude of patterns in consumption development, world developments will be briefly summarized by separately inspecting five groups of countries. The discussion will mainly focus on the period after 1970, that is, an era when the post-war consumption growth had, for the most part, ceased in the Western industrialized nations.

Western Europe and Anglo-American countries

Traditionally, Western industrialized countries are divided into wine, beer, and spirit countries by the dominant beverage. This division still works today, and can be effectively used to analyse consumption trends. It is a central element in discussion of homogenization. Homogenization, as it appeared up to the late 1970s, meant that differences between national consumption levels diminished, and beverage preferences changed so that the traditionally dominant beverage lost popularity in relative terms (Sulkunen 1983). The question here is whether such a homogenization continued into the 1980s.

The homogenization hypothesis appears to be supported in the group of countries with the highest alcohol consumption—the *wine-drinking countries*. In France, a decline in alcohol consumption began as early as the 1950s, and

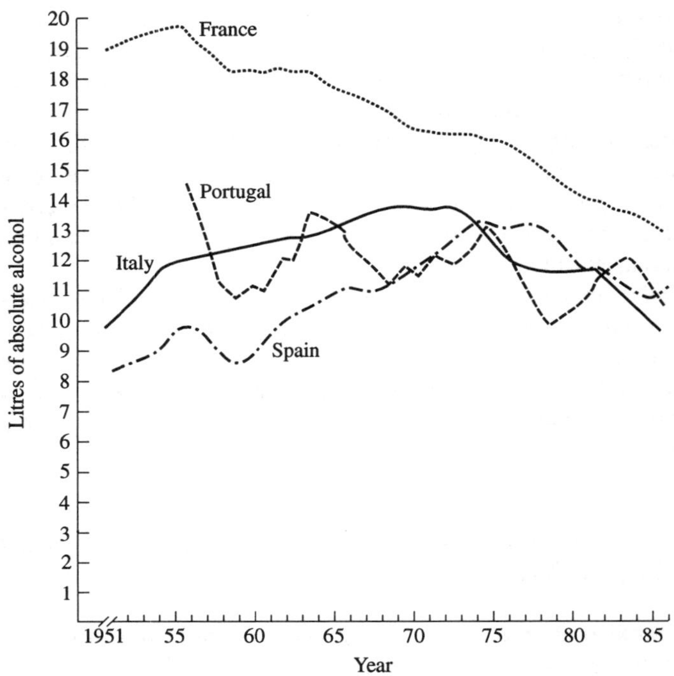

Fig. 1.1 Wine-drinking countries. Annual total per capita consumption in litres of absolute alcohol in France, Portugal, Italy, and Spain: 1951–85, expressed as 3-year moving averages.

Source: based on data in Pyörälä (1990).

later other wine countries followed, although at a slower pace. A detailed analysis of Mediterranean wine-drinking countries (Pyörälä 1990) shows that part of the decrease in wine consumption was substituted by other beverages, particularly beer. As consumption statistics from wine countries often reflect variation in production rather than variation in actual consumption, statistical series may fluctuate widely on an annual basis. It is advisable, therefore, for the figures to be smoothed out. This has been done in Fig. 1.1, with data taken from the study by Pyörälä (1990). Despite the continuous decline in consumption, France is still the leading country in world alcohol consumption statistics, excluding very special cases like Greenland.

Defining trends in alcohol consumption is a risky business. However, the author of a recent Italian study (Rossi 1992) has been so bold as to estimate that aggregate alcohol consumption in Italy by the year 2000 will be around 7.5 litres of 100 per cent alcohol per capita, instead of the approximately 9 litres level of today. This decrease would be due to a continued decline in wine-drinking, which would be only partly compensated by an increase in beer consumption. In Italy, the main argument behind this forecast is the decreasing popularity of wine, and the increasing popularity of beer, among young people. Similar observations have been made in other wine-drinking countries, for example, a recent French study points out that urban youth are the avant-garde in abandoning traditional wine-drinking (Aigrain *et al.* 1991).

Countries where *beer* has been the dominant beverage are mainly those of Central Europe and North America. Some traditional spirit-drinking countries, like Finland and Sweden, have joined the ranks of beer-drinking countries since the 1970s. The consumption level in these countries has usually been lower than in wine-drinking areas. The beer-drinking countries with the highest consumption, like Germany and Belgium, have reached overall consumption levels similar to wine-drinking countries and now show a fairly stable picture. The beer-drinking countries have shown no common consumption trend since the 1970s. Some of them, like Australia and the United States, show a slight decline, whereas others, like the newcomer Finland, belong to the small group of countries where alcohol consumption has been increasing in the last few years.

The last group, the *spirit-drinking* countries, is today small in number and have low consumption levels. Among Western industrialized countries only Iceland and Norway would still be regarded as spirit-drinking. In Iceland, the 1989 reform liberalizing beer sales led to a decrease in the share of spirits in aggregate alcohol consumption (Olafsdottir 1991). The former German Democratic Republic was, in 1989, the leading spirit-drinking country in the world.

Changes in beverage preferences can be illustrated with triangular diagrams (Fig. 1.2), originally used by Sulkunen (1983). (Note that Fig. 1.2 includes world-wide data.) In Fig. 1.2a, the three smaller triangles at the corners are areas where the share of one beverage type (wine, beer, or spirits) exceeds 50 per cent of aggregate alcohol consumption. The central triangle is a no man's land, where none of the three beverage types has more than half of the total consumption. Changes in preferences can be shown by locating countries in the triangle at different points in time, and connecting these locations with a line. Thus, in Fig. 1.2a, showing changes from the early 1950s to the early 1970s, there is a general tendency for movement from the corners towards the centre, that is, the position of the dominant beverage type was strong in the early 1950s but weakened rapidly until the 1970s. Figure 1.2b shows the development in two 9-year periods in the 1970s (dashed line) and 1980 (solid line). The wine-drinking countries in the lower left corner have continued the move towards the centre but are still located in the wine triangle. The central tendency is also visible in the top triangle of beer-drinking countries. The structural changes in preference have been the greatest in the spirit-drinking countries, and have continued the move away from spirits, a shift which began in the 1950s, and continued through later decades.

Finally, one should note that the decline of wine and rise of beer in wine-

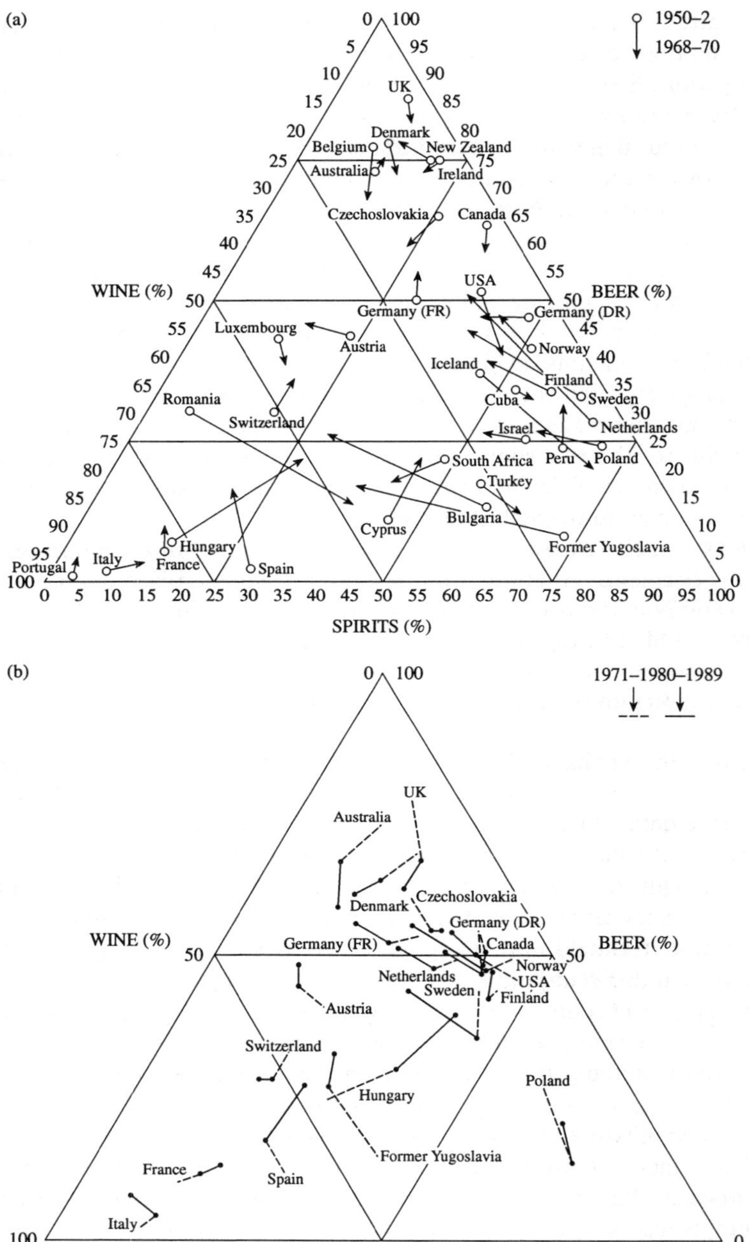

Fig. 1.2 Distribution of annual average alcohol consumption by beverage type in selected countries: 1950–89. (For explanation, see text.)

Source: (a) Sulkunen (1983). (b) Data from DDA.

drinking countries, paralleled an increasing wine consumption in all beer- and spirit-drinking countries in Western Europe. This, together with the diminishing differences in overall consumption levels, seems to constitute evidence for the convergence hypothesis. It must be remembered, however, that the Western industrialized world comprises only 10 per cent of mankind, even though responsible for the highest figures in the consumption statistics. What happens in the majority of countries in the world may be a quite different story.

Eastern Europe

Although data on Eastern Europe are available from official sources, they should be interpreted with reservation. This is particularly true of the former Soviet Union, where the extensive unrecorded consumption of alcohol makes official figures almost useless, in large measure as a consequence of the 1985 alcohol reform which led to a huge production of home-made alcohol and an extensive use of non-beverage alcohol (see, for example, Tarschys 1993). It is difficult in such circumstances to arrive at reliable estimates of the true consumption level. Attempts have been made based on police records, and also on the use of mortality statistics (Nemtsov and Nechaev 1991).

The general conclusions for the former Soviet Union thus remain vague. A guess at the present level of alcohol consumption would be between 8 and 10 litres per capita for the Eastern European countries of this group (Treml 1991; B. M. Levin and M. B. Levin 1988; Simpura 1992). The 1990 estimate for Moscow, on the basis of indirect evidence from mortality statistics by Nemtsov and Nechaev (1991), was about 11 litres per capita. This is roughly the same as the figures for 1984, the year prior to the alcohol reform. In the former Soviet Union, the highest consumption levels have been systematically reported for the most western areas, the Baltic states. The 1985 reform led to a short period of decreasing alcohol consumption until about 1988. Thereafter, unrecorded production probably compensated for an increasing part of the supply which had been cut off by the new administrative measures. Therefore, the present level of consumption may well be the same as before the attempted restrictions. To make matters even more complicated, the official consumption figures for the years before 1985 may have been deliberately modified downwards.

As for the other Eastern European countries, the data is in some cases more reliable. Sudden changes have taken place in Poland, where alcohol issues have played a role in the political processes. After a long period of increasing consumption, the country experienced a rapid decline from almost 9 litres of 100 per cent alcohol per capita to 6.5 litres in the early 1980s. At the beginning of the 1990s, a liberalization of the alcohol sales system was leading the country again towards the level of 9 litres (Wald *et al.* 1993).

Alcohol preferences in Eastern Europe vary as much as in the West. The former Soviet Union, the three Baltic countries Estonia, Latvia, and Lithuania, and Poland, have traditionally been spirit-drinking countries. Changes in preferences have been small in this group. Czechoslovakia is, after Germany, the leading beer-drinking country in the world, and nothing seems to threaten the position of beer in that national setting. In south-eastern Europe, the share of wine becomes more important, although not equalling the Mediterranean wine-drinking countries. Indeed, as mentioned earlier, the official consumption figures in this region report a decline in the share of wine in aggregate alcohol consumption, and here too beer-drinking is increasing.

Japan

Outside the European cultural circle, Japan is the country providing the most accurate data of alcohol consumption (Tsunoda *et al.* 1992; Shimizu 1990). A very low level of aggregate alcohol consumption in the early 1950s (less than 2 litres per capita), grew slowly but continuously until the late 1980s. The consumption doubled in the 25-year period from 1955 to 1980 (Suwaki 1985). With a present consumption level around 6.5 litres per capita, Japan is one of the few countries in the world showing an increase in alcohol consumption over recent years (see Fig. 1.5). This increase has been accompanied by changes in beverage preferences. Beer, in particular, is becoming more popular compared with the local traditional beverages. It should be noted, however, that consumption has grown in all beverage categories. Formerly, spirits were indisputably the dominant type but today beer has reached an equal share. The level of consumption, 6.5 litres per capita, is the same as in Sweden, for instance, and does not fall far behind the US or UK levels.

Japan is an interesting case with regard to the homogenization hypothesis. This country, with a strongly embedded cultural tradition in drinking, has experienced a rapid Westernization of economic and social life (Kono and Takano 1992). Thus, Japan might serve as an example of what may be happening in the other rapidly industrializing countries of South-East Asia. The other side of the coin is the acculturation of drinking habits in populations of Japanese origin in the United States, which have been studied extensively in the last few years (Izuno *et al.* 1992; Tsunoda *et al.* 1992). The results of these studies seem to indicate that a simple acculturation model is not sufficient. The processes of change have varied in different locations. In Japan, the addition hypothesis appears to be valid, and Western patterns have not pushed aside old traditions.

Latin America

Contrary to the stable or downward trend in alcohol consumption in the industrialized world, developing countries mainly show a rapid increase in consumption levels (Smart 1991). This is true for Latin America in particular, as seen in the Dutch Distillers' Association data. Unfortunately, the information on developing countries is scattered and accuracy may often be questionable. Thus, for instance, the Dutch data only covers part of Latin America, and even for those few countries which are given an entry, information on the consumption of spirits is usually unavailable. Keeping this in mind, one must view with caution the observation that Latin American countries (Brazil, Cuba, and Paraguay, with only Cyprus standing between the last two) have leading positions in the statistics on growth rate of alcohol consumption from 1970 to 1990 (DDA 1992). Another source (Smart 1991) covers developments in the 1970s only, but includes information on almost all Latin American countries. Of the 21 countries in the world which had a consumption increase of more than 40 per cent, six were in Latin America. It should be noted that many of those 21 countries were small states which experienced immense growth in tourism in the 1970s.

Latin American countries still have fairly low consumption levels compared to the industrialized world. The average consumption for the 10 Latin American countries included in the DDA (1992) was below 4 litres per capita. Although consumption of spirits is often missing from these figures, it is evident that the level of consumption is far behind the Western European level of 8 litres per head or more. Because of missing data, nothing much can be said about beverage preferences. Fairly high rates have been reported for increase of beer consumption in the 1980s. This may partly reflect a move towards commercially produced alcohol from unrecorded and home-made alcohol. For wine, consumption figures in wine-producing Latin American countries show a constant decline since the mid 1970s. DDA (1992) gives estimates for the consumption of spirits for some Latin American countries for the late 1980s. Today, the share taken by spirits is negligible in Argentina, about 25 per cent in Chile and Mexico, and as high as 33 per cent in Brazil.

Africa and Asia

Turning to those areas where three-quarters of the world's population lives, alcohol consumption data becomes increasingly problematic. The review by Smart (1991) gives information on 48 countries in Africa and 28 countries in Asia. The per capita consumption estimates for 1980 were 2.73 litres for Africa and 2.11 litres for Asia. Even if one takes into account the huge proportion of children in these populations, it remains evident that consumption levels in most African and Asian countries are well behind those of Western industrialized nations. Smart (1991) concludes that 'there is evidence of a relationship between advanced economic development and alcohol consumption levels'. That means, of course, that there is considerable variation among the African and Asian countries. Up to now only a few of these countries exceed 4 litres per capita consumption.

On the other hand, African and Asian countries are potential sites for increasing alcohol consumption, although it is almost impossible to say anything about consumption trends (Partanen 1991). Part of this potential has already been realized through moves towards commercially produced alcohol, and beer in particular (Partanen 1991; Kortteinen 1989*a*,*b*; Maula *et al.* 1989). However, domestic production is still the dominant channel of availability in most of these countries. Partanen (1991) gave an estimate for the distribution of alcohol consumption in Kenya in 1978. At that time, commercially produced beer accounted for 16 per cent of total consumption and industrial spirits and wine had a share of only 1 per cent. Home-brewed beer (46 per cent), and illegally distilled alcohol (37 per cent), completely dominated the market. A report on Tanzania (Kilonzo and Pitkänen 1992) reminds us that there is considerable regional variation within developing countries—consumption in a northern region was estimated to be four times higher than the average consumption for the whole country.

A technical note on the quality of data

There are numerous difficulties in using alcohol consumption data for international comparisons. Some of these problems become particularly difficult in the longitudinal perspective. Remarks have already been made on these issues, but it will be useful at this juncture to summarize briefly the main difficulties.

First, the definition of what is an alcoholic beverage varies from country to country, and may change over time. In some countries, legislation determines which beverages will be called alcohol beverages and thus should be included in the official statistics. In other countries, the definitions may be based on less formal rules. The most serious problems here are posed by low-alcohol beers. The Dutch Distillers' Association statistics, for instance, do not set any lower limit of alcohol content in their definition of beer (DDA 1992).

Second, the conversion factors used to transform consumption into litres of 100 per cent alcohol raise complicated issues. This problem relates both to the determination of consumption levels, and to the classification of countries into beer, wine, and spirit countries. Evidently, the conversion factors must vary in different countries. Moreover, the factors for a country change over time, as the consumer preferences move towards stronger or milder brands within a broader category. For instance, the increase of wine consumption in Finland has included a shift from fortified wines to natural wines. In some countries, these changes have been accounted for in the reporting of consumption figures. The standard international statistical sources do not, however, usually reveal which conversion factors have been employed for different countries and different years.

Third, it is sometimes difficult to tell whether the figures in international consumption statistics concern production or consumption. This is a problem in estimating wine consumption in particular, as the fluctuations in production due to weather may be large. The discussion in this chapter is, however, mainly based on consumption data. The DDA (1992) explicitly states that its country-by-country time series data concern consumption, not production.

Fourth, unrecorded consumption is a major problem in developing countries and also in Eastern Europe. The problem, however, is far from trivial in other parts of the world. Home-brewed beer, home-made wine for personal use, and home-distilling occur to some degree virtually everywhere. In the industrialized world, imports by travellers from trips abroad may be a significant source of alcohol. Finally, the use of non-beverage alcohol or surrogates also plays a role. Estimates for the volume of unrecorded consumption are difficult to determine. As an example, studies made in the Nordic countries (Österberg 1987; Reinås 1991), indicate that the share of unrecorded consumption may vary between 15 and 50 per cent of the actual aggregate alcohol consumption. Also, there may be fluctuations in the volume of unrecorded consumption within countries over time.

Long waves of alcohol consumption?

These purported long waves are supposed to cover centuries rather than decades, so that the periodicity of these waves 'seems to be about three generations—seventy years or so' (Room 1991). In the ISACE study on alcohol control experiences in seven countries, the hypothesis of long waves was taken as the starting point for describing consumption trends (Mäkelä *et al.* 1981). The long waves described there started in the mid 19th century, when alcohol intake was high in most countries in Europe and in North America (Mäkelä *et al.* 1981):

> At the turn of the century, there was a decline in alcohol consumption which continued until the period between the two world wars. . . . Between World War II and the 1970s, consumption increased in almost all countries providing reasonably accurate statistics, . . . In most countries, the rate of increase in consumption slowed at some point in the 1970s, and in some countries consumption levelled off or slightly declined.

Using the concept of long waves is a helpful presentational device for an everyday description of changes in alcohol consumption. So far, however, the idea is familiar to researchers only, and in public opinion and political debate even the existence of the post-war consumption growth may still be largely unknown. In present everyday explanations, the short-term memories of changes in alcohol consumption are conveniently attributed to economic fluctuations or increasing international contacts. In the model of long waves, however, the core idea is that there are changes which cannot be explained with reference to any obvious factor, 'such as buying power, the amount of leisure time, social misery, or industrialization and urbanization' (Mäkelä *et*

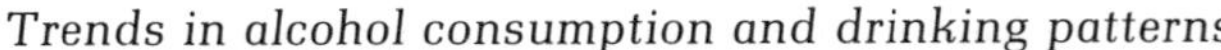

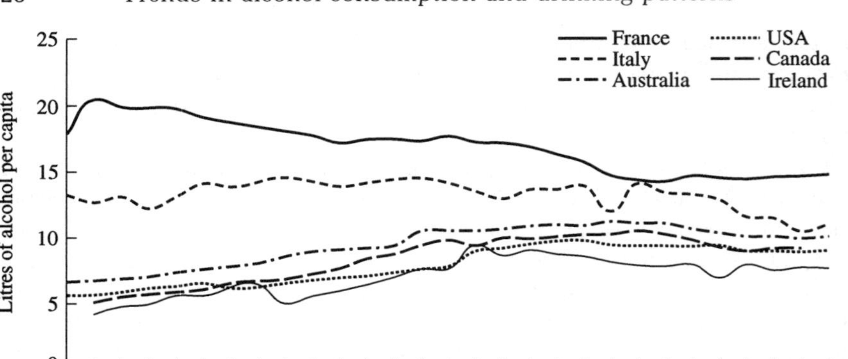

Fig. 1.3 Countries with decreasing alcohol consumption: 1961–90.
Source: DDA (1992).

al. 1981). Room (1991) proposes that these waves of consumption reflect a kind of dialectic social learning process. Learning from experience but also forgetting and learning again, may partly explain the unexpected turns in the attitudes of populations towards drinking and alcohol control measures. It remains an open question why and how such processes should spread their effect over a large number of countries or even world-wide.

What has happened with the long waves after the mid 1970s? For most countries, the available time series are too short or too inaccurate to be used for a test of the hypotheses. For the industrialized countries, the question is more feasible and culminates in the idea of a possible inflection point in the 1970s or 1980s. To illustrate this contention, data from industrialized countries are shown in Figs 1.3–1.5, dividing countries into three categories by the dominating trend in the 1980s. These figures, based on the data in DDA (1992), already show that the industrialized countries provide a multitude of trends instead of a single and homogeneous pattern. The notion that trends in countries with similar alcohol preferences should resemble each other, is also challenged to some extent. The Mediterranean wine countries, of course, show much similarity.

Some of the industrialized countries showed a declining curve after a peak in consumption around the year 1980 (for example, the United States, Canada, and Australia, in Fig. 1.3). Up to now, the United States is the most thoroughly analysed case in this group (Clark and Hilton 1991; Room 1991). Researchers refer to an attitudinal and cultural change as the main explanation. Similar explanations have been proposed for Canada (Smart 1989). For many countries, and in particular those in Central Europe, the consumption level seems remarkably stable (Fig. 1.4). Finally, there are a few countries with consumption growth in the 1980s (Fig. 1.5). These are quite

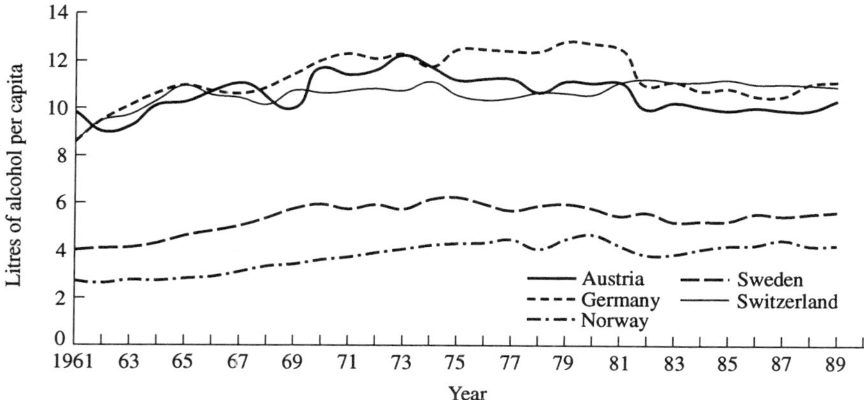

Fig. 1.4 Countries with stable alcohol consumption: 1961–91.
Source: DDA (1992).

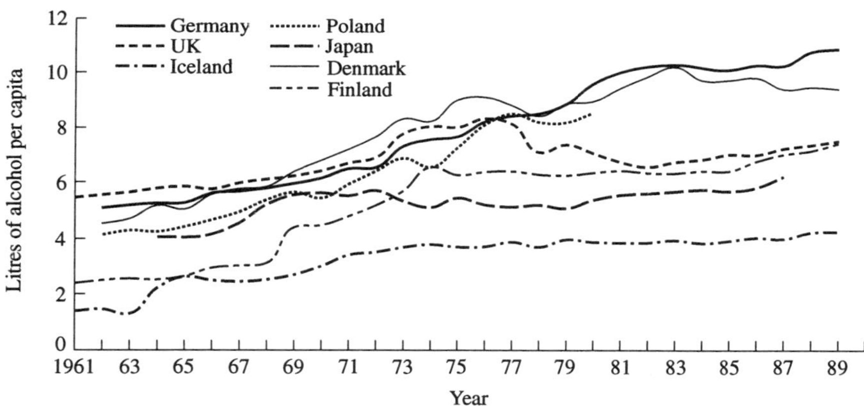

Fig. 1.5 Countries with increasing alcohol consumption: 1961–89.
Source: DDA (1992).

different cases, and the explanations for the growth vary from political and societal changes to economic factors and changes in alcohol control systems. However, these fluctuations are mostly short-term phenomena.

Finally, the idea should be explored as to whether the long waves in the Western industrialized countries are also felt in the developing world. This possibility has been intimated by Smart (1991), but his data does not cover the 1980s, and the inferences therefore remain somewhat open. The question concerning the existence of world-wide long waves must, for the present, be left unsolved.

The role of drinking patterns in changes of aggregate alcohol consumption

What happens behind the consumption curves? This question relates to two different issues. One is the qualitative side of drinking, or cultural drinking patterns and related changes. The other, to be discussed later, concerns the attempt to explain changes in alcohol consumption in the context of more general social changes and economic and political factors. The discussion below is based on data from industrialized countries only.

In the ISACE study, the main issue was the increase of alcohol consumption in the post-war era up to the mid 1970s. In the description of change, new groups of drinkers, new drinking situations, and changes in individual drinking habits were presented as components of the process. 'When new demographic groups enter the drinking scene, established drinkers are confronted with new types of drinking company and situations. And new drinking situations and new cominations of persons drinking together obviously give rise to new ways of drinking' (Mäkelä *et al.* 1981). This quotation emphasizes the fact that the proposed components of change are closely intertwined. Today, the task of describing shifts in drinking patterns is even more complicated, as there is not only consumption growth but also unchanged or declining consumption levels which demand explanation.

A decomposition model for changes in alcohol consumption

To account for all the components proposed in the ISACE study would require a lot more research. For instance, the homogenization hypotheses of beverage preferences is closely related to the use of alcoholic beverages at meals. In wine-drinking countries, much of the decline in consumption is due to the weakening ties between wine and meals. In Central Europe, the opposite tendency of increasing wine consumption largely reflects changes in beverage preferences at meals (Hupkens *et al.* 1993).

In this chapter, a more mechanistic method of decomposing alcohol consumption will be discussed. The level of per capita alcohol consumption at a given point in time can be presented as a product of three factors referring to drinking patterns: (1) the proportion of drinkers in the population (D, in Fig. 1.6); (2) average frequency of drinking (F); and (3) average intake of alcohol per drinking occasion (I) (for more details see Simpura 1980, 1987, chapter 6).

If changes in the three factors over time are relatively small, it can be shown that the proportional change in consumption per capita is approximately the sum of the proportional changes in the three factors. Put simply, changes in alcohol consumption levels result from changes in the abstinence rates, drinking frequency, and intake per occasion. All these three elements change simultaneously and they may change in opposite directions.

C = consumption per capita

I = average intake of alcohol per occasion

F = average frequency of drinking (occasions per year)

D = proportion of drinkers in the population

$C = I * F * D$

$$dC \approx dI + dF + dD$$

Fig. 1.6 A decomposition of changes in alcohol consumption.

So far, this decomposition approach has only been applied systematically to the Finnish drinking habits data for the period since 1968 (Simpura 1987). Over a period of consumption growth (1968–76), it was at first a rise in drinking frequency, and later a decrease in abstinence rates and an increase in intake per occasion, which contributed to consumption growth. In a later period of stable consumption (1976–84), changes in all three factors remained small. It should be noted that a stable consumption level could also have been achieved by changes in opposite directions in the three factors. Knowledge of the role of the three factors may be relevant in policy planning and to educational efforts.

1. Abstinence From the epidemiological point of view, abstainers have traditionally been regarded as a resource for new recruits to the populations of drinkers. Recently, however, there has been increasing evidence that abstainers include former drinkers. These 'neo-abstainers' consist of several subgroups, the most important being the health-conscious former drinkers, and former heavy drinkers who take abstinence as the central goal of their lives. So far, few studies have contained detailed analyses of the flow to and from the files of abstainers (Sulkunen 1987).

The definitions of abstinence or non-drinking vary considerably in published research. Table 1.1 contains some research results on abstinence rates. The abstainers here are mainly those who did not report any drinking in the previous 12 months. Some results based on different definitions (for example, 'never drink', 'no drinking in the last week', etc.), are also indicated. It is difficult to detect any remarkable systematic differences in abstinence rates, either by national beverage preferences or by the average level of consumption. On the contrary, it is perhaps surprising that countries at very different consumption levels may have such similar abstinence rates. The scarce data available seem also to indicate that abstinence rates are relatively stable within each country if no radical contextual changes in conditions take place.

This apparent stability in abstinence rates is, of course, important from the point of view of the decomposition model. The low abstinence rates in many countries indicate that the reserves for potential 'new consumers' have almost been exhausted there, and the contribution made by neo-abstainers cannot be detected in these crude results.

Figure 1.7 gives the proportions of total abstainers in 1990 from a recent all-European consumption survey (Reader's Digest 1991): the problems of

Table 1.1 Rates of abstinence among adult population: mid 1970s–late 1980s in certain countries

Country	Year	Percentage abstaining			Age range	Source
		M	F	Total		
Countries with increasing consumption						
Finland	1976	9	20		15–69	Simpura (1987)
	1979	10	23		20–69	Hauge & Irgens-Jensen (1989)
	1984	12	27		15–69	Simpura (1987)
	1985[b]	14	29		15–64	Berg *et al.* (1991)
	1991	13	21		15–64	Berg *et al.* (1991)
Iceland	1979	12	27		20–69	Hauge & Irgens-Jensen (1989)
	1984	(8)[a]	(18)		20–59	Helgason (1988)
UK	1978	(6)	(11)		18+	Wilson (1980)
England & Wales	1987[b]	(5)	(8)		18+	Goddard & Ikin (1988)
Wales	1988	(6)	(12)		18–64	Bennett *et al.* (1991)
Denmark	1985	(3)	(7)	5	16+	Hansen & Andersen (1985)
	1990			5	16+	Schmidt (1991)
Japan	1976[b]	(16)			?	Shimizu (1990)
Tokyo	1979	(18)				Shimizu (1990)
Tokyo	1984	(5)				Shimizu (1990)
Countries with stable consumption						
Switzerland	1975	8	17	12	15–74	Fahrenkrug (1989)
	1981	7	18	13	15–74	Fahrenkrug (1989)
	1987	14	31	22	15–74	Fahrenkrug (1989)
Norway	1979	11	20		20–69	Hauge & Irgens-Jensen (1989)
	1985	12	19		18+	Nordlund (1987)
Sweden	1979	8	15		20–69	Hauge & Irgens-Jensen (1989)
Spain	1980			17	18–75	Enriquez (1984)
Seville	1987	8	22		18+	Gili *et al.* (1989)

Table 1.1 *continued*

Country	Year	Percentage abstaining			Age range	Source
		M	F	Total		
Countries with decreasing consumption						
Australia	1976			(8)	16–65	Armyr *et al.* (1982)
	1981			(11)	16–65	Armyr *et al.* (1982)
	1982[c]			(12)	16–65	Armyr *et al.* (1982)
Canada	1978	11	19		15+	HW (1989)
	1985	14	21		15+	HW (1989)
		15	23		15+	HW (1989)
	1989	17	28		15+	Eliany *et al.* (1990)
France						
Languedoc–Rousillon	1986			(15)	15+	Balmés *et al.* (1989)
USA	1979	24	40		18+	Clark & Hilton (1991)
	1984	24	36		18+	Clark & Hilton (1991)

Definition of abstinence: 12 months before the study without drinking alcohol.
[a] Figures in parenthesis are based on other definitions of abstinence (see text).
[b] The first study during the period of increasing consumption.
[c] The first year of decreasing consumption.

defining 'never drinking' are visible here. Respondents in Spain, Portugal, and Greece may have interpreted the question differently from those in most other countries. The rates for Belgium and Luxemburg are unexpectedly high. The findings are similar to those from results from another survey covering all European Union countries (Hupkens *et al.* 1993). In that survey, a sample of the population over 15 years of age was interviewed in 1988. The largest deviations from the abstinence rates in Fig. 1.7 were found for Spain (24 instead of 36 per cent in Fig. 1.7), and Belgium (14 instead of 22 per cent). With the exception of the United Kingdom (18 instead of 14 per cent) and Ireland (30 instead of 25 per cent), the Hupkens *et al.* 1988 study reported lower abstinence rates than the 1990 study represented in Fig. 1.7. In general terms, however, the slightly surprising finding that abstinence rates may be higher in wine-drinking countries than elsewhere was repeated.

2. Drinking frequency Comparable data on drinking frequency are also difficult to obtain. Only the results from the 1990 European consumer survey data are presented here (Reader's Digest 1991) (see Fig. 1.8). Roughly, the rates for daily drinkers follow the consumption levels. The rates for Italy and Portugal are perhaps unexpectedly high.

The data from other surveys suggest that changes in drinking frequency are

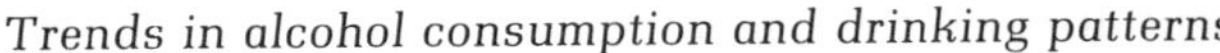

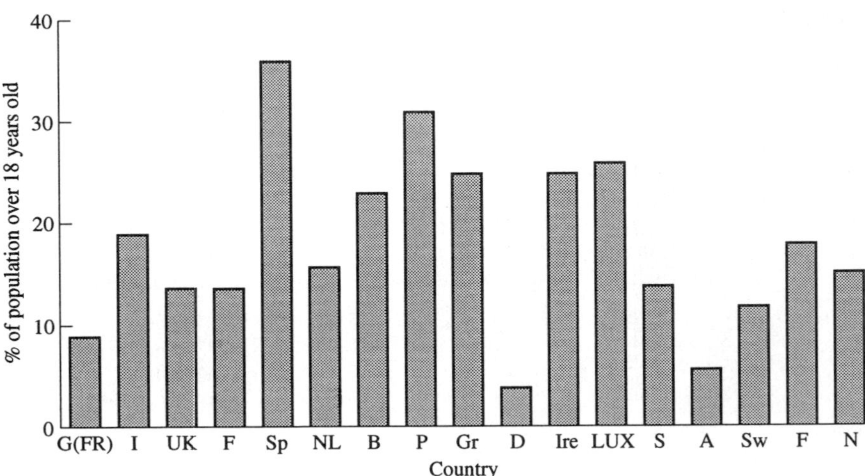

Fig. 1.7 Abstainers in Europe: 1990.
Source: Readers' Digest (1991).

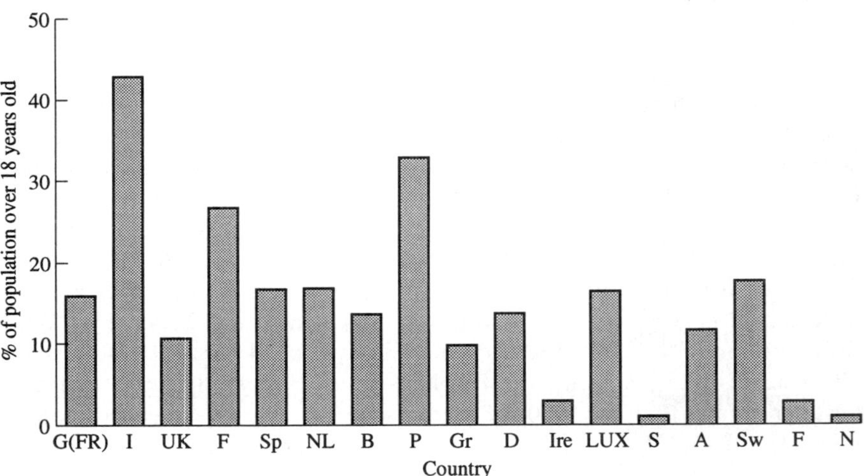

Fig. 1.8 Daily drinkers in Europe: 1990.
Source: Readers' Digest (1991).

more likely to occur than changes in abstinence rates. Surveys conducted in the United States show a decline in the rate of daily drinkers around 1980, at the time when consumption level was beginning to decrease (Hilton 1991). Similarly, there is evidence that the increase of alcohol consumption in

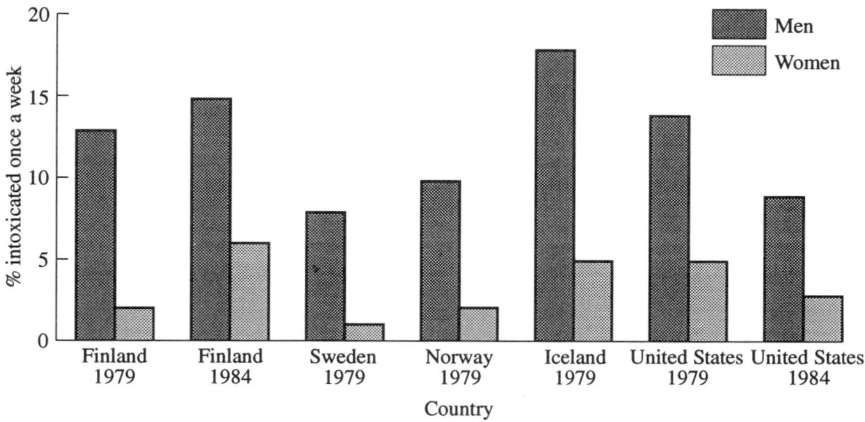

Fig. 1.9 Frequency of intoxication in selected countries: 1979–84.
Source: see references in Table 1.1.

Finland in the late 1980s took place through increased drinking frequency (Berg *et al.* 1991).

3. Intake per occasion and intoxication The third component in the decomposition of changes in consumption is the mean intake per occasion. Again, no systematic review of research results is available.

The frequency of heavy intake is another question of interest. Investigation into the experience of subjectively defined intoxication is rare in surveys outside the Nordic countries and North America, and Fig. 1.9 gives results from these areas. However, data concerning relevant trends for other countries in the 1980s should be available in the near future.

A useful and interesting time series on the frequency of intoxication has been derived from Swedish studies of military conscripts since the mid-1970s (between 97 and 98 per cent of men in Sweden are conscripted). These figures, presented in Table 1.2, indicate a steady decline in the frequency of intoxication.

During this period (1976–88), overall alcohol consumption in Sweden was essentially unchanged. A slight decline of consumption in the early 1980s was so small that it should not have had any radical effect on drinking patterns in general. Against that background, the results on frequency of intoxication in Table 1.2 are important as they show that self-reported drinking behaviour may change significantly in conditions of stable alcohol consumption.

Trends of drinking patterns in sociodemographic groups

The second perspective on drinking patterns and level of alcohol consumption, concerns the distribution of consumption among sociodemographic

Table 1.2 Frequency of intoxication among Swedish military conscripts: 1976–88

Answer category	1976	1977	1978	1979	1980	1981	1982	1983	1984	1985	1986	1987	1988
About once a week	19.4	20.2	18.4	16.5	12.6	10.6	9.7	6.9	6.5	6.1	5.3	6.2	6.2
About once a month	41.7	42.4	43.1	42.2	40.2	36.9	36.9	35.1	35.0	37.1	35.8	36.1	38.5
Less often	26.8	25.8	25.7	27.6	32.6	35.2	36.7	39.2	39.2	39.3	38.8	37.2	39.1
Never	10.7	10.5	10.3	11.0	13.5	16.2	15.8	18.0	17.3	15.9	15.7	15.0	15.1
Non-response	1.4	1.1	2.5	2.8	1.1	1.0	0.9	0.9	1.9	1.6	4.4	5.5	6.2
Number	52 361	52 129	47 659	49 658	49 902	54 363	51 932	52 011	49 358	35 278	46 646	40 533	41 125

Source: SCIAD (1991).

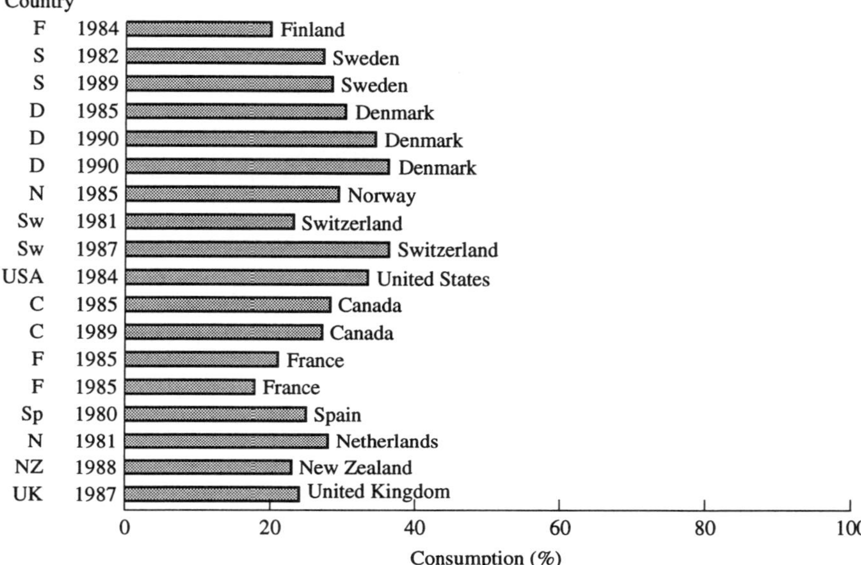

Fig. 1.10 Women's share of alcohol consumption in selected countries: 1980–90. See text for further details.

Source: see references in Table 1.1.

groups. Practical examples include the question of whether women contribute more or less to alcohol consumption, or whether one can talk about generations of drinking, like the 'wet generation' in Finland, which was thought to be responsible for the consumption increase of the 1980s (Sulkunen 1983). Investigation of such avant-garde groups is a worthwhile task for research, and is relevant to policy formulation.

In many countries, women are a favourite target group for alcohol education, and they are often thought to have increased their drinking over recent periods more than men. The available information on changes in drinking patterns shows, however, that the share of women in aggregate alcohol consumption is remarkably stable, and there is very little evidence that changes in women's drinking patterns differ from those of the male population (Fig. 1.10). (Note that for many countries, the data reproduced in Fig. 1.10 are secondary calculations derived from published results and may contain a wide margin of error.)

Data on trends in this instance are again available for only a few countries, and comparability over years may be questionable. The most reliable data probably derive from Sweden, where they are available for the years between 1982 and 1989. During that period, women's share of alcohol consumption fluctuated between 27 and 31 per cent. A preliminary interpretation could be that the share taken by women in aggregate alcohol consumption is relatively stable in the absence of major social change. As a consequence, the much discussed possibility of increasing female drinking is more a question of perception than of prevalence.

Another favourite target group are adolescents. The dramatic changes of alcohol consumption in wine-drinking countries have been attributed largely to changes in young persons preferences. This concerns not only beverage preference, but also other aspects of drinking. The traditional patterns of drinking mainly at meals is contested by leisure drinking which often leads to intoxication (Pyörälä 1991). Drinking frequency may, however, be lower with these new patterns. However, it is likely that the consumption level with the new drinking patterns is lower than with the traditional patterns for older age groups. It should be emphasized that the observed changes in young people's drinking patterns are not sudden, but take a decade or more to achieve a clearly visible effect.

An emerging group of drinkers in the industrialized countries are the elderly. Their drinking patterns have varied considerably in different countries. In the Mediterranean region, older males have been a traditionally heavy drinking group. Elsewhere in the Western world, older people have so far constituted the lightest drinking segment. As the population in the industrialized world is ageing, patterns among the elderly become more important. Changes in demographic structures will make it more difficult to analyse and understand long-term variation in the level of alcohol consumption.

It is already commonplace to calculate the mean population consumption figures for the population over 15 years of age. With the demographic changes awaiting the industrialized world, one should consider whether the elderly above 70 or 75 years of age should also be excluded from the denominator in calculations of mean consumption. In the developing countries, the problems of accounting for changes in demographic structure pose even greater problems.

The ongoing Collaborative Alcohol-related Longitudinal Project (Fillmore *et al.* 1991), has already provided further important information on the nature of changes in alcohol consumption, both at individual and aggregate levels. The results complicate the picture by pointing out that social class has a different relevance for changes in alcohol consumption in different age groups. Briefly, it appears that among young people there is a great deal of social group specificity in drinking patterns and consumption levels, whereas the elderly show remarkable social group similarities.

The information above suggests that some features of drinking habits may have changed greatly, even if consumption levels and beverage preferences have been relatively stable. The available data do not allow more detailed conclusions.

Substitution or addition?

In the context of sudden changes in alcohol availability, the question of substitution and addition has come to the fore (Mäkelä 1983). In a discussion of long-term trends in aggregate alcohol consumption, questions on the distinction between additive and substitutional effects are complicated. The issue of substitution and addition has policy relevance, as many decision-makers seem to hope that harmful drinking patterns can be substituted by less harmful ones, but without affecting the economic interest connected with the level of alcohol consumption.

Little discussion has so far taken place on the meaning of addition and substitution as bearing on differences between sociodemographic groups, or relevant changes in the three components of the decomposition model described above.

Models for explaining changes in aggregate alcohol consumption

There are three major factors that have been used to explain changes in aggregate alcohol consumption. They are related to different time perspectives. The most popular explanatory models emphasize economic factors in relation to medium- and short-term changes. In discussion on long-term trends, cultural explanations and the role of structural changes in society become more prominent. Industrialization, for instance, is often referred to as an underlying factor influencing alcohol consumption. Finally, changes in systems of alcohol sales and production produce short-term effects which may also have influences over the long run.

1. Economic explanations

The review of trends in alcohol consumption given earlier in this chapter provides instances to mesh with each of these explanatory models. Unfortunately, there seems to be little systematic attempt to use appropriately different explanations for different types of trend. So, for example, economic factors serve to explain the growth of alcohol consumption in Japan or Finland in the late 1980s, both of which are exceptions to the most common trends in the Western industrialized world. However, economic factors are also used to explain consumption growth in the developing countries. In the latter case at least, one should consider whether economic explanations should defer more to structural changes in the society at large. Following this line of thinking, one could also say that the decline of alcohol consumption in wine-drinking European countries is partly due to structural-economic changes which slowly destroy the cultural background with favoured extensive wine consumption.

Economic explanations typically refer to income and purchasing power on the one hand, and to prices and price elasticities on the other. At the latter point, a new problem is emerging as non-alcoholic beverages are increasingly visibly competing with alcohol. The substitution effects and cross-elasticities between alcohol and non-alcoholic beverages should be taken in to the econometric research agenda.

2. *Cultural explanations*

Changes in culture are probably most relevant to long-term trends. As was stated above, the discussion on long waves of alcohol consumption arose from the notion that there are changes which do not follow the fluctuation of economic influences. Industrialization, together with the consequent cultural changes, or changes in the moral climate and attitudes, provide the best examples. Westernization and commercialization of traditional life styles in the developing world, or strengthened moral concerns in the United States, provide further instances. As mentioned earlier, the studies of declining wine consumption in France suggest that the decrease is connected with industrialization, the well-educated urban young being the trend setters abandoning wine drinking (Aigrain *et al.* 1991).

An important aspect of industrialization is what is termed the normalization of alcoholic beverages as commodities. This was reflected in an analysis of the development of alcohol consumption in the post-war era (Mäkelä *et al.* 1981):

> The disreputability of alcohol was fading, age and sex segregation was breaking down, and drinking became integrated with other social activities. . . . There was also a corresponding normalization of alcoholic beverages as economic commodities. Alcohol became increasingly intermingled with other products . . .

The normalization process has been strengthened in the Nordic countries as a consequence of their wish to join the European Union. In the last decade, however, there are already some signs of an opposite process. The change in the moral climate in the United States could be interpreted as a turn in the direction of 'de-normalization' of alcohol. Similarly, one might wonder whether a process of de-normalization is also making slow inroads in wine-drinking countries. In general, these signs are still weak and no broad move towards de-normalization can as yet be anticipated.

3. *Explanations based on changes in alcohol sales systems*

In recent years the impact of public policy has been most visible in the case of the former Soviet Union and its 1985 alcohol reform (Treml 1991; Lagerspetz 1992; Seps 1992; Mikalkevicius and Šinkunas 1992). Changes in Iceland after the 1989 beer liberalization should also be mentioned (Olafsdottir 1991).

Large-scale reforms as occurred in the former Soviet Union have, in addition, more longstanding influences on alcohol consumption, and thus the policy explanation involves features of cultural change as well as the immediate impact of the policy intention. A number of comparatively minor public policy operations with short-term effects can easily be identified in industrialized countries.

The idea of normalization of alcohol as a commodity has been extended to control policies (Mäkelä *et al.* 1981). In the last few years, such normalizing tendencies have gained ground in a number of countries. In Poland, the recent political fluctuations have loosened the former control system and, as a consequence, alcohol consumption showed a rapid rise (Wald *et al.* 1993; Moskalewicz and Świątkiewicz 1992). In the United States, some of the remaining alcohol monopoly states have partly or wholly abandoned this system (Holder and Janes 1989). This is, of course, a development which goes against the tightening moral attitudes towards alcohol in the country as a whole.

In the field of alcohol control policy, signs of de-normalization are still few. The most striking example is France, with the new erestrictive legislation on alcohol advertising.

Conclusions

The following conclusions can be drawn from the topics discussed in this chapter.

1. In the industrialized world, the almost universal upward trend in consumption ceased in most, but not all countries, by the early 1980s.
2. The signs of any new trend, perhaps one of diminishing consumption, are very weak in the industrialized world. Rather, the present state of affairs is characterized by contradictory tendencies.
3. As there is no common trend, so is there no one common explanation for the trend in alcohol consumption seen over recent decades. Parallel and intersecting explanations are needed, and good examples are available to support very different models of explanation.
4. A remarkable event in the world-wide perspective is, however, the continuing decline of alcohol consumption in wine-drinking countries. This decline is being felt in practically all Mediterranean wine countries. As these countries are at the top of the international consumption league, this suggests that homogenization of consumption levels is continuing.
5. In many countries of the developing world, alcohol consumption is increasing. This may partly be a consequence of a move toward commercial beverages, and there is still in these regions a large potential for consumption growth. Developments in these regions cannot be explained

merely by reference to possible overall trends of alcohol consumption in the industrialized world.

References

Aigrain, P., Boulet, D., Lambert, J. L., and Laporte, J. P. (1991). La consommation du vin en France: evolutions tendancielles et diversite des comportements [The consumption of wine in France: evolutionary tendencies and diverse patterns]. *Revue de l'Economie Meridionale*, **39**, 19–52.

Armyr, G., Elmér, Å., and Herz, U. 1982). *Alcohol in the world of the 80s*. Sober, Stockholm.

Balmés, J.-L., Boulet, D., and Picheral, H. (1989). Approche des processus d'alcoolisation: L'exemple du Languedoc–Roussillon. [The first signs in the process of alcoholization]. *Journal d'Alcoologie*, No. 2, 99–113.

Berg, M.-A., Peltoniemi, J., and Puska, P. (1991). Suomalaisen aikuisväestön terveyskäyttäytyminen. Kevät 1991. [Health behaviour among the Finnish adult population. Spring 1991], Report No. B3. National Public Health Institute, Helsinki.

Bennett, P., Smith, C., and Nugent, Z. (1991). Patterns of drinking in Wales. *Alcohol and Alcoholism*, **26**, 367–74.

BAC (Brewers' Association of Canada) (1992). *International Survey. Alcoholic beverages, taxation and control policies*, (8th edn). Brewers' Association of Canada, Ottawa.

Bruun, K. *et al.* (1975) *Alcohol Control Policies in Public Health Perspective*, Vol. 25. Finnish Foundation for Alcohol Studies, Helsinki.

Clark, W. G. and Hilton, M. E. (ed.) (1991). *Alcohol in America*. State University of New York, Albany, NY.

DDA (Dutch Distillers' Association) (1992). *World drink trends*. Dutch Distillers' Association and NTC, Henley-on-Thames, UK.

Eliany, M., Giesbrecht, N., Nelson, M. Wellman, B., and Wortley, S. (ed.) (1990). *National alcohol and other drugs survey, 1989*. Health and Welfare Canada, Ottawa.

Enriquez de Salamanca, R. (1984). *Estudio de los habitos de consumo de alcohol de la poblacion adulta española* (Study of the drinking habits of the adult Spanish population] Ministerio de Sanidad y Consumo, Madrid.

Fahrenkrug, H. (1989). Swiss drinking habits: results of surveys in 1975, 1981 and 1987. *Contemporary Drug Problems*, Summer, 201–25.

Fillmore, K., Hartka, E., Johnstone, B. M., Leino, E. V., Motoyoshi, M., and Temple, M. T. (1991). The collaborative alcohol-related longitudinal project: preliminary results from a meta-analysis of drinking behaviour in multiple longitudinal studies. *British Journal of Addiction*, **86**, 1203–10.

FFAS (Finnish Foundation for Alcohol Studies). (1977). *International statistics on alcoholic beverages*. Production, sale and consumption, 1950–72. Finnish Foundation for Alcohol Studies, Helsinki.

Gili, M., Giner, J., Lacalle, J. R., Franco, D., Perea, E., and Dieguez, J. (1989). Patterns of consumption of alcohol in Seville, Spain. Results of a general population survey. *British Journal of Addiction*, **84**, 277–85.

Goddard, E. and Ikin, C. (1988). *Drinking in England and Wales in 1987*. HMSO, London.

Godfrey, C. (1989). Factors influencing the consumption of alcohol and tobacco: the use and abuse of economic models. *British Journal of Addiction*, **84**, 1123–38.

Hansen, E. J. and Andersen, D. (1985). *Alkoholforbrug og alkoholpolitik* [Alcohol consumption and alcohol policy]. Institute for Social Research, Copenhagen.

Hauge, R. and Irgens-Jensen, O. (1987). *Alkoholen i Norden* [Alcohol in the Nordic countries. Report from the Scandanavian Drinking Survey 1979]. Supplement for *Alkoholpolitik*, *Tidskrift för Nordisk Alkoholforskning*, Helsinki.

HW. (1989). *Alcoholism in Canada*. Health and Welfare Canada, Ottawa.

Helgason, T. (1988). Áfengisneysluvenjur og einkenni um misnotkun 1974 og 1984 [Drinking habits and symptoms of alcohol abuse in Iceland in 1974 and 1984]. *Læknablaðið*, **74**, 129–36.

Hilton, M. (1991). Trends in U.S. drinking patterns. Further evidence from the past twenty years. In *Alcohol in America*, (ed. W. G. Clark and M. E. Hilton), pp. 121–38. State University of New York, Albany, NY.

Holder, H. and Janes, K. (1989). Control of alcohol beverage availability: state alcoholic beverage control systems having monopoly functions in the United States, *State monopolies and alcohol prevention*, (ed. T. Kortteinen), Report No. 181, pp. 355–460. Social Research Institute of Alcohol Studies, Helsinki.

Hupkens, C. L. H., Knibbe, R. A., and Drop, M. J. (1993). Alcohol consumption in the European Community: uniformity and diversity in national drinking patterns. *Addiction*, **88**, 1391–1404.

Izuno, T. *et al*. (1992). Alcohol-related problems encountered by Japanese, Caucasians and Japanese-Americans. *International Journal of the Addictions*, **27**, 1389–1400.

Kilonzo, G. P. and Pitkänen, Y. T. (eds). (1992). *Pombe. Report of the alcohol research project in Tanzania, 1988–90*, Report B/24. Institute of Development Studies, University of Helsinki.

Kono, H. and Takano, T. (1992). Patterns and problems of alcohol consumption in Japan. *World Health Forum*, **13**, 326–9.

Kortteinen, T. (1989*a*). *Agricultural alcohol and social change in the Third World*. Finnish Foundation for Alcohol Studies, Helsinki.

Kortteinen, T. (ed.) (1989*b*). *State monopolies and alcohol prevention*, Report No. 181. Social Research Institute of Alcohol Studies, Helsinki.

Lagerspetz, M. (1992). Estonia: changing problems in a re-emerging state. In *Social problems around the Baltic sea*, (ed. J. Simpura and C. Tigerstedt), No. 21, pp. 23–38. The Nordic Council for Alcohol and Drug Research, Helsinki.

Levin, B. M. and Levin, M. B. (1988). *Alkogol'nava situaciya—1988* [Alcohol situation—1988]. Institute of Sociological Research, USSR Academy of Sciences, Moscow.

Mäkelä, K. (1983). The uses of alcohol and their cultural regulation. *Acta Sociologica*, **26**, 21–31.

Mäkelä, K., Room, R., Single, E., Sulkunen, P., and Walsh, B. (1981). *Alcohol, society and the state*, Vol 1. Alcohol Addiction Foundation, Toronto.

Maula, J., Lindblad, M., and Tigerstedt, C. (eds). (1989). *Alcohol in developing countries*. Proceedings from a meeting, No. 18. The Nordic Council for Alcohol and Drug Research, Helsinki.

Mikalkevicius, A. and Šinkunas, S. (1992). Ideology and alcohol problems in Lithuania. In *Social problems around the Baltic Sea*, (ed. J. Simpura and C. Tigerstedt), No. 21, pp. 53–68. The Nordic Council for Alcohol and Drug Research, Helsinki.

Moser, J. (1992). *Alcohol problems, policies and programmes in Europe*. WHO, Regional Office for Europe, Copenhagen.

Moskalewicz, J. and Świątkiewicz, G. (1992). Social problems in the Polish political debate. In *Social problems around the Baltic Sea*. The Nordic Council for Alcohol and Drug Research NAD, Helsinki.

Nachrichten für Aussenhandel [*Export News*]. (1992). Bier ohne Alkohol kommt an [Non-alcoholic beer is coming]. 19 May, 6.

Nemtsov, A. V. and Nechaev, A. K. (1991). Alkogol'naya situaciya v Moskv'e v 1983–1990 gg (The alcohol situation in Mosvow in the years 1983–1990). *Social'naya i Klinicheskaya Psikhiatriya*, No. 1, 75–83.

Nordlund, S. (1987). *Data om alkohol og andre stoffer* [Data on alcohol and other substances], Report No. 1. National Institute for Alcohol Research (SIFA), Oslo.

Olafsdottir, H. (1991). I forandringens tid: Islandsk alkoholpolitikk i 1980-årene [In changing times: Icelandic Alcohol Policy in the 1980s]. *Nordisk Alkoholtidskrift*, **8**, 342–51.

Österberg, E. (1987). Recorded and unrecorded alcohol consumption. In *Finnish drinking habits*, (ed. J. Simpura), pp. 17–36. Finnish Foundation for Alcohol Studies, Helsinki.

Partanen, J. (1991). *Sociability and intoxication*. Finnish Foundation for Alcohol Studies, Helsinki.

Pyörälä, E. (1990). Trends in alcohol consumption in Spain, Portugal, France and Italy from the 1950s until the 1980s. *British Journal of Addiction*, **85**, 469–77.

Pyörälä, E. (1991). *Nuorten aikuisten juomakulttuuri Suomessa ja Espanjassa* [Drinking culture among young adults in Finland and Spain], Report No. 183. Research Institute of Alcohol Studies, Helsinki.

Reader's Digest. (1991). *Eurodata: A consumer survey of 17 European countries*. Reader's Digest Association, London.

Reinås, K. T. (1991). *Alkoholens kilder. Nordmenns totala alkoholforbruk i 1989* [The sources of alcohol. The aggregate consumption of alcohol by Norwegians in 1989]. National Directorate on Alcohol and Drugs, Oslo.

Room, R. (1991). Cultural changes in drinking and trends in alcohol problems indicators: Recent U.S. experience. In *Alcohol in America*, (ed. W. G. Clark and M. E. Hilton), pp. 149–63. State University of New York, Albany, NY.

Rossi, D. (1992). *Alcool: consume e politiche in Europa* [Alcohol: consumption and politics in Europe]. Edizioni Otet, Rome.

Salomaa, J. (1990). *Alkoholin kulutus eräissä OECD-maissa vuosina 1960–1988* [Alcohol consumption in some OECD member countries 1960–1988], Report No. 16. Economic Research and Planning Department, Finnish Alcohol Company, Helsinki.

Schmidt, D. (1991). *Danskernes brug af rusmidler* [Use of intoxicants in Denmark], Report No. 15. Reports on Prevention and Hygiene, National Board of Health, Copenhagen.

Seps, Dz. (1992). Alcohol problems in the Latvian cultural and political context. In *Social problems around the Baltic Sea*, (ed. J. Simpura and C. Tigerstedt), No. 21. NAD, Helsinki.

Shimizu, S. (1990). An alcohol social system: drinking culture and drinking behaviors in Japan. *Seisin Hoken Kenkuy*, **36**, 85–100.

Simpura, J. (1980). Decomposition of changes in aggregate consumption of alcohol in Finland 1968, 1969 and 1976. *Journal of Studies on Alcohol*, **41**, 572–6.

Simpura, J. (ed.) (1987). *Finnish drinking habits. Results from interview surveys held in 1968, 1976 and 1984*. Finnish Foundation for Alcohol Studies, Helsinki.

Simpura, J. (1992). Social and political preconditions of preventing alcohol problems in the changing Europe. In *L'alcologia in Europa. Verso soluzione comunitarie*, (ed. I. Vantini *et al.*), pp. 104–14. Editrice Compositori, Bologna.

Single, E., Giesbrecht, N., and Eakins, B. (1981). *Alcohol, society and the state*, Vol. 2. Alcohol Addiction Foundation, Toronto.

Smart, R. G. (1989). Is the postwar drinking binge ending? Cross-national trends in per capita alcohol consumption. *British Journal of Addiction*, **84**, 743–8.

Smart, R. G. (1991). World trends in alcohol consumption. *World Health Forum*, **12**, 99–103.

Sulkunen, P. (1983). Alcohol consumption and the transformation of living conditions. A comparative study. In *Research advances in alcohol and drug problems*, (ed. R. J. Gibbins *et al.*), Vol. 7, pp. 247–97. Plenum, New York.

Sulkunen, P. (1987). Abstinence. *Finnish drinking habits*, (ed. J. Simpura), pp. 37–54. Finnish Foundation for Alcohol Studies, Helsinki.

Sulkunen, P. (1989). Drinking in France 1965–1979. An analysis of household consumption data. *British Journal of Addiction*, **84**, 61–72.

Suwaki, H. (1985). Japan. International review series: Alcohol and alcohol problems research. *British Journal of Addiction*, **80**, 127–32.

SCIAD (Swedish Council for Information on Alcohol and Other Drugs (1991). *Report 1991. Trends in alcohol and drug use in Sweden*. Swedish Council for Information on Alcohol and other Drugs, Stockholm.

Tarschys, D. (1993). The success of a failure: Gorbachev's alcohol policy, 1985–88. *Europe–Asia Studies*, **45**, 7–25.

Treml, V. G. (1991). Drinking and alcohol abuse in the USSR in the 1980s. In *Soviet social problems*, (ed. A. Jones *et al.*), pp. 119–36. Westview, Boulder, CO.

Tsunoda, T. *et al.* (1992). The effect of acculturation on drinking attitudes among Japanese in Japan and Japanese Americans in Hawaii and California. *Journal of Studies on Alcohol*, **53**, 369–77.

Vanston, N. (1991). Patterns and trends in alcohol consumption. A statistical survey. *Expert meeting on the negative social consequences of alcohol use*, pp. 33–46. Oslo, 27–31 August. Norwegian Ministry of Health and Social Affairs, in collaboration with the UN Office at Vienna Centre for Social Development and Humanitarian Affairs, Oslo.

Wald, I. *et al.* (1993). Alcohol policy in the light of social changes. In *Experiences with community action projects: new research in the prevention of alcohol and other drug problems*, (ed. T. K. Greenfield and R. Zimmerman), CSAP Monograph. No. 14, pp. 88–94. US Department of Health and Human Services, Rockville, MD.

Wilson, P. (1980). *Drinking in England and Wales*. HMSO, London.

2. Individual risk and population distribution of alcohol consumption

Paul H. H. M. Lemmens

Introduction

The finding that more than 90 per cent of all liver cirrhosis cases in the French département of Ille-et-Vilaine could be attributed to alcohol consumption is evidence of the significant role of alcohol in the aetiology of this disease (Pequignot *et al.* 1978). However impressive such a percentage, it does not provide information on the proportion or types of drinkers who will *not* be affected. Similarly, even though the risk of dying of cirrhosis among alcoholics is estimated to be up to 20 times higher than among non-alcoholics (Brody and Mills 1978), only about 10 per cent of clinically diagnosed alcoholics will actually develop the disease (Lelbach 1975). Evidently, the individual's overall consumption is not solely responsible for the negative effects of drinking. Genetic, biological, and psychosocial factors interact to co-determine whether a person will experience negative consequences of their drinking within a certain time period. Moreover, drinking itself is a complex, and often irregular behaviour, consisting of more than one parameter. The individual pattern may change many times over the course of a lifetime. The variation in vulnerability and drinking behaviour makes assessment of individual exposure to alcohol and prediction of its outcomes difficult, but it does not necessarily imply that indices of aggregate consumption and indicators of negative effects of consumption will be similarly irregular and unpredictable. In fact, national per capita consumption figures and indicators of alcohol-related harm tend to be fairly stable or change gradually over time, and individual differences and variations seem to balance each other out up to some point. The relationship between aggregate level indicators of risk factors, such as per capita alcohol consumption, and the prevalence or incidence of problems in society related to this risk factor, has always been of major epidemiological interest.

Evidence from ecological designs in epidemiology, concerning such aggregate relationships between consumption and health indicators, is of limited value with respect to questions of causation. For instance, the negative association between per capita wine consumption and incidence of coronary heart disease in the Western world (St. Leger *et al.* 1979) should not be taken to imply that wine consumption can prevent myocardial infarctions. Still, ecological designs do have their specific merit. They can give an indication of a possible relationship between risk factor and outcome, which, in studies of populations relatively homogeneous with regard to the risk factor, would go unobserved (Rose 1985). As more and more results from multivariate case-control and prospective longitudinal studies on alcohol become available, one might ask what is the significance of alcohol-related risks established at the individual level for society at large? For a better understanding, it is necessary to investigate how the established relationships at the individual level combine at the population level. The section to follow deals with the impact overall level of exposure can be expected to have on occurrence of alcohol problems in a population for four types of dose-response relationships. An important variable determining rates of harmful consequences to be expected at the aggregate level is the distribution of alcohol consumption in the population. In a later section (p. 42) a summary is given of discussions about a distribution model of alcohol consumption. The assessment of population-level outcome as a function of the relative risk and the population distribution of the risk factor leads up to the discussion on pp. 54–57 of the so-called prevention paradox, which highlights one of the dilemmas of primary prevention, whether to focus on overall drinking or on excessive consumption.

Exposure to alcohol: relative risks

The concept in epidemiology that captures the conditional probability for an individual of experiencing a negative effect of exposure to a disease factor in a certain period of time is the relative risk. Usually assessed in case-control or prospective studies, dose-response relationships between consumption level and some type of harm give information on the risk at different levels of consumption. In a formal sense, the incidence of a particular alcohol-related outcome in a population can be seen as the product of two variates, the risk function for that outcome and the population distribution of alcohol consumption (Kleinbaum *et al.* 1982). In this section a summary is given of the consequences of these combinations for the relationship between incidence and consumption in the population at large. It should be kept in mind that what follows is a formal description. Other factors, such as measurement issues, social stratification, number of abstainers, and drinking pattern, also cause variation in outcome (incidence), and a simple risk function of average annual alcohol consumption probably will not cover the entire phenomenon. For the sake of simplicity, it is assumed that these other factors are held constant. In the examples below, it is furthermore assumed that the period over which consumption is operationalized, is the same for the studies assessing risk and population distribution.

Combinations of risk functions and consumption distributions

Several risk functions are realistically possible in the case of (total volume of) alcohol consumption. In Fig. 2.1 some empirical examples are given. The particular curves are chosen because they seem reasonable approximations of ideal models, such as the linear (Fig. 2.1a), the convex or exponential function (Fig. 2.1b), a threshold (Fig. 2.1c), and a U-shaped model (Fig. 2.1d). The inclusion of any of the four examples does not imply that the role of alcohol has been established beyond any doubt. In addition, the standard error of the relative risk estimates is sometimes quite large and not constant over the entire consumption scale.

It has been shown for the linear risk case that the incidence in the population is dependent only upon total consumption but independent of the particular distribution of consumption (Skog 1991). Thus, with a linearly increasing risk (relative risk of abstainers set at 1, no threshold), any consumption by any member, either a heavy drinker or a very light one, has the same effect on population incidence. In all other cases, the incidence in the population depends in varying degrees on the way consumption is distributed in the population.

In the case of a strongly convex function (for example, in Fig. 2.1b), minute changes in distribution, especially when they occur in the tail of the consumption distribution, will have large effects on the incidence. For instance, on the basis of the risk curve in Fig. 2.1b and the consumption distribution in their control (population) group, Péquignot *et al.* (1978) estimated that if the 2.5 per cent heaviest drinkers in Ille-et-Vilaine would limit their drinking to about 12 glasses per day (population average would only fall with about 2 per cent), the total number of cirrhosis cases in the region would drop to 63 per cent of its original number (an empirical example of the effect of a change in distribution on liver cirrhosis mortality can be found in Norström 1987). The effects on incidence for risks other than the strongly convex cirrhosis case are less dependent upon the tail of the consumption distribution.

The U-shaped risk function, apparent in many epidemiological studies on total mortality is a special case. Obviously, the minimal risk for an individual is not abstention (or non-exposure) but some intermediate, light, or moderate level. Because of this non-monotonic relationship between individual risk and consumption, there is also an optimum mean population level of consumption at which incidence will be lowest. Because of the often large dispersion and positive skewness of alcohol consumption distributions (most people drink much less than average), this optimum population mean level is expectedly lower than the optimum individual level (Skog 1991). The larger the dispersion

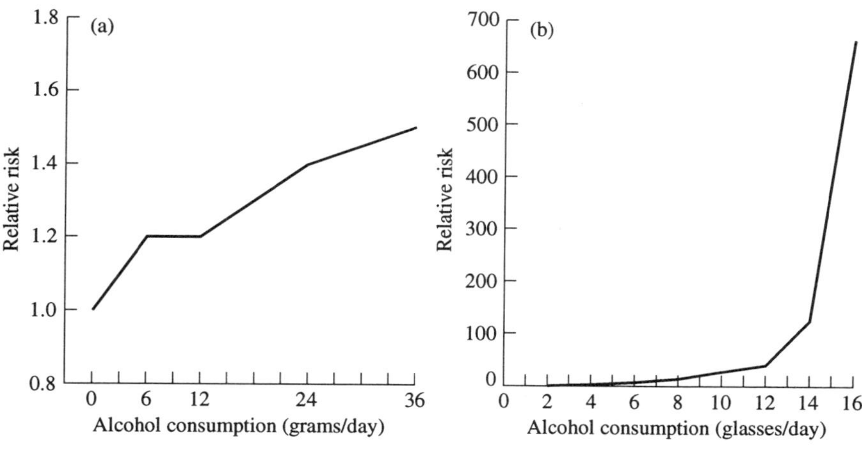

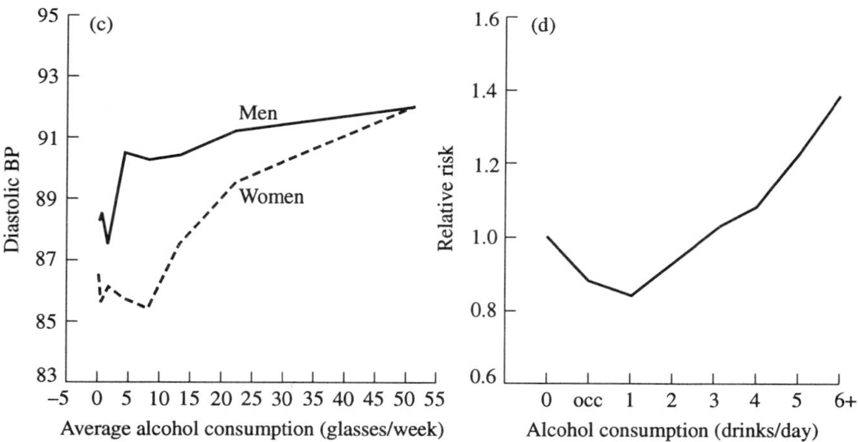

Fig. 2.1 Four examples of empirically established dose-response relationships between alcohol consumption and four alcohol-related outcomes in the general population. (a) Risk of breast cancer as established in a meta-analysis. *Source:* Longnecker *et al.* 1988. (b) Risk of liver cirrhosis for male sample in a French département, case-control design. *Source:* Pequignot *et al.* 1978. (c) Relationship between diastolic blood pressure and consumption of alcohol for adult men and women in a Michigan town, age–weight adjusted figures. *Source:* Harburg *et al.* 1980. (d) Total mortality risk of male abstainers (0), occasional (occ), and regular drinkers, aged 40–59 years. *Source:* Bofetta and Garfinkel (1990).

relative to the mean, the larger this difference between the individual and population optimum will be. In conclusion, for all non-linear dose-response relationships, whether developments in rates of specific harm in a society will closely follow changes in total or mean consumption will depend on the particular shape of the consumption distribution, the topic of the next section.

The above examples over-simplify the situation in many respects. Apart from variation in distribution of consumption across substrata, it should be kept in mind that risk functions may not be equal for all segments of the population. Men and women not only differ in body mass and body water, resulting in a stronger impact of the same dose of alcohol, but there is evidence of a greater female susceptibility to alcohol's negative effects due to other factors as well (Gomberg 1989). Another concern when dealing with empirical assessments of risk is that they are most often based on self-reports of consumption in the recent past, leaving little room for the inclusion of longer-term effects of alcohol. This emphasis on recent consumption may cause a bias in the estimated risks, underestimating the effects of alcohol for those who had decreased their consumption in the period before assessment, and thereby overestimating the effect for those drinking at relatively low, stable levels. A further complication is that aspects of an individual's drinking pattern (stability, frequency) may produce a reporting bias due to selective forgetting (Lemmens *et al.* 1992). Similarly, when estimates of consumption are not based on identical self-report methods in both risk and population studies, biased estimates of incidence may result as well. Since epidemiology is usually concerned with assessment of the general level of exposure to an environmental agent, consumption in risk studies are usually averaged over some period of time, without paying much attention to the drinking pattern. A fourth concern when combining results from different epidemiological studies is this difference in drinking pattern. It is not unlikely that cases stem from a population that is more homogeneous in drinking pattern than the controls. Naturally, there is a positive relationship between frequency of drinking and total quantity, but given a certain overall volume, the blood alcohol level (peak exposure) resulting from a pattern with high frequency may be quite lower than one with a high quantity per occasion.

The distribution of alcohol consumption

Before the 1950s in the United States, particularly after repeal of prohibition, alcohol consumption was not considered an important factor in causing diseases such as liver cirrhosis and cancer. The reasons for the high prevalence of health problems among alcoholics had to be found in their bad nutritional status. Overall level of consumption was of little relevance for the medical practice or for the prevention and treatment of alcoholism (Katcher 1993). The emergence of the epidemiological paradigm in the post-war years, linking disease with environmental causes, has broadened the 'infections and deficits' orientation of medicine to include environmental risk factors. This shift toward a more general risk approach has ramifications for a public health policy, including the one on alcohol.

The main argument of Brunn *et al.* (1975) was that control of alcohol availability had become a public health issue because: 'changes in the overall consumption of alcoholic beverages have a bearing on the health of the people in any society'. The authors argued that total consumption was an important indicator of the magnitude of alcohol-related problems in society. A crucial element in their conclusion was the 'relative invariance' of the distribution of total volume of consumption, which established a predictable, positive association between mean consumption and excessive use. Specifically, the percentage of the drinking population consuming more than 100 ml of pure alcohol per day (about eight glasses) appeared to be proportional to the square of the mean consumption (Bruun *et al.* 1975, p. 36). Since excessive use was regarded as the main determinant of alcohol-related disease, this relative invariance was a necessary bridge between normal (means) and excessive consumption, or between social drinking and abuse. The claims regarding the nature of a so-called single distribution model of consumption have changed over the years. The relationship between normal drinking and alcohol-related harm in the Ledermann (1956) model was fixed, relatively invariant (Bruun *et al.* 1975). In a weaker version, the model was 'sometimes true' (Skog 1981). In the next section a brief review of the single-distribution model, its criticisms, and modifications is presented.

The Ledermann model

Several scientific studies that correlated regional statistics on overall volume of consumption and excess mortality in France before, during, and after World War II, led Ledermann to hypothesize a very strong relationship between overall consumption in a population and excessive use (see Skog 1982, for a historical overview of Ledermann's work). In his view, no qualitative distinction between normal use and alcoholic consumption levels could be made, but the differences were quantitative and gradual. He suggested, in mathematical terms, a restricted log-normal distribution model of alcohol consumption, now known as the Ledermann (1956) formula. The formula enabled him to estimate prevalence of heavy use; that is, the proportion in a population with an average daily consumption of alcohol exceeding a particular level. Since the formula has only one unknown parameter, per capita consumption, it was fairly easy to implement. As a logical consequence Ledermann inferred that, 'If this connection cannot be broken', prevention of alcohol-related disease had but one option: '. . . the suppression of alcohol in all the forms in which it is consumed' (Ledermann 1964, p. 8). Thus, given the invariance in relation between mean and heavy drinking, treatment or prevention focusing on alcoholics only would not suffice. In a sense, the

Ledermann model has given the control-of-supply model of prevention a statistical, scientific argument, as opposed to the moralistic legitimacy of earlier prohibition (Walsh and Hingson 1987). In this approach to prevention, a reduction of total volume of consumption is seen as the prime target of a primary prevention strategy. Per capita consumption is regarded not only as an indicator of harm but as a principal factor in the epidemiology of alcohol-related problems: prevention measures will be successful only when they succeed in bringing down average consumption (see, for example, Kendell 1984).

Ledermann's model has been implemented internationally by Canadian researchers who tested the model on empirical samples (for instance, de Lint and Schmidt 1968; Smart and Schmidt 1970; de Lint 1974). Initial enthusiasm was later tempered by studies criticizing Ledermann's assumptions as well as the data that were used for empirical testing. Still others did not find conclusive evidence of a close fit between the lognormal and empirical distributions (see Skog 1983 for an overview). Although the strict Ledermann formula could not be sustained, enough evidence remained for Bruun *et al.* (1975, p. 32) to conclude that: 'differences as to dispersion between populations with similar levels of consumption are quite small'. Using data from several subpopulations from six different countries, they arrived at the conclusion that the proportion of heavy consumers in a population of drinkers is approximately proportional to the square of the mean consumption. Even though rejecting Ledermann's quasi-mathematical model, most of its implications remained pertinent.

Even this weaker version of the distribution model has been criticized (see Duffy 1986 for a summary), for example, the interpretation of change in distribution from analyses of cross-cultural data. Cases with populations with an upward trend in consumption are fairly well documented (see Skog 1985*a*), with change in distribution roughly as expected on the basis of a general shift of the entire drinking population. However, Lemmens (1991) has noted that few empirical examples are available in which the developments in heavy drinking during an overall downward trend, will be of the same, albeit reversed, magnitude as in the case of an upward trend. There is one real and verifiable example reported by Kendell *et al.* (1983), based on surveys conducted in Scotland in 1978 and 1982. In line with the single distribution prediction, the study found that a decline in overall consumption had been accompanied by similar developments at all consumption levels, which was slightly stronger at the highest levels. The result of the study may be biased, however, because non-drinkers in 1978 were excluded from the 1982 survey, as a result of which light drinkers may have been under-represented (Altman 1991).

Another type of criticism has come from Duffy and Cohen (1978) who showed that even small differences in the (log) dispersion parameter between two populations that have equal means would result in large differences in estimates of excessive use. By stressing the relative invariance of (log) dispersion, one neglects the sometimes large differences between populations in heavy drinking prevalence. Indeed, examples show large differences between estimates of excessive use given a certain mean. However, when adopting a view of the entire (empirical) range of population means, one could defend that 'a doubling of the average consumption must lead to a full quadrupling of the proportion of heavy consumers' (Skog 1985*b*, p. 92), defined as over 100 ml pure alcohol daily, even though the standard error of the estimated rate is as high as 32 per cent. It may appear that the argument is between those asserting the bottle to be half empty and those claiming it to be half full.

Question marks have been put beside the alleged unimodality of the consumption distribution. For instance, Miller and Agnew (1974) raise the point that, even if factors creating a change in mean consumption of the non-alcoholic population do not affect the alcoholic population, this effect may go unobserved in general population surveys because of the large differences in size of the two populations. A bimodal distribution model is compatible with the classic disease model, which contends that the drinking behaviour of the majority of the population is governed by different mechanisms than the small minority of diseased alcoholics. Similar to the bimodal argument is the criticism that the population as a whole is not homogeneous, a basic assumption of the Ledermann model. In support of this, many empirical examples are cited in which a change in mean consumption is not reflected in a similar change in all subpopulations (Duffy 1991). These criticisms will be elaborated upon with recent empirical data on pp. 48–50, after a discussion of the most recent development, Skog's theory of collectivity of drinking cultures.

Collectivity of drinking cultures

Discarding the mathematically strict Ledermann formula and the idea of a fixed distribution, but trying to account for the regularities in distribution, Skog (1985*b*) has proposed a theory of drinking behaviour in terms of: (a) a process of social interaction or diffusion (Skog 1980), and (b) the multiplicative character of the process underlying change in consumption. As a point of departure he presented the plot, shown in Fig. 2.2, depicting 5 percentile values with mean consumption for 21 subpopulations. In his view, a change in mean consumption in a population of drinkers is the reflection of a shift in consumption by all types of drinkers, at all levels in that population (although, of course, not every drinker). In the plot, this is characterized by a positive slope of regression for all percentile values considered. This collective shift is brought about by the pressure experienced in a person's local environment, a pressure that is dependent on 'the extent to which his consumption level deviates from that of his friends' (Skog 1980, p. 75). The size and structural features of a person's network are seen as important predictors of speed and extent of diffusion. Independent factors causing change in consumption, such as availability or price, are mediated and synchronized through collective,

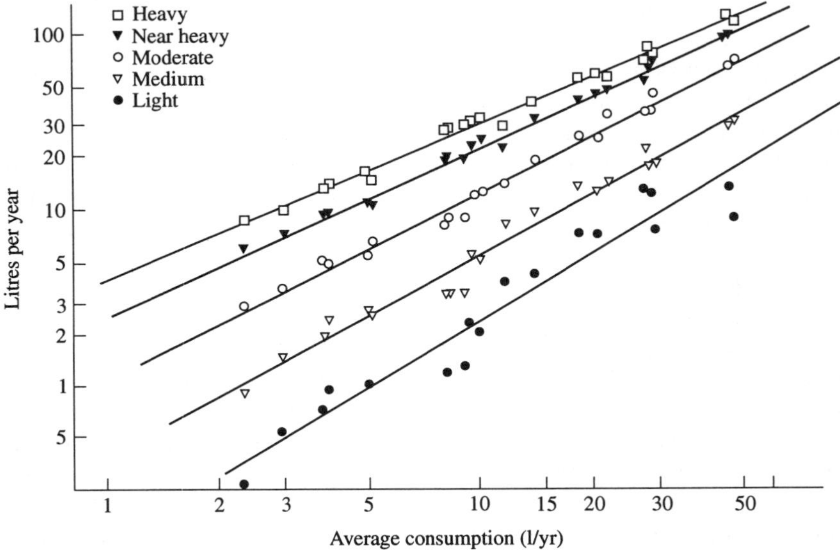

Fig. 2.2 Relationship between average consumption and the consumption level of selected drinking groups, defined by percentile values, in 21 general population surveys. The straight lines are least square regressions for each percentile point. *Source:* from Skog (1985*b*).

interactive channels. A large change in overall consumption is the result of such chain reactions within the entire population.

In his second hypothesis, Skog assumes that the pressure on an individual to change drinking behaviour results in a change that is proportional to the initial, baseline level (C_{t1}). In technical terms: $C_{t+1} = \alpha C_{t1}^{\beta}$. This proportional change also predicts a linear relationship between successive, logarithmic percentile and mean values, as in Fig. 2.2. Again, in technical terms: $C_p = \alpha_p M^{\beta p}$, where M is the mean and C_p the value of the percentile considered. An additional observation was that the size of the β_p-parameter seemed to decline with increasing percentile (see Tan *et al.* 1990 for a formal statistical treatise).

Lemmens *et al.* (1990) have tried to answer the question whether the empirical relation between alcohol distributions over time can be described by a log-linear, multiplicative model as suggested by Ledermann, and in a less formal sense by Skog. Using a statistical procedure called empirical probability plotting, Lemmens *et al.* (1990) showed that the relationships between Dutch male and female consumption distributions assessed in surveys conducted in 1970, 1981, and 1985 were indeed linear. Hence, they confirmed Ledermann's and, again in a less formal way, Skog's interpretation of regularity: up to a shift in scale and location, respectively the β and α in the

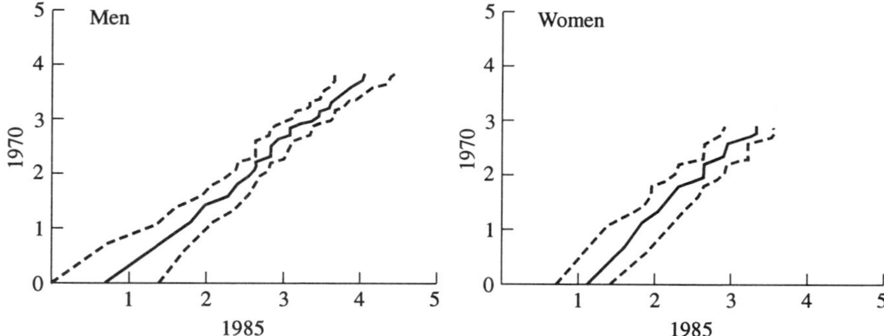

Fig. 2.3 Empirical probablity plots with 0.95 confidence band (– – – –) of the male and female distributions in the year 1970 (y-axis), with the respective 1985 distributions as reference (glasses per week, on a log scale). Average consumption in 1985 was about twice that of 1970.

Source: Lemmens *et al.* (1990).

above formula, there is no detectable or apparent difference between distributions (logarithmic data) in the three years. In the example given in Fig. 2.3, any observable deviation from a straight line, either convex or concave, would contradict the idea of regular, multiplicative change. As one can quickly verify, the variation from a straight line does not seem to be systematic. Visual inspection of the plots strongly suggest linearity of the relationship over the years. It appeared impossible, however, to estimate the exact magnitude of these parameters of change, and statistical uncertainty as to the exact nature of the change remains (Tan *et al.* 1990). The results support the hypothesis of proportional change of consumption distributions, irrespective of their exact distributional form (whether gamma, Weibull, or log-normal). Lemmens (1991) has extended comparisons over time with data from the United States, United Kingdom, Germany, and Switzerland, which, more or less, confirm the above outcome. Both Skog's and Lemmens' *et al.* empirical results thus affirm the idea of regularity across time and across (sub)populations. However, one should be careful with generalizations, since the results of the comparisons are highly dependent on the methods that are used to measure consumption, and, secondly, because longitudinal comparisons of distributions with large differences in the mean are still sparse.

Social interaction theory, as presented by Skog, offers a promising theoretical framework for the explanation of the observed regularities in overall consumption. It would be interesting to expand this line of research further and see whether it would be possible to predict developments in consumption (or patterns) in the population, either diverging and converging, from data on social integration, patterns of communication, and diffusion. As an example, one might consider testing whether differences in social interaction between the sexes could account for the diverging trends (1958–81) in male and female abstention rates in the Netherlands. Similarly, it would be interesting to investigate the possible role of communication patterns or indicators of social equality in the variation in male/female abstention ratio across regions in the Netherlands.

Homogeneity of the population

With adoption of a general distribution model of total consumption (such as the single distribution model: Schmidt and Popham 1978), relative high stress is put on the concept of homogeneity of the population with regard to drinking behaviour and the effects of consumption. Criticism has often concentrated on this concept because of its generalistic character (Parker and Harman 1978). Homogeneity implies, among other things, that all individuals in a population are exposed to the same stimuli that influence their drinking, that the upper limit of consumption is more or less the same for all, and that the alcohol is metabolized in a similar fashion. Although quite usual in formal statistics, this restriction is often hard to test empirically. With regard to alcohol, subpopulations have been found to differ in several of the above aspects. It is, nevertheless, difficult to specify the fundamental variables determining homogeneity. In practice, consumption distributions usually depict per drinker consumption, because variation in the number of non-drinkers is not necessarily related with per drinker consumption. For instance, abstention rates across regions of the United States are not positively related to per drinker consumption. In fact, in 1984, the driest regions showed the highest per drinker consumption (based on sales statistics: Hilton 1988). Another important distinction is between male and female populations. Women evidently differ from men in alcohol metabolism, mainly due to differences in body fluid and weight, with a ratio of about 1.4 to 1 in blood alcohol concentration resulting from consumption.

The notion of social contagion (Ledermann 1956) or social interaction mechanism (Skog 1985*b*), through which change in a population or group occurs collectively, is based on the idea that due to mutual influences, the population as a whole moves up and down the consumption scale. In practice, one would expect that no group would be exempt from the pressure to change, since all groups are more or less connected. Thus, in a society with changing consumption one would expect no large groups or subpopulations to be obvious exceptions of the general trend. A question that has been asked is about how general the central tendencies are: whether all social strata or groups change in the same way when overall consumption rises or declines? And a related question is whether a rise or decline in prevalence of heavy drinking is dependent on, or associated with, overall consumption level only? Several examples to the contrary have been given. Using very large samples, Tuck (1980) found no association between total consumption in the United Kingdom between 1974 and 1978 and the number of *daily* drinkers. The large increase in total consumption in the period was caused by an increase in the number of drinkers at moderate frequencies. Duffy (1991), using similarly large UK samples, covering the years 1979 to 1989, reports a small, positive association between average frequency and total consumption. However, an equally small but negative correlation was found between total consumption and daily drinking. This result has lead both authors to conclude that the distribution model is inadequate for description of the *drinking frequency distribution*. Duffy (1991, p. 7) remarked that '. . . changes in average consumption being due to changes in the frequency pattern of lower-frequency drinkers'. In the same report, subpopulations defined by sex and age were found to differ with respect to trends. The negative association between developments in the proportion of daily drinkers among younger and older women drew particular attention.

Others have reported on a negative relationship between a change in average consumption and a change in prevalence of heavy drinking. For a longitudinal series in the Netherlands covering the period 1958–81, Knibbe *et al.* (1985) report a tripling of mean consumption in the general population. Most subpopulations considered showed similar increases in mean consumption such that their ranking did not change. However, for young men and for non-religious men a decline in or unchanged average consumption was accompanied by an increase in heavy consumption. Extended with data from a general population survey in 1989, the same Dutch series permit a crude comparison between an indicator of heavy drinking and average consumption over four periods, five age groups, and in two cohort comparisons, for men and women separately (Neve *et al.* 1993). In general, the relationship is indeed positive but there are some exceptions where the relationship is negative, indicative of a reversed development. Mainly for the male subsamples in the period and cohort comparisons, there are a few instances where an increase in mean is not accompanied by an increase in heavy drinking. This suggests that, particularly between 1981 and 1989, drinking among men has become more homogeneous, and that distributions in different strata may vary over time. Per capita consumption may not always accurately mirror or reflect changes that take place in subpopulations. For instance, Romelsjö (1987) has reported that the decrease in Swedish consumption over the years 1976–84 was higher in the highest socio-economic status category, and in the younger age groups, and among men. This has lead to smaller differences in consumption between social strata in Sweden.

In line with the basic idea of social interaction and using about 25 panel studies from 14 different countries, Fillmore *et al.* (1994) have recently tried to predict changes in drinking pattern (that is, frequency, quantity per occasion, and stability of heavy drinking) at the individual group level (defined by sex and age) with changes in aggregate indices (per capita consumption measured at the population level). Their meta-analysis of per capita change and change in sex-by-age groups showed differential change in these groups, and the authors conclude that 'aggregate level changes in per capita consumption do not carry equal weight among all groups in society'. They report, for instance, that a large change in per capita consumption is associated with a change in frequency especially in the female samples, and with a change in quantity especially in the younger subpopulations. Their results indicate that developments within societies are not as homogeneous as a generalistic model would suggest. A remarkable outcome of the work of Fillmore *et al.* (1991) is that, although there is a positive relationship between prevalence of heavy drinking and per capita consumption in their meta-sample, which is in line with the collective hypotheses—chronicity of heavy drinking is not related to per capita consumption. The topic of stability of heavy drinking will be discussed in more detail on pp. 52–54.

A final and perhaps most convincing example of how a change in prevalence of heavy drinking is not reflected in a change in per capita consumption, has been given by Norström (1987). He reports that after the abolition of the Swedish Bratt alcohol rationing system, a change in distribution has taken place without an obvious change in per capita consumption. Apparently, the abolition of this system, in which each individual had a personal monthly quota, had a different impact on light to moderate drinkers, at one end, and heavy drinkers, at the other. In effect, the abolition has meant a price increase for lighter or moderate drinkers (those drinking less than their quota) and a decrease of restrictions for the heavier consumers, who were able to drink over the previous limit. The result has been that the dispersion of the distribution increased dramatically. The abolition was a 'natural' experiment which may be difficult to repeat. It is tempting to infer from its result that a sudden and vast change in a single factor that is known to affect drinking behaviour (that is, price, availability) may change the distribution in a different way than when a multitude of natural and slow changes are in effect. Such an effect of policy on different types of drinkers should be considered before a policy measure is introduced.

As it appears, then, there are differences between social strata within populations, as there are differences between countries (that is, regionally separated populations), which may increase or decrease over time. Societies obviously differ with regard to the consumption of their drinking patterns, often referred to as drinking cultures. Some are more homogeneous in their drinking than others, which may show larger inequality of consumption (for example, France and Norway, as presented in the Lorentz index in Skog 1985*a*). There has been a tendency in some of the advocates of the single distribution theory to disregard this diversity and concentrate on overall and general developments.

Triviality and causality

A recurring issue in the discussion on the distribution model concerns its possible triviality. It can be argued that *of course* there is a relation between

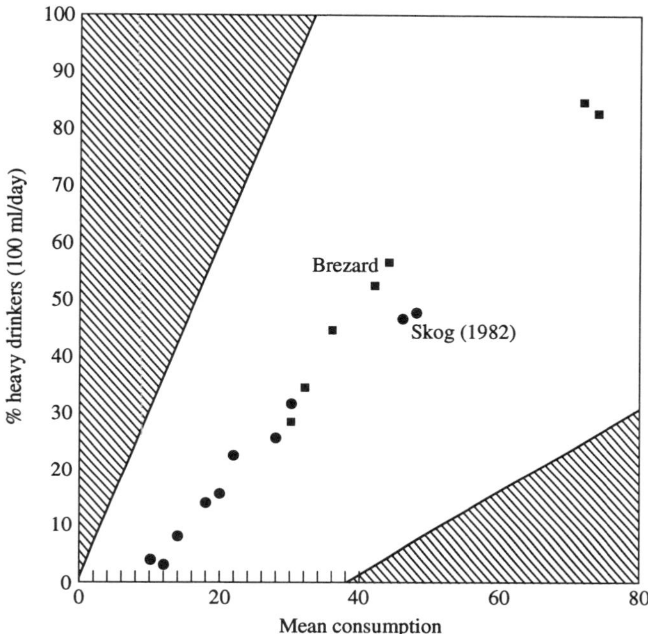

Fig. 2.4 Relationship between mean consumption and proportion of heavy drinkers. Shaded areas represent physiological impossibilities (right lower corner: consumption limit set at 500 ml 100% alcohol per day), and logical restrictions (left upper corner: according to Markov rule). The points are data from several surveys from Brezard and Skog.

Source: Skog (1982, fig. 10).

mean and proportions at high (that is, much larger than the mean) levels, since the mean is a composite of all values and the correlation between sample averages and proportions of heavy drinkers is expectedly positive (Alanko 1991). The question is not whether there is such a relationship, but whether the relationship is of any consequence or relevance. Crucial in this respect are the direction of causality and the degrees of freedom a distribution model has. In other words, how invariant is the relationship between mean and dispersion. Regarding the latter, Skog (1982) has given the formal margins within which the relationship may vary. Figure 2.4 shows the so-called Markov rule of inequality (upper area) and what is a physiological reality, an upper bound of 500 ml of pure alcohol on average per day. Clearly, the margins are very large compared to the empirical examples, which seem to float somewhere midstream. But, as already mentioned before, some have argued that even within this restricted empirical range, the differences may not be regarded as small (Duffy and Cohen 1978).

One of the confusing elements in the discussion over the single distribution is the causal direction. Because of Bruun's finding of only a slightly decreasing (log)dispersion with increasing average, others have been inclined to interpret this in a causal sense as: 'the mean determines the tail' (Rose and Day 1990), since the mean varies while the (log)dispersion remains about the same. Critics of this (for example, Duffy 1986; Alanko 1991) have maintained that overall consumption should be regarded a result, as the sum of all individual drinking, rather than an independent factor, and that the average or total consumption is falsely taken as a causal agent. In a formal statistical sense 'parameters known to be true of the population do not determine the attributes of the individuals . . . but . . . the properties of the individuals determine the parameters of the population' (Alanko 1991). Skog (1984*a*) has tried to reconcile this micro/macro-level contradiction by referring to wetness as a social fact transcending individual relevance, exerting coercive power, and as having a constraining influence on the individual. A person is confronted directly with the drinking of others in his or her environment, but also indirectly through the fiscal regulations and economic effects, or via the medical consequences of drinking. From this perspective, it is quite legitimate to view such social facts, even though originating in individual behaviour, as having an independent effect on individual behaviour, to study their relationships and contingencies, without a direct reference to individual-specific behaviour or perceptions from which they originate. This reciprocal nature of events is well accepted and studied in economics.

As a result of the large changes in overall consumption of alcohol in Norway in the past 120 years, Skog (1984*a*) speculated on the origins of long-term change in consumption. In this study he suggests a general mechanism of social interaction which would be (more or less) sufficient to explain long-term variations in aggregate consumption. The only conditions for this 'random' wave-like pattern he has observed (Norway, 1850–1980) are random, individual fluctuations, and a social interaction network characterized by long-range indirect ties. No additional external social forces are necessary to produce change at the aggregate level. Provocative as it is academically, the case of Norway is a single one, which may not be wholly representative. As in Norway, per capita consumption in the Netherlands dropped dramatically during the first half of the 20th century, but this decline does not seem to have been preceded by a clear increase in the latter half of the 19th century. Furthermore, it is difficult to conceive of social networks of the type suggested as being historically invariant, and the reciprocal nature of events (social facts) makes it difficult to assign a causal direction to any single relationship.

Similar alcohol distributions; differences in long-term exposure

In the beginning of this chapter it was emphasized that liver cirrhosis is not solely dependent on recent total consumption, but also on drinking patterns over longer periods. It seems well established that risk for cirrhosis should incorporate at least two main determinants, quantity and duration of (heavy) drinking (Lelbach 1975). Ideally, not only present but also past behaviour should accumulate into a composite measure, that takes latency of potential harmful effect into account. How past drinking combines into a present risk can only be determined empirically. Assessment of lifetime consumption retrospectively is, however, problematic, and only a few attempts have been made to validate an instrument for a non-clinical population (Skinner and Sheu 1982; Sobell *et al.* 1988). From what is known, it seems that individual drinking behaviour is not very stable in time, and this presents special problems for researchers. For example, heavy drinkers at one time may have become abstainers at another and vice versa, without any apparent change in aggregate consumption. Hence, two populations may look similar at the aggregate level, but they may be composed of individuals with different drinking histories (Skog and Duckert 1993). There is relatively little general population research available which may give us information about individual drinking patterns over longer periods of time since cohort studies in this area are sparse. Fillmore (1987) reported for general male US samples that chronicity of problem drinking was highest in middle age. So, even though prevalence at one point in time is probably highest among young US men, remission from high, and thus risky, levels is also more likely in this age group. These lifetime variations are not equal for all populations. Populations characterized by similar per capita consumption and distributions, may be composed of individuals with quite different accumulated risks. The fluctuations in drinking status and pattern over the life course could explain in part the large discrepancies found between the problem drinking category in the general population and alcoholics in treatment populations with regard to age composition, interrelatedness, and severity of problems (Fillmore and Midanik 1984).

Describing fluctuations in drinking over time is complicated, and not only because of measurement error. By means of a structural equation model at three time points, Tan (1989) has presented some evidence of a relatively large stability of drinking status in a representative sample of 40- to 60-year-old men from a small Dutch town, while adjusting for this measurement error and taking effects on drinking of age, occupation, and marital status into account. He reported a correlation between consumption scores as high as 0.89 between 3 points in time (covering 10 years). Predictability of consumption category was thus quite high, even though the sample's average increased over the years by more than 300 per cent. Other sources, however, report that chronicity of heavy drinking is by no means a homogeneous phenomenon across time (Skog and Duckert 1993), subpopulations (Cahalan and Room 1974), or countries (Fillmore *et al.* 1991).

In spite of the lack of lifetime consumption data Skog (1984*b*) estimated a risk function for cirrhosis mortality which could incorporate the accumulating detrimental effect of heavy drinking. Skog's final model was a generalized exponential risk for cirrhosis as a function of a cumulative lifetime consumption measure to which weights were applied that decreased sharply over time. The application of weights allowed, for instance, for the empirical observation of a decreasing risk when a person reduces his volume or abstains from further drinking. At the aggregate level, this latency became apparent in lagged effects of a rise in per capita consumption on cirrhosis mortality, but it was also shown to take into account the sharp fall in cirrhosis incidence rates after a sudden decline in per capita consumption of relatively 'wet' countries (Popham 1970; Skog 1980; Norström 1987). More work on the relationship between lifetime drinking careers and individual risk is needed to test this and other derived models and to assess the effect of drinking career on incidence of other alcohol-related effects.

The prevention paradox

What are the implications of the above issues for a public health strategy toward alcohol-related problems? After having established a risk factor in epidemiological research, the goal of a primary prevention strategy is to prevent an increase of the part of the population that is at risk, or to bring about a decrease in the population exposed to high levels of the risk factor. It usually involves some sort of screening of the, not necessarily entire, population for the particular risk factor, followed by treatment or counselling of a selected group of persons. In this approach, the focus is on subjects that are at the *highest risk*. Another available option for a prevention strategy is the reduction of exposure to the risk factor for the *entire population*. Which method is the most effective for a particular outcome will depend on the interaction between risk function and distribution of the risk factor in the population, as was sketched on pp. 39–42.

For alcohol problems characterized by linear increasing risks, the factor determining incidence is the mean consumption, regardless of distribution. That is, every sip adds to the risk, whether taken by a light or a heavy drinker. Therefore, a particular decrease in consumption by *any* member in society will affect the incidence rate in a similar fashion. In such a case, any approach effectively reducing total consumption would be indicated. Most empirical evidence, however, suggests some kind of exponential function with or without a threshold. As has been outlined pp. 41–42, the distribution of consumption then becomes a factor influencing incidence rate. The impact of the shape of the distribution will vary with the particular outcome considered. It is this variation that gives rise to the so-called 'prevention paradox', which refers to the seemingly contradictory situation that although heavy drinkers are at a (much) higher individual risk for a particular drinking problem, most of the people who actually experience the alcohol-related problem cannot be

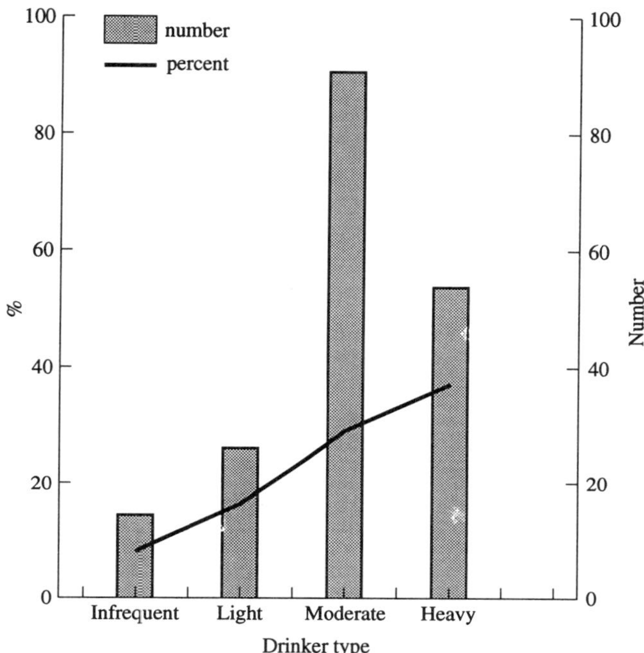

Fig. 2.5 Percentage in each drinker category reporting drinking alcohol during a 6-hour period prior to their injury that led to their visit to the emergency room of a general county hospital in California (solid line and left scale). The bars represent the corresponding numbers (those reporting drinking prior to event) in the sample (right scale).

Source: Cherpitel (1993).

considered heavy drinkers at all. In Fig. 2.5 this is exemplified with data from Cherpitel's (1993) emergency room study. The slope in Fig. 2.5 gives an indication of the possible involvement of alcohol in the total number of injuries reported to an emergency room in a county hospital in California. As can be interpretated from the slope, the proportion of injured persons reporting drinking prior to the injury increases with the usual consumption category of the injured person. Although not assessed multivariately, this increase in proportion signifies alcohol as a possible risk factor in accidents. The drinking categories were defined by a usual or customary consumption measure, consisting of a frequency and quantity component of drinking in the previous month. The important role of alcohol in injury is also apparent in the over-representation of heavy drinkers among those injured, either with or without prior alcohol involvement, which is more than twice the proportion in the general population (19 versus 9 per cent). Although more heavy drinkers get hurt and the risk for an alcohol-related injury appears to increase with consumption, the bars in Fig. 2.5 shows that about two-thirds of all people with a possible alcohol-related injury are nevertheless non-heavy drinkers. It is clear that most of the people with a possible alcohol-related injury are moderate drinkers, and less than one-third are actually heavy drinkers.

The term 'prevention paradox' was originally proposed by Rose (1981) in an article on prevention of coronary heart disease, in which he showed that a preventive effort that would be successful in substantially lowering cholesterol levels in the high-risk group, would still be less effective in minimizing the overall incidence of coronary heart disease than a campaign that would be able to establish even a marginal downward shift of the risk factor in the total population. Krietman (1986) has given empirical evidence of a similar situation when considering certain alcohol-related social problems. He showed that an approach toward a safer limit with even reasonable success would have only a marginal effect on the incidence of social problems. Considering the safe limits proposed by the Royal College of Psychiatrists (1986), he found that most problem drinkers in two British surveys were to be found below these limits. In two 'wet' samples of company directors and brewery workers maximum reductions in the subsample of problem drinkers of not more than 60 per cent is original size could be attained, if one were to use a 'safe limit' of total consumption. Other examples come from Moore and Gerstein (1981), who report that most event-based alcohol problems, such as the above injury example, are to be found among moderate drinkers.

Because the outcome is highly dependent on the factual risks and consumption levels, the prevention paradox may seem simply a game of numbers, definitions, and assumptions. Nevertheless, it does have real ramifications for a prevention strategy. As a general rule, it can be concluded that for some alcohol problems a prevention focus on heavy drinkers may not be warranted or deemed most effective. Although the distribution of consumption is a principal determinant in the equation joining incidence of harm and per capita consumption, the emphasis on the relationship between mean and excessive use may not always be expedient. For a function with increased risk at relatively lower levels of consumption, as may well be the case for event-based problems, a rather low limit is indeed set for the effect of primary prevention that is directed at specific target groups of excessive drinkers. In these instances, a public policy directed at all or lower consumption levels and reaching moderate drinkers may be indicated. For alcohol problems with other risk functions, such as strongly concave ones or those with a large threshold, the situation may be different. In these cases, the pay-off in terms of a direct decline in problem or disease incidence as a result of a general reduction of consumption may not be as great, and an approach that targets excessive drinking, frequency of intoxication, or context may be called for, or at least may be equally effective.

Because of the observed regularities in the distribution of consumption, however, the difference made here between a prevention focus on heavy drinking and general or overall consumption may be superfluous. If it would appear that a change in drinking level of the majority of drinkers would, as a matter of fact, be accompanied by a change in consumption of those drinking at the tail end, or vice versa, the distinction made in the paradox would be dispensable. However, the example of Sweden shows that strong policy measures that affect groups of drinkers differently can change the distribution in an unexpected way. Even in the case of regularity, the question of which strategy is more effective in establishing the desired change in consumption, one that is directed at the total volume of consumption or one that targets specific drinkers or aspects of the drinking pattern, remains difficult to answer. Given the state of affairs at this point it is hard to predict realistically the effects of specific measures. What can be learned by studying empirical risk functions and prevention campaigns is what the limitations of the different approaches are.

An issue, recently raised, might further refine the above paradox. It concerns the way drinking problems are operationalized. Mäkelä (1991) contended that the questions on drinking problems used in surveys fail to discriminate between minor and severe consequences of drinking, since they typically do not inquire about the frequency of occurrence of these problems. He argued that the problems among the heavy drinkers are probably of a greater intensity and frequency than the same type of problems reported among moderate and lighter drinkers. Treating all black-outs or social problems as equal, whether it occurs in an infrequent or a heavy drinker would obscure the real magnitude of problems caused by the heavier drinking pattern. To bridge these 'two worlds of alcohol problems' (Room 1977), Mäkelä proposed a synthesis of the epidemiological and the clinical tradition. The former stresses general drinking practices but often overlooks the grave clinical evidence of alcoholism and dependence, while the latter treats sick individuals, unaware that one is watching only the tail end of a continuum.

Conclusion

This chapter has observed that a slight change in distribution can have a large impact on mortality in the case of exponentially increasing risk, but also that the margins of prediction of a change in distribution at the tail end from a change in per capita consumption are quite large. For certain other categories of harmful consequences of drinking, the phenomenon referred to as the prevention paradox seems to de-emphasize heavy drinking as the principal factor relating total volume and harm. In both instances, however, the distribution of consumption is an important concept when shifting the perspective to issues of public health. Its mean indicates overall exposure of a population to a risk factor, its dispersion yields information as to the proportion exposed to high levels. The distribution of consumption also shows regularities which are meaningful for those considering a prevention policy. The so-called wetness of a drinking culture has an impact on where and when people are allowed to drink and actually drink. That the relationship between wetness and individual drinking is of a reciprocal nature should not be used to denounce the scientific relevance of the construct. Wetness or total consumption in a population will, of course, explain only a fraction of the variation in rates of negative effects. Parameters, such as stability of drinking careers or frequency of drinking and intoxication, also determine the empirical association between total consumption and harm, and prevention should not focus singularly on total consumption. Future research into the social contexts that facilitate change in consumption of either heavy drinkers or social drinkers might add to the knowledge of regularities at the aggregate level, and may increase the possibilities of effective ways of prevention.

References

Alanko, T. (1991). Per capita consumption and rate of heavy use of alcohol: on evidence and inference in the single distribution debate. Paper presented at the seminar *Single population theories in epidemiology*, 4 October. Social Statistics Section and the Addictions Forum, Royal Statistical Society.

Altman, D. G. (1991). *Practical statistics for medical research.* Chapman & Hall, London.

Bofetta, P. and Garfinkel, L. (1990). Alcohol drinking and mortality among men enrolled in an American Cancer Society propsective study. *Epidemiology*, **1**, 342–8.

Bruun, K., *et al.* (1975). *Alcohol control policies in public health perspective*, Vol. 25. Finnish Foundation for Alcohol Studies, Helsinki.

Brody, J. and Mills, G. (1978). On considering alcohol as a risk factor in specific diseases. *American Journal of Epidemiology*, **107**, 462–7.

Cahalan, D. and Room, R. (1974). *Problem drinking among American men.* Rutgers Center of Alcohol Studies, New Brunswick, NJ.

Cherpitel, C. J. (1993). Alcohol and injuries: A review of international emergency room studies. *Addiction*, **88**, 923–38.

de Lint, J. (1974). The epidemiology of alcoholism: the elusive nature of the problem, estimating the prevalence of excessive use and alcohol-related mortality, current trends and the issue of prevention. In *Alcoholism: A medical profile*, (ed. N. Kessel, A. Hawker, and H. Chalke). Edstall, London.

de Lint, J. and Schmidt, W. (1968). The distribution of alcohol consumption in Ontario. *Quarterly Journal of Studies on Alcohol*, **298**, 968–73.

Duffy, J. (1986). The distribution of alcohol consumption: 30 years on. *British Journal of Addiction*, **81**, 735–42.

Duffy, J. (1991). *Trends in alcohol consumption patterns, 1978–1989.* NTC Publications Ltd, Henley-on-Thames.

Duffy. J. and Cohen, G. (1978). Total consumption and excessive drinking. *British Journal of Addiction*, **73**, 259–64.

Fillmore, K. (1987). Prevalence, incidence, and chronicitiy of drinking patterns and problems among men as a function of age: A longitudinal and cohort analysis. *British Journal of Addiction*, **82**, 77–83.

Fillmore, K. and Midanik, L. (1984). Chronicity of drinking problems among men: A longitudinal study. *Journal of Studies Alcohol*, **45**, 228–36.

Fillmore, K. M., Golding, J. M., Leino, E. V., Ager, C. R., and Ferrer, H. P. (1991). Proportions of chronic heavy drinking among persons at risk and in the total population and postulated explanations from aggregate data accounting for cross-study differences. Paper presented at the *17th Annual Alcohol Epidemiology Symposium* , June. Sigtuna, Sweden.

Fillmore, K. M., Golding, J. M., Leino, E. V., Ager, C. R., and Ferrer, H. P. (1994). Societal level predictors of groups' drinking patterns: A research synthesis from the collaborative alcohol-related longitudinal project. *American Journal of Public Health*, **84**, 247–53.

Gomberg, E. (1989). *Alcohol and women.* Rutgers Center of Alcohol Studies, New Brunswick, NJ.

Harburg, E., Ozgoren, F., Hawthorne, V. M., and Schork, M. A. (1980). Community norms of alcohol usage and blood pressure: Tecumseh, Michigan. *American Journal of Public Health*, **70**, 813–20.

Hilton, M. (1988). Regional diversity in United States drinking practices. *British Journal of Addiction*, **83**, 519–32.

Katcher, B. S. (1993). The post-repeal eclipse in knowledge about the harmful effects of alcohol. *Addiction*, **88**, 729–44.

Kendell, R. E. (1984). The beneficial consequences of the United Kingdom's declining per capita consumption of alcohol in 1979–82. *Alcohol and Alcoholism*, **19**, 271–6.

Kendell, R. E., De Roumanie, M., and Ritson, E. (1983). Effect of economic changes on Scottish drinking habits, 1978–1982. *British Journal of Addiction*, **78**, 365–79.

Kleinbaum, D. G., Kupper, L. L., and Morgernstern, H. (1982). *Epidemiologic research. Principles and quantitative methods.* Van Nostrand Reinhold, New York.

Knibbe, R., Drop, M., van Reek, J., and Saenger, G. (1985). The development of alcohol consumption in the Netherlands: 1958–1981. *British Journal of Addiction*, **80**, 411–19.

Kreitman, N. (1986). Alcohol consumption and the prevention paradox. *British Journal of Addiction*, **81**, 353–63.

Ledermann, S. (1956). *Alcool, alcoolism, alcoolisation*, Vol. I. PUF, Paris.

Ledermann, S. (1964). Can one reduce alcoholism without changing total consumption in a population? Paper presented at the *27th International Congress on Alcohol and Alcoholism.* Frankfurt-am-main, Germany.

Lelbach, W. (1975). Quantitative aspects of drinking in alcoholic liver cirrhosis. In *Alcoholic liver pathology*, (ed. J. Khanna, Y. Israel, and H. Kalant), pp. 1–8. ARF, Toronto.

Lemmens, P. (1991). Measurement and distribution of alcohol consumption. Dissertation, University of Limburg.

Lemmens, P., Tan, E., and Knibbe, R. (1990). Comparing distributions of alcohol consumption: empirical probability plots. *British Journal of Addiction*, **85**, 751–8.

Lemmens, P., Tan, E., and Knibbe, R. (1992). Measuring quantity and frequency of drinking in a general population. A comparison of 5 indices. *Journal of Studies on Alcohol*, **53**, 476–86.

Longnecker, M. P., Berlin, J. A., Orza, M. J., and Chalmers, T. C. (1988). A meta-analysis of alcohol consumption in relation to risk of breast cancer. *Journal of the American Medical Association*, **260**, 652–6.

Mäkelä, K. (1991). Impact of changes in availability of alcohol of heavy and dependent drinkers. Paper presented at the *International Symposium on Drug Dependence*. Mexico City.

Miller, G. and Agnew, N. (1974). The Ledermann model of alcohol consumption. *Quarterly Journal of Studies on Alcohol*, **35**, 877–98.

Moore, M. and Gerstein, D. (1981). *Alcohol and public policy: Beyond the shadow of prohibition*. National Academy Press, Washington, DC.

Neve, R., Diederiks, J. P. M., Knibbe, R. A., and Drop, M. J. (1993). Developments in drinking behavior in the Netherlands from 1958 to 1989. A cohort analysis. *Addiction*, **88**, 611–21.

Norström, T. (1987). The abolition of the Swedish rationing system: Effects on consumption distribution and cirrhosis mortality. *British Journal of Addiction*, **82**, 633–41.

Parker, D. A. and Harman, M. S. (1978). The distribution of alcohol consumption model of prevention of alcohol problems. A critical assessment. *Journal of Studies on Alcohol*, **39**, 377–99.

Péquignot, G., Tuyns, A., and Berta, J. L. (1978). Ascitic cirrhosis in relation to alcohol consumption. *International Journal of Epidemiology*, **7**, 113–20.

Popham, R. (1970). Indirect methods of alcoholism prevalence estimation: A critical evaluation. In *Alcohol and alcoholism*, (ed. R. Popham). University of Toronto Press.

Romesljö, A. (1987). Epidemiological studies on the relationship between a decline in alcohol consumption, social factors and alcohol-related disabilities in Stockholm county and the whole of Sweden. Dissertation. Sundbyberg, Sweden.

Room, R. (1977). Measurement and distribution of drinking patterns and problems in general populations. In *Alcohol related disabilities*, (ed. G. Edwards, M. M. Gross, M. Keller, J. Moser, and R. Room), WHO, Offset Publication No. 32, pp. 61–87. World Health Organization, Geneva.

Rose, G. (1981). Strategy of prevention: Lessons from cardiovascular disease. *British Medical Journal*, **282**, 1847–51.

Rose, G. (1985). Sick individuals and sick populations. *International Journal of Epidemiology*, **14**, 32–8.

Rose, G. and Day, S. (1990). The population mean predicts the number of deviant individuals. *British Medical Journal*, **301**, 1031–4.

Royal College of Psychiatrists (1986). *Alcohol: Our favourite drug*. Tavistock, London.

Schmidt, W. and Popham, R. E. (1978). The single distribution theory of alcohol consumption. *Journal of Studies on Alcohol*, **39**, 400–19.

Skinner, H. and Sheu, W.-J. (1982). Reliability of alcohol use indices. *Journal of Studies on Alcohol*, **43**, 1157–70.

Skog, O.-J. (1980). Social interaction and the distribution of alcohol consumption. *Journal of Drug Issues*, **10**, 71–92.

Skog, O.-J. (1981). Alcoholism and social policy: Are we on the right lines. *British Journal of Addiction*, **76**, 315–21.

Skog, O.-J. (1982). *The distribution of consumption. 1: A critical discussion of the Ledermann model*, (mimeographed series No. 64). National Institute for Alcohol Research (SIFA), Oslo.

Skog, O.-J. (1983). *The distribution of consumption. 2: A review of the first wave of empirical evidence*, (mimeographed series No. 67). National Institute for Alcohol Research (SIFA), Oslo.

Skog, O.-J. (1984*a*). *The long waves of alcohol consumption*, (mimeographed series

No. 78). *National Institute for Alcohol Research* (*SIFA*), *Oslo*.

Skog, O.-J. (1984*b*). The risk of function for liver cirrhosis from lifetime alcohol consumption. *Journal of Studies on Alcohol*, **45**, 199–208.

Skog, O.-J. (1985*a*). *The distribution of alcohol consumption. III: Evidence of a collective drinking culture*, (mimeograph series No. 8/85). National Institute for Alcohol Research (SIFA), Oslo.

Skog, O.-J. (1985*b*). The collectivity of drinking cultures: A theory of the distribution of alcohol consumption. *British Journal of Addiction*, **80**, 83–99.

Skog, O.-J. (1991). Epidemiological and biostatistical aspects of alcohol use, alcoholism, and their complications. In *Windows on science*, **40**, (ed. P. C. Erickson and H. Kalant). ARF, Toronto.

Skog, O.-J. and Duckert, F. (1993). The development of alcoholics' and heavy drinkers' consumption: A longitudinal study. *Journal of Studies on Alcohol*, **54**, 178–88.

Smart, R. G. and Schmidt, W. (1970). Blood alcohol levels in drivers not involved in accidents. *Quarterly Journal of Studies on Alcohol*, **31**, 968–71.

Sobell, L., Sobell, M., Leo, G., and Cancilla, A. (1988). Reliability of a timeline method: Assessing normal drinkers' reports of recent drinking and a comparative evaluation across several populations. *British Journal of Addiction*, **83**, 393–402.

St. Leger, A. S., Cochrane, A. L., and Moore, F. (1979). Factors associated with cardiac mortality in developed countries with particular reference to the consumption of wine. *Lancet*, **i**, 1017–20.

Tan, E. (1989). Lisrel, with special attention for a longitudinal study of alcohol consumption. Paper presented at the *Kettil Bruun Society Symposium*, 11–16 June. Maastricht, the Netherlands.

Tan, E., Lemmens, P., and Koning, A. (1990). Regularity in alcohol distributions: implications for the collective nature of drinking behaviour. *British Journal of Addiction*, **85**, 745–50.

Tuck, M. (1980). *Alcoholism and social policy* (Home Office Research Study No. 65). HMSO, London.

Walsh, D. C. and Hingson, R. W. (1987). Epidemiology and alcohol policy. In *Epidemiology and health policy*, (ed. S. Levine and A. M. Lilienfeld), pp. 265–91. Tavistock, London.

3. Alcohol consumption and social consequences, dependence, and positive benefits in general propulation surveys

Lorraine T. Midanik

I was some months into the hunt when, pushed to the edge of patience by too many too-careful answers, I heard myself demand of a major figure in alcohol research, 'How much can I safely drink before I begin to encroach upon certain areas of risk such as cancer, heart disease and liver disease? How much can I safely drink without impairing my intellectual capacities or taking years off my life? Given the state of the art, what is the best course for a person to follow?' I think these are fair, legitimate questions, and I feel that the people who work in the field of alcohol ought to be willing to respond. If there's a danger, I want to know about it, and if I can drink with impunity, I want to know about that, too, because I love to drink (Gross 1983, p. xiii).

Introduction

These salient questions posed by Leonard Gross in 1983 have been and will continue to be of concern to many drinkers. Yet, most social scientists working in alcohol research remain hesitant to respond to questions concerning what amounts of alcohol will put someone at risk for alcohol problems. The underlying reasons for this reluctance are both methodological and political. The studies located for this review of the relationship between alcohol use and consequences of drinking on an individual level not only vary greatly by how alcohol use and alcohol problems are measured (or not measured) but also by what analytical techniques were used (or not used) to answer specific research questions. The non-comparability among the studies both within and across countries makes definitive statements about the risks of consequences due to certain levels of alcohol intake or patterns of alcohol use quite problematic. Moreover, the very definition and recognition of what are said to be the 'consequences of alcohol use' are themselves a result of a complex interplay between political, cultural, and contextual factors.

This chapter focuses on consequences of drinking (social consequences, dependence, and positive benefits) and seeks to extend both the original work presented in Bruun *et al.*'s *Alcohol control policies in public health* (1975) and Mäkelä's (1978) extensive review of the research in this area. In the last 15 years, additional studies have been conducted which examine closely the relationship of alcohol use and the consequences of drinking on an individual level. In addition to reviewing these recent studies, this paper will also explore several other important issues relevant to this topic including how alcohol use as a risk factor has been measured and the relative importance of total annual consumption versus patterns of use in predicting consequences of drinking.

There are relatively few large-scale surveys that examine alcohol use and alcohol-related consequences together (see Table 3.1). Most social scientists who work with alcohol studies in general populations are concerned with the prevalence of different categories of alcohol consumption (for example, abstainer, light, moderate, heavy), patterns of alcohol use (for example, frequent, heavy drinking), and the prevalence of different categories or specific types of alcohol-related problems (Mäkelä 1978). Assessment of all of these components together is rare.

In addition to methodological and political concerns, another explanation for why alcohol use and alcohol-related consequences are not usually analysed simultaneously in great depth is the implicit assumption that since the relationship between the two is generally positive, it is not useful to go beyond simple correlations and cross-tabulations. But as Mäkelä (1978) points out, these types of analyses '. . . tell rather little about how decisive actual intake is as a determinant of adverse consequences'.

This chapter is presented in six sections. The first includes a discussion of the central methodological issues inherent in the analysis of alcohol use and alcohol-related consequences. This includes how alcohol consumption and consequences of drinking have been defined in the literature as well as how respondents attribute their problems to their alcohol use. The second section is a discussion of the general findings on alcohol use and consequences of drinking. This section draws on a review of the international literature on the relationship of alcohol use and consequences by type of problem: social consequences and dependence symptoms. In some cases, researchers have combined all problems into one index with a specified cut-off point; in other studies, problem items have been disaggregated into areas such as work and family problems. A general review of the work on positive consequences of drinking is also included. The third section reviews research which has assessed the shape of the risk function for various consequences of drinking. This approach, adapted from research on physical harm due to drinking, has been conducted primarily in the Scandinavian countries and provides an opportunity to assess the probability of reporting different types of consequences given specific levels of alcohol use.

The fourth section focuses on the few studies which have used both total annual intake and patterns of alcohol use as predictors of consequences. Some of this research seeks to compare these two measures, while in other studies drinking patterns are seen as mediating variables. The fifth section examines specific variables which influence and in some cases, mediate the relationship of alcohol use and social consequences—such as age and gender. The final section summarizes the findings of the literature review and proposes recommendations for future research. This paper can provide a basis from which researchers working with alcohol survey data will further explore and specify the relationship of yearly intake, patterns of alcohol use, and how these factors effect different consequences of drinking.

Methodological issues

In classic epidemiological research, a risk factor is defined as exposure to a specific condition that increases the probability of developing disease. The most cited example in the epidemiological literature is smoking and lung cancer. Even when other factors, such as environmental conditions, genetic susceptibility, and demographic characteristics are controlled, the positive association between cigarette smoking and lung cancer has remained strong. Longitudinal studies support the association as causal.

The alcohol field presents significant challenges to the traditional epidemiological approach. First, alcohol consumption is related to multiple outcomes—many of which are social as opposed to physical. Secondly, drinking patterns are quite varied thus leaving the question open concerning whether regular doses (heavy or otherwise) of ethanol are potentially more risky than heavy sporadic drinking. Hence, the measurement of alcohol use becomes a crucial factor in establishing risk.

There have been several ways alcohol consumption has been measured in general population surveys which include volume, heavier drinking patterns, typologies that delineate several types of drinking patterns, and frequency and typical quantity of drinking measures assessed separately. Despite the variety of ways that alcohol use can be assessed, there has been a strong emphasis on volume measures to establish thresholds above which individuals have a high probability of problems.

Volume alone has been measured in four different ways: usual quantity/frequency measures (beverage specific and a global measure), a graduated frequency measure, all drinking occasions in the last 7 days, and a survey period estimate method. Measures of heavier drinking patterns have been derived from the frequency of drinking five or more, or eight or more drinks on one occasion over some time period (usually weekly), as well as from more 'subjective' measures such as self-reported frequency of drunkenness or intoxication and frequency of feeling 'high' or 'tight'. Thus, it is with caution that one compares these studies.

Measures of alcohol problems or consequences also differ—particularly across countries. In some studies, a global index of social consequences or dependence symptoms is derived from a simple count of problems with a cut-off point dividing severe from less severe reports of problems. Sometimes problem items in these studies are weighted, but in most cases they are not. Other researchers have specified categories of problems (for example, work problems), and the analyses are conducted separately on several types of social consequences. Even within these global indexes or specific problem indexes, the analytical techniques used vary from cross-tabulations of drinker categories (defined as abstainer, light, moderate, and heavy drinkers) to number of problems reported, to logistic modelling to plot risk curves for various types of consequences. Here again, comparisons among studies are problematic and conclusions may only be drawn with caution.

In addition, there is the need to consider how respondents attribute problems to their alcohol use. Because none of the studies contain a measure of the prevalence of social problems in general, for example, family problems not attributed to alcohol, researchers have no way of knowing whether or not respondents erroneously attribute some or all of their social problems to their alcohol use.

The general relationship between alcohol use and its consequences

Studies included in this chapter are primarily national samples undertaken since 1978 which include an analysis of the relationship of alcohol use to alcohol problems. Table 3.1 presents the studies by author, type of sample, measures used to alcohol use, and alcohol problems within each country.

Social consequences

Alcohol-related social problems have been measured in at least two different ways: (1) specific problems, and (2) global measures as an overall index of social consequences associated with alcohol use. The variation in how these indices have been conceptualized is evidenced in their titles, for example, Social Consequences Index (Hilton 1991*a*,*b*; Clark and Midanik 1982), Negative Experiences (Jasinski 1989), Lack of Demeanor and Non-Fulfillment of Social Roles (Fillmore *et al.* 1992), and Social Disapproval (Knupfer 1984).

In the United States since 1978, the relationship between alcohol use and global indexes of alcohol-related problems has been assessed in both the 1979 and the 1984 national alcohol surveys. Clark and Midanik (1982) developed an index based on any positive response to items related to spouse problems, friends/relatives problems, police and accident problems, and job problems

Table 3.1 Studies of alcohol consumption and alcohol problems

Country and source	Sample	Consumption measure	Problem measure
England and Wales			
Breeze (1985)	NS[a] 1982 I[b], $N=1994$ Women	All drinking occasions last 7 days	Psychological dependence, physical dependence, drunk and hangover symptoms
Goddard and Ikin (1988)	NS 1987 I, $N=3930$	All drinking occasions last 7 days	Psychological dependence, physical dependence, drunkenness, drunken driving
Finland			
Mäkelä and Simpura (1985)	NS 1979 M[c], $N=1793$ Current drinkers	Typical QF[d] by beverage type	Hangover symptoms, accident, health, reckless behaviour, belligerence, drunken driving, positive effects, control worries, social reactions: family, doctor, work, police, friends
Hauge and Irgens-Jensen (1986, 1987, 1990)	NS 1979 M, $N=1793$ Alcohol consumers	Typical Qf by beverage type; frequency of intoxication	As above
Saila (1987)	NS 1976 I, $N=2942$ NS 1984 I, $N=3870$	SPE[e]	Quarrels, drinking and driving, damage to belongings, loss of money, fight, accident, victim of cheating/robbery/ theft, hangover symptoms, beneficial effects
Mäkelä and Mustonen (1988)	NS 1984 I, $N=2866$ Current drinkers	SPE[e] grouped into 7 classes	Positive effects, behavioural concomitants of drinking, single drinking occasions, health, social reactions

Iceland			
Hauge and Irgens-Jensen (1986, 1987, 1990)	NS 1979 M, $N=1742$ Alcohol consumers	Typical QF by beverage type; frequency of intoxication	Hangover symptoms, accident, health, reckless behaviour, belligerence, drunken driving, positive effects, control worries, social reactions: family, doctor, work, police, friends
Norway			
Hauge and Irgens-Jensen (1986, 1987, 1990)	NS 1979 M, $N=1378$ Alcohol consumers	Typical QF by beverage type; frequency of intoxication	As above
Poland			
Moskalewicz and Swiatkiewicz (1986)	NS 1984 $N=624$ 'Lucky drinkers'	Average annual consumption; intoxication	Positive experiences
Jasinski (1989)	NS (quota sampling) 1980 (lifetime) I, N 1980 N=1972 1985 N=1808	Frequency of drinking spirits last 3 months and last drinking occasion	Positive and negative experiences [both surveys use quota sampling]
Scotland			
Kreitman and Duffy (1982)	Random Sample (1978) I, $N=287$ Company directors, Senior executives Volunteer Sample (1978) I, $N=247$ Shop-floor workers in breweries and distilleries	1-week retrospective diary: total consumption and 4 drinking pattern variables	General health, alcohol dependence syndrome, marital and family problems, work problems, public order

Table 3.1 *continued*

Country and source	Sample	Consumption measure	Problem measure
Sweden			
Hauge and Irgens-Jensen (1986, 1987, 1990)	NS 1979 M, $N=1582$ Alcohol consumers	Typical QF by beverage type; frequency of intoxication	Hangover symptoms, accident, health, reckless behaviour, belligerence, drunken driving, positive effects, control worries, social reactions: family, doctor, work, police, friends
United States			
Clark and Midanik (1982) Clark (1982)	NS 1979 I, $N=1772$	Beverage-specific quantity, graduated frequencies: no. of drinks/month (5 categories)	Belligerence, child-raising concerns, money, problems with spouce, friends/relatives, police, job; loss of control, dependence symptoms, binge drinking, health worries
Knupfer (1984)	9 population samples combined (county and natl) 1977–9 M+I, $N=7347$	Frequency of drunkenness (5+, 8+, feeling high, feeling drunk, combined index: 2 of the 4)	Indices of Social Disapproval and Personal Concer
Grant and Harford (1990)	NS 1984 I, $N=2167$ (downweighted total sample)	Av. ethanol (oz) consumed per day during past year: from beverage-specific quantity items related to typical amount of drinking on recent occasions and frequency of heavier drinking occasions	DSM-III-R Alcohol Dependence based on 8 of the 9 dependence criteria

Harford *et al.* (1991)	NS 1984 I, $N=2167$ (downweighted total sample)	Av. ethanol (oz) consumed per day during past year; monthly frequency of intoxication (subjective)	Dependence Symptoms Index ($n=12$); dependent = 3 or more symptoms; Alcohol-related problems: legal (4), belligerence (2), physical health (3), work/financial (5), social/family (12) problems = 1 or more vs none in 5 groups
Hilton (1991*a*)	NS 1984 I, $N=3185$ Current drinkers	Heavy drinking: 5 or more drinks per occasion or 8 or more drinks per day at least once a week	Dependence Symptoms Index ($n=13$); moderate – 3 or more, high = 4 or morc; Consequences Index ($n=32$); moderate = 4 or more, high = 8 or more
Hilton (1991*b*)	NS 1984 I, $N=118$ Heavy drinkers (drinks 8 or more drinks on one occasion three times/week or more)	Monthly Volume; Frequency of Drunkenness, frequency of 8 or more drinks/day	Consequences Index ($n=32$); high-problem group = 8 or more, low-problem group = 1–7
Fillmore *et al.* (1992)	Meta-analysis of 21 studies: 1960–82 (see Fillmore *et al.* 1991)	Frequency of drinking/month, quantity drinking/typical occasion	Physiological consequences, mental, and existential problems, casualty problems, lack of demeanour and non-fulfilment of social roles, negative personal reasons

[a] NS, national survey.
[b] I, personal interview.
[c] M, mailed questionaire.
[d] QF, quantity/frequency volume measure.
[e] SPE, survey period estimates, (see Simpura 1987).

and looked at the prevalence of this global measure by approximate number of drinks per month by gender. As expected, while only 9 per cent of males and 5 per cent of females reported any social consequences related to drinking in the last 12 months, the percentage dramatically increased for both men and women as the number of drinks per month increased: 27 per cent of men and 37 per cent of women who drank over 120 drinks per month reported at least one social consequence. Hilton (1991*a*,*b*) conducted two analyses of the 1984 US national alcohol survey which focused on the relationship between alcohol use and alcohol-related problems. His first analysis on heavier drinkers only (eight or more drinks per day at least three times a week) yielded a rather small sample size ($N=118$). From a list of 32 questions concerning negative consequences of drinking, he developed two groups: a high problem group (eight or more consequences) and a low problem group (less than eight consequences). Hilton found that the higher problem group scored higher on three measures of alcohol use (frequency of eight or more drinks per day, volume of alcohol consumed per month, and frequency of self-reported intoxication). Using logistic regression, he found that none of the demographic variables were related to problem status and that frequency of eight or more drinks per day was only weakly related.

Hilton's second analysis compared heavier drinking patterns (monthly frequency of 5+ drinking occasions and monthly frequency of 8+ drinking days) with demographic variables to predict social consequences. Although, overall, the total variance explained in each model was moderate (17 per cent for the model with 5+ drinking occasions variable included: 23 per cent for the 8+ drinking days included), the measures of heavier drinking were the best predictors of social consequences and, of the two, the 8+ measure was stronger.

Jasinski's (1989) analysis of two Polish national drinking surveys in 1980 and 1985 took a different approach to this issue. This study included global indexes of both negative and positive experiences associated with alcohol and assessed their relationship separately and together with mean annual alcohol consumption, mean annual consumption of spirits, and percentage of persons who on the last occasion of drinking spirits had blood alcohol concentrations of over 0.05 (defined as intoxicated). As expected, at each level the higher the score on the index of bad experiences, the higher the level of mean annual alcohol consumption. The higher the mean annual alcohol consumption, the more likely the respondents reported both negative and positive consequences associated with alcohol.

Finally, Knupfer (1984) used a meta-analytic approach to combine several data sets to assess alcohol use and alcohol problems in nine population samples (one national and eight county samples). She developed a two-part Social Disapproval Index which indicates if someone had been critical of the respondent's drinking. The more stringent the definition of heavier alcohol use, the higher the proportion reporting social disapproval. For example, 66 per cent of those who report having eight or more drinks on one occasion three or more times a week, report at least one negative response (43 per cent if the cut-off point is three or more).

Since 1978, several studies have been published that have compared alcohol consumption levels with reports of *specific categories* of negative consequences. Many of these studies have categorized annual intake into light, moderate, and heavier groups and then looked at the proportion of specific problems reported within these categories (Goddard and Ikin 1988; Saila 1987; Harford *et al.* 1991). Similar to the studies using global measures, these studies found that as intake increases, so do self-reports of all kinds of problems.

Alcohol dependence

The classification of alcohol problems typically gets dichotomized: problems arising from the external environment (social consequences) and problems within the individual associated with excessive or chronic use of alcohol. Alcohol researchers, primarily from the disciplines of sociology or public health, have tended to call individual problems 'dependence symptoms'. Alcohol researchers from the disciplines of medicine, psychology, and psychiatry have frequently argued that there is a core set of dependence dimensions derived from several sources, for example, DSM-III-R, ICD-10, which define the Alcohol Dependence Syndrome. With these sets of items, an accurate clinical diagnosis can be made. Most of the research in this area used 'dependence symptoms'.

When dependence is conceptualized as disaggregated symptoms, the research varies from positive associations between consumption and dependence to more complex analyses that address rather specific research questions. Research studying positive responses to dependence items (physical or psychological effects of drinking) by type of drinker (light, moderate, heavy) or by annual alcohol intake has consistenly shown higher alcohol dependence rates for heavier drinkers or for higher average consumption (Breeze 1985; Goddard and Ikin 1988; Clark and Midanik 1982; Harford *et al.* 1991; Fillmore *et al.* 1992; Hauge and Irgens-Jensen, 1986, 1987; Krietman and Duffy 1982; Mäkelä and Simpura 1985). Few researchers have gone beyond cross-tabulations or correlations to address more complex research questions.

Hilton (1991*b*), for example, used measures of heavier drinking (monthly frequency of 5+ drinking occasions and monthly frequency of 8+ drinking days) along with demographic variables to assess their ability to predict dependence. Both indicators of heavier drinking within each model were the best predictors of dependence with the 8+ measure providing a stronger predictive value than the 5+. Grant and Harford (1990) using the same dataset, developed DSM-III-R criteria and assessed the relationship of dependence and ethanol consumption for a group of heavier drinking respondents (consumed five or more drinks at a sitting at least once in the last year). Although overall the relationship of ethanol and dependence was strong for this sample, the association was strongest for the younger groups and was progressively weaker for the older respondents.

Hauge and Irgens-Jensen (1986) compared annual alcohol intake and frequency of intoxication in terms of their predictive value for two dimensions of dependence symptoms (hangover symptoms and control worries). They concluded that incidents of intoxication were most closely associated with hangover symptoms, while overall intake was a better predictor of control worries.

Positive consequences of drinking

Little research has been done on the positive effects of drinking even though the positive effects of alcohol use have been measured in US alcohol surveys from the 1960s to the present (Cahalan *et al.* 1969). Only six studies (Scandinavian countries and Poland) have examined the relationship between alcohol use and positive benefits of drinking (Hauge and Irgens-Jensen 1990; Mäkelä and Mustonen 1988; Mäkelä and Simpura 1985, Jasinski 1989; Moskalewicz and Swiatkiewicz 1986; Saila 1987).

There is a general positive relationship between reports of positive consequences and alcohol use from studies conducted in Finland (Saila 1987) and in four Scandinavian countries (Hauge and Irgens-Jensen 1990). Moskalewicz and Swiatkiewicz (1986) examined only those drinkers in Poland who reported no negative effects from drinking during the year preceding the survey ('lucky drinkers') who comprised slightly more than 20 per cent of their sample. Overall, these lucky drinkers consumed less than other drinkers, and there was a strong positive relationship between the amount drunk and the number of positive consequences. Further, drinking to intoxication was not an unusual event. The authors conclude (p. 16) that the '. . . context of drinking, expectations towards alcohol and other factors not seized by the inquiry, play a significant role'.

Some studies examined alcohol use and reports of positive consequences of drinking *and* reports of negative consequences. Jasinski's (1989) analysis of Polish drinking found that as annual alcohol consumption rises, so do reports of *both* positive and negative consequences. In Finland, Mäkelä and Simpura (1985) found that at all levels of consumption, more people reported benefits of drinking than control worries or negative social reactions to drinking, however, in the highest consumption group, the balance between negative and positive effects evens out. Mäkelä and Mustonen (1988) reported that positive effects of drinking increase at a more rapid rate at the lower end of alcohol use compared to institutional reactions against drinking which increase faster at the upper ranges of alcohol use. Hauge and Irgens-Jensen (1990) also found that the more an individual reports positive consequences of drinking, the more likely negative consequences of drinking will also be reported.

Hauge and Irgens-Jensen (1990) found that frequency of intoxication was more strongly correlated with positive consequences than yearly alcohol consumption. Further, the differences in reports of positive consequences between the four Scandinavian countries studied are smaller when frequency of intoxication is held constant compared to holding consumption constant. Mäkelä and Mustonen (1988) compared two transformations of annual alcohol intake to assess the predictive value of both positive and negative consequences of drinking. They found that the logarithm of annual alcohol intake was the best predictor of benefits of drinking while the square of annual alcohol intake best predicted reactions against drinking by institutional agents.

Hauge and Irgens-Jensen's (1990) work represents the final type of analysis in this area which compares four Scandinavian countries in terms of their annual alcohol use, intoxication frequency, and reports of positive consequences. Their results show that positive consequences, while significantly correlated with yearly alcohol consumption, were more strongly related to intoxication frequency.

Alcohol use as a risk for social consequences

It is possible to examine the probability of occurrence of specific consequences or types of consequences at given levels of alcohol use. The relationship between alcohol consumption and some specific consequence can be expressed as a function of consumption level (for example, risk of cirrhosis) or as a U-shaped or J-shaped curve (for example, coronary heart disease). Mäkelä and Mustonen (1988) proposed that the risk function for social consequences should also vary by condition and by culture. Consequences due to drinking can then be associated with low, moderate, or high levels of alcohol use and provide data on a threshold for any alcohol-related problem.

Primarily, studies of the shape of risk curves have been conducted in the Scandinavian countries. Mäkelä and Simpura (1985), using data from a representative mailed questionnaire of adults in Finland in 1979, used logistic modelling to assess the probability of specific types of consequences. By examining the slopes of the logit models, they found that social reactions to drinking grew more rapidly with increasing consumption than the probability of belligerence or drunken driving (behavioural concomitants of drinking) and accidents or health problems (direct causal consequences of drinking). They found that at all levels of consumption positive effects are more common than control worries or negative social reactions to drinking. At the highest level of consumption, approximately the same number of drinkers are worried about their drinking as report positive benefits. They also note that informal social reactions and personal concerns about drinking begin to occur at much higher levels than reactions from institutional agents, yet as consumption increases, institutional reactions increase more rapidly. For all consumption levels, more people are concerned about their drinking than report control reactions.

Mäkelä and Mustonen (1988) using Finnish interview data collected in 1984 not only assessed the risk function of alcohol use but attempted to find a suitable transformation of annual intake of alcohol for each of their 24 logit models of experiences related to drinking. They found that the logarithm of annual alcohol intake, as compared to untransformed data or the square of annual intake, is the best predictor of positive consequences of drinking, whereas the square of annual alcohol intake is the best predictor of institutional reactions against drinking. This finding implies that at lower drinking levels positive consequences increase faster whereas institutional reactions increase more rapidly at higher drinking levels. Moreover, annual intake of alcohol (untransformed) is the best predictor of most indicators of behavioural concomitants of drinking and consequences of single drinking occasions. By plotting the risk curves for both positive and adverse consequences of drinking, Mäkelä and Mustonen (1988) illustrate that while two indicators of positive consequences begin to level out at the highest consumption levels, adverse consequences increase at a more rapid pace. The risk curve for getting arrested by the police mirrors that of positive experiences related to drinking.

In an analysis which compares four Scandinavian countries (Iceland, Finland, Norway, and Sweden), Hauge and Irgens-Jensen (1986, 1990) assessed the relationship of annual intake with control worries, hangover symptoms, reckless behaviour, and positive consequences. Although the intent of their analyses was to compare rates of problems among the four countries while holding alcohol consumption constant and to assess the relationship of alcohol use, frequency of intoxication, and consequences of drinking among the countries, Hauge and Irgens-Jensen also developed risk curves for each of the four indices for each country. Because they did not use logistic modelling techniques, their results cannot be directly compared to the research previously discussed. For each type of consequence, there appears to be some variation in each of the curves among the countries. For example, there appears to be a very strong linear relationship between alcohol consumption and reckless behaviour for Iceland, whereas the curves for Norway and Finland are slower in lower consumption categories, and increase rapidly in the higher consumption categories. As was the case in the work previously described, there does not seem to be a threshold effect. Problems are reported at virtually all levels of alcohol consumption; there does not seem to be a specific amount which marks the 'danger zone' above which problems begin to occur.

The potential for a broader application of risk function analysis is great, including an examination of the shape of the risk curves cross-culturally. For example, is the risk curve in the United States for institutional reactions similar to that of Finland, or do reactions from formal agents begin at lower levels of consumption in the United States compared to Finland? Also, given the general lowering of per capita consumption, a longitudinal approach would be of great interest. For example, does the risk curve for behavioural concomitants in 1979 look similar to the ones generated in both 1984 and 1990 and again, is this phenomenon similar across countries?

Annual intake, drinking patterns, and consequences of drinking

Annual alcohol intake (total volume) and drinking patterns have been used to assess the relationship between alcohol use and consequences. Drinking patterns have been sometimes defined as mediating the relationship between total alcohol use and consequences. Another approach is to assess which variable better predicts specific drinking problems. Three studies which specifically address the relationship between patterning of drinking, annual intake, and reports of social consequences are described here.

Using a random sample of company directors and senior executives and a sample of shop-floor workers of breweries and distilleries in Edinburgh, Krietman and Duffy (1982) assessed whether drinking pattern variables (maximum daily consumption, maximum session consumption, maximum rate, number of drinking days) mediated the relationship between volume (intake the last 7 days) and five categories of consequences (general health, alcohol dependence syndrome, family, work, and social problems). Initially, there was a strong positive relationship between consumption and consequences. This relationship became non-significant when patterns were entered into the model for work and health consequences (for company directors) and for social and work consequences (for production workers). Kreitman and Duffy (1982) conclude that in four of the five types of consequences studied, style of drinking has a mediating effect but that for certain types of consequences, drinking patterns may be more important than total consumption.

Hauge and Irgens-Jensen (1986) looked at alcohol use and reports of control worries, hangover symptoms, and reckless behaviour in four Scandinavian countries. Within each country there was a positive relationship between annual consumption and each category of negative consequences. However, countries with higher total consumption did not necessarily have higher rates of negative consequences when compared to countries with lower total consumption. This finding lead the researchers to look at patterns of drinking (feeling of being intoxicated and higher quantities of alcohol consumed on one occasion). Both the reported frequencies of intoxication and larger quantities per occasion were higher in Finland and Iceland as compared to Norway and Sweden. When the frequency of intoxication is held constant, the differences between the countries in terms of alcohol problems is minimal. Based on a series of correlational and regression analyses, Hauge and Irgens-Jensen (1986) conclude that the frequency of reported experiences of intoxication is a more significant predictor of problems than annual consumption of alcohol.

Finally, Clark (1982) used the US 1979 national alcohol survey to assess frequency of drunkenness and amount of drinking as predictors of social consequences of drinking, dependence symptoms, and loss of control over drinking. He found that both the drunkenness measure and the volume measure had a modest independent effect on drinking problems when the effect of the other predictor variable was controlled. He argues that asking the frequency of drunkenness directly as opposed to inferring it from self-reports of heavy episodic drinking is preferable, and that respondents can best report their own impairment since body size, tolerance to alcohol, and the rapidity of drinking can affect the degree of drunkenness attained.

Mediating/confounding variables

A consistent finding in the alcohol epidemiological literature is that there are vast differences in drinking across specific demographic subgroups, for example, men report more alcohol use and more alcohol problems than women, younger people report more alcohol use and alcohol problems than older people (Clark and Hilton, 1991). This section will examine the influence of gender, age, and other mediating and confounding variables to explain the relationship between alcohol use and alcohol problems. Emphasis will be placed on studies which have assessed the impact of alcohol intake and/or drinking patterns on multiple groups of consequences for specific demographic subgroups using multivariate models.

Age In an analysis of ethanol and dependence (DSM-III-R), Grant and Harford (1990) found that age was the most powerful modifier when other demographic variables were controlled. For 20-year-olds, the estimated odds for dependence was 1.85 compared to 1.29 for 60-year-olds. Age was also a significant modifier of the relationship of ethanol and impaired control over drinking and tolerance and/or withdrawal (components of dependence) with risk decreasing with age. Hilton (1991*a*) also found age to be a significant negative predictor of both dependence symptoms and consequences in multiple regression models which included monthly frequency of 5+ drinking occasions. In their analysis of alcohol intake and experiences related to drinking in Finland, Mäkelä and Simpura (1985) found that most categories of consequences can be predicted by annual intake or by annual intake and age. For example, younger people report more concomitant behaviour and drinking, for example, recklessness, belligerence, and drunken driving. Younger people also more frequently report positive benefits of drinking as well as more worries about their drinking.

In contrast to the studies just presented, Hauge and Irgens-Jensen (1987), who analysed data from four Scandinavian countries, found that when annual consumption and intoxication frequency were held constant, the effect of age on consequences of drinking is limited. Age is of little significance with respect to control worries, perhaps reflecting the belief that this type of consequence is more dependent on longer-term drinking. Age is of greater significance with respect to other types of negative experiences. Older people are more likely to have experienced health problems and social reactions to their drinking; younger people are more likely to report hangover symptoms and reckless behaviour.

Gender Since there are marked differences between male and female alcohol consumption and self-reports of alcohol-related problems, one would expect that gender would be an important factor in dependency. However, Harford *et al.* (1991) found that gender was not an important modifier of the relationship between ethanol use and dependence. Yet, the risk of reporting a physical problem due to drinking was higher for women (risk for health problems increased by 0.51 compared to 0.20 for each additional ounce of ethanol consumed daily for men). Further, the risk of physical problems were more closely related to intoxication for women than for men. It is important to note that gender was also not a significant modifier of the relationship of ethanol and other social consequences of drinking.

Perhaps one explanation of Harford *et al.*'s (1991) findings is that the impact of gender should be assessed as an interaction with age as Mäkelä and Simpura (1985) suggest. For example, in their analysis of Finnish data, Mäkelä and Simpura (1985) found considerable variation in age groups between men and women concerning social reactions to drinking. In the younger age groups, disapproval of drinking from friends is equally likely for men and women, but in the older age groups, criticisms from friends are more likely for men. This differs for disapproval of drinking from relatives in which the gender differences are stronger for both age groups. Moreover, in an analysis which holds annual intake constant, Mäkelä and Simpura (1985) found that with the exception of drunken driving, there were no gender differences in reports of consequences of drinking.

Finally, Knupfer's (1984) analysis of the relationship between frequency of intoxication and indices of personal concern about drinking and social disapproval indicates that when more stringent criteria are applied to intoxication measures (8+ drinks once a week or more), women's reports of both personal concern and social disapproval are higher than rates among men. When the criteria for intoxication are less stringent, the frequency of a positive response on either index is lower for women compared to men.

Other variables Grant and Harford (1990) found that other socio-demographic variables, such as gender, ethnicity, marital status, and education, were not identified as important mediating variables. However, in their analysis of component subscales of the DSM-II-R, they found that higher levels of education were more strongly associated with daily ethanol intake and both 'continued drinking despite consequences' and 'giving up important activities in favor of drinking' (two subscales). Grant and Harford (1990) argue that heavier drinking by those in higher social positions may be less tolerated. This view differs from Mäkelä (1978), who argued that individuals in lower social positions are more likely to be sanctioned for their heavier drinking behaviour.

Finally, Hauge and Irgens-Jensen (1986) illustrate the importance of cross-cultural factors in assessing the relationship between alcohol consumption, frequency of intoxication, and consequences of drinking among four Scandinavian countries. Although they found differences in rates of negative consequences among the four countries, the findings indicate that these differences disappear when intoxication frequency was held constant. This implies that cultural variation in drinking pattterns is perhaps a major variable in comparing problem rates across countries.

Conclusions

1. There is a consistent, positive relationship between alcohol use (annual alcohol intake) and alcohol problems. This includes both social consequences, alcohol dependence, and positive consequences of drinking. This relationship holds for broader, global measures as well as for specific categories of alcohol problems.
2. There is little evidence that discernible threshold effects exist for consequences of drinking.
3. By using logit analysis and examining the shape of alcohol risk curves for various consequences of drinking, it is clear that the probability of having an alcohol-related consequence varies by type of consequence, age, and culture. Institutional reactions appear to occur more rapidly at higher consumption levels as compared to other types of experiences.
4. There is evidence that patterning of drinking is as important, and in some cases, more important than annual intake as a predictor of alcohol problems.
5. The transformation of alcohol intake may vary by the experience to which it is being predicted. In the Finnish data, the logarithm of annual intake was the best predictor of positive consequences of drinking while the square of

annual intake was a better predictor of negative reactions to drinking by institutional agents.

6. As annual intake increases, so do reports of *both* negative and positive consequences of drinking.
7. Age is significant specifically in terms of reports of dependence. The relationship between ethanol consumption and dependence is strongest for the younger age groups.
8. Gender is surprisingly less important as a confounding variable. At very high levels of consumption, there are few differences between men and women.
9. Future research needs to continue to specify the relationship between annual intake, drinking patterns, and different types of alcohol problems. Particular attention should be placed on replicating research conducted in the Scandinavian countries to assess its application to other countries.

Acknowledgements

This research was supported by a National Alcohol Research Center Grant (AA-05595) from the US National Institute on Alcohol Abuse and Alcoholism to the Alcohol Research Group, Berkeley, California. The author wishes to thank Andrea Mitchell and Beth Thomas for their help in locating the materials for this paper.

References

Breeze, E. (1985). *Women and drinking*. Office of Population Censuses and Surveys, Social Survey Division. HMSO, London.

Bruun, K., *et al.* (1975). *Alcohol control policies in public health perspective*, Vol. 25. Finnish Foundation or Alcohol Studies, Helsinki.

Cahalan, D. (1970). *Problem drinkers*. Jossey-Bass, San Francisco.

Cahalan, D., Cisin, I. H., and Crossley, H. M. (1969). *American drinking practices*. Rutgers Center of Alcohol Studies, New Brunswick, NJ.

Clark, W. B. (1982). Frequency of drunkenness in the U.S. population. *Journal of Studies on Alcohol*, **43**, 1267–75.

Clark, W. B. and Hilton, M. E. (ed.) (1991). *Alcohol in America*. State University of New York, Albany, NY.

Clark, W. and Midanik, L. (1982). Alcohol use and alcohol problems among U.S. adults: Results of the 1979 National Survey. Alcohol and health monograph. 1, *Alcohol consumption and related problems*, Publication No. (ADM) 82–1190, pp. 3–52. US Department of Health and Human Services, Rockville, MD.

Fillmore, K. M., Hartka, E., Johnstone, B., Leino, V., Motoyoshi, M., and Temple, M.

(1991). A meta-analysis of life course variation in drinking, *British Journal of Addiction*, **86**, 1221–68.

Fillmore, K. M., Golding, J. M., Leino, E. V., Motoyoshi, M., Ager, C. R., and Ferrer, H. P. (1992). Relationships of measures of alcohol consumption with alcohol-related problems in multiple studies: A research synthesis from the Collaborative Alcohol-Related Longitudinal Study. Paper presented at the *18th Annual Meeting of the Kettil Bruun Society, Alcohol Epidemiology Symposium*, 1–5 June. Toronto, Canada.

Goddard, E. and Ikin, C. (1988). *Drinking in England and Wales in 1987*. Office of Population Censuses and Surveys, Social Survey Division. HMSO, London.

Grant, B. F. and Harford, T. C. (1990). The relationship between ethanol intake and DSM-III-R alcohol dependence. *Journal of Studies on Alcohol*, **51**, 448–56.

Gross, L. (1983). *How much is too much? The effects of social drinking*. Random House, New York.

Harford, T. C., Grant, B. F., Hasin, D. S. (1991). The effect of average daily consumption and frequency of intoxication on the occurrence of dependence symptoms and alcohol-related problems. In *Alcohol in America. Drinking practices and problems*, (ed. W. B. Clark and M. E. Hilton), pp. 213–37. State University of New York, Albany, NY.

Hauge, R. and Irgens-Jensen, O. (1986). The relationship between alcohol consumption, alcohol intoxication and negative consequences of drinking in four Scandinavian countries. *British Journal of Addiction*, **81**, 513–24.

Hauge, R. and Irgens-Jensen, O. (1987). Age, alcohol consumption and the experiencing of negative consequences of drinking in four Scandinavian countries. *BJA*, **82**, 1101–10.

Hauge, R. and Irgens-Jensen, O. (1990). The experiencing of positive consequences of drinking in four Scandinavian countries. *British Journal of Addiction*, **85**, 645–53.

Hilton, M. E. (1991*a*). Higher and lower levels of self-reported problems among heavy drinkers. In *Alcohol in America. Drinking practices and problems*, (ed. W. B. Clark and M. E. Hilton), pp. 238–48. State University of New York, Albany, NY.

Hilton, M. E. (1991*b*). Demographic characteristics and the frequency of heavy drinking as predictors of self-reported drinking problems. In *Alcohol in American. Drinking practices and problems*, (ed. W. B. Clark and M. E. Hilton), pp. 194–212. State University of New York, Albany, NY.

Jasinski, J. (1989). Good and bad experience related to drinking. Some findings of the 1980 and 1985 Polish Drinking Surveys. Paper presented at the *15th Annual Alcohol Epidemiology Symposium*, 11–16 June. Maastricht, the Netherlands.

Knupfer, G. (1984). The risks of drunkenness (or, *Ebrietas Resurrecta*). *British Journal of Addiction*, **79**, 185–96.

Krietman, N. and Duffy, J. (1982). Beyond consumption: The effect of drinking patterns on the consequences of drinking. Paper presented at the *8th annual Meeting of the Kettil Bruun Society, Alcohol Epidemiology Symposium*. Helsinki, Finland.

Mäkelä, K. (1978). Level of consumption and social consequences of drinking. In *Research advances in alcohol and drug problems*, (ed. Y. Israel *et al.*), Vol. 4, pp. 303–48. Plenum, New York.

Mäkelä, K. and Mustonen, H. (1988). Positive and negative experiences related to drinking as a function of annual alcohol intake. *British Journal of Addiction*, **83**, 403–8.

Mäkelä, K. and Simpura, J. (1985). Experiences related to drinking as a function of annual alcohol intake and by sex and age. *Drug and Alcohol Dependence*, **15**, 389–404.

Moskalewicz, J. and Swiatkiewicz, G. (1986). Lucky drinkers. Paper presented at the *IGCAS conference, Drinking Patterns and Drinking Problems*, 22–26 September. Zaborow, Poland.

Saila, S. L. (1987). The consequences of drinking. In *Finnish drinking habits. Results from interview surveys held in 1968, 1976 and 1984*, (ed. J. Simpura), Vol. 35, pp. 150–66. Finnish Foundation for Alcohol Studies, Helsinki.

Simpura, J. (ed.) (1987). *Finnish drinking habits. Results from interview surveys held in 1968, 1976 and 1984*, Vol. 35. Finnish Foundation for Alcohol Studies, Helsinki.

4. Alcohol and risk of physical harm

Peter Anderson

Introduction

To understand the relationship between alcohol consumption and harm it is necessary to identify studies which contain a quantitative measure of individual alcohol consumption and a measure of individual harm in relation to alcohol consumption. From these studies, graphs can be constructed which plot risk curves for the relationship between drinking and harm for a full range of alcohol consumption.

In terms of physical harm, reviews of epidemiological studies have largely discussed the role of alcohol as a risk factor for cirrhosis of the liver, cancers, and cardiovascular disease (Anderson *et al.* 1993; Duffy 1992*a*; Rydberg *et al.* in press; Holman and Armstrong 1990; Verschuren 1993). This paper reports on some of these studies and presents a number of risk function curves on the relationship between alcohol consumption and harm.

The measurement of alcohol consumption

Methods of determining levels of drinking include direct interviews, with or without independent confirmation, self-completed questionnaires, and data taken from medical notes. A few workers attempt to assess lifetime exposure but most enquire about drinking over the past month, year or five years. However, since most physical harm is likely to be due to long-term alcohol use it is important to make some assessment of lifetime drinking. The obvious question: 'How long must I drink at this level to put myself at how much risk?' cannot be answered by available data. Many prospective studies have not been designed to provide information about the risks associated with alcohol; this partly accounts for lack of detailed consumption data.

Different methods have been used to measure alcohol consumption, including quantity frequency questionnaires and drug methods (Duffy 1992*b*). In the quantity frequency questionnaire, respondents are asked about their drinking of each of three types of alcoholic beverages, beer, wine, and spirits. For each beverage type, the usual frequency of drinking over a one month, three month, or other time period is recorded. The usual quantity of each beverage type drunk on each occasion is also noted. Although quantity frequency questionnaires are commonly used, there are difficulties with its interpretation. First, it is not all together clear how respondents understand the questions, which seem to require the reporting of the most common frequencies and quantities rather than the averages which may be greater. A second difficulty concerns respondents being restricted to the response categories listed on the questionnaire. Under-reporting in this instance is best allowed for by providing very high response categories.

A second method to measure alcohol consumption is to use the diary method based on consumption during a specified number of days of the week prior to interview (Duffy 1992*b*). The main difficulty of this approach relates to variabilities in individual consumption. For example, if week-to-week variation in the amount of alcohol consumed is relatively large, then the ordering of individuals by reported alcohol consumption using this method will not reflect their ordering over a longer time period. This could have the effect of giving false information on the association between consumption and outcome variables and the magnitude of the association. In particular, the risk in the consumption categories relative to the zero consumption category will be biased towards a relative risk of 1.0. These biases will be exaggerated, the shorter the time period used for description of drinking occasions.

Measurement differences can also affect the comparison of results between different studies (Duffy 1992*b*). Differences in response biases or under-reporting between studies, as might occur when analysing studies from different countries, can lead to different descriptions and sizes of the dose-response relationship. A difference in the description of the dose-response relationship is particularly likely to be found in studies using different measurement methods in countries which show appreciable temporal variation in levels and patterns of individual drinking. Quantity frequency measurements are less likely to be affected by within-individual temporal variation than last weeks' diary method of consumption and so should produce a more stable ordering of individuals by their consumption level, with less misclassification.

The under-reporting of consumption by individuals, that is known to occur in population surveys, has considerable implications for epidemiological studies (Duffy 1992*b*). In general, relationships between alcohol consumption and the risk of harm will be 'too steep'. In other words, the level of risk associated with a particular amount of alcohol consumption will, in fact, correspond to a greater amount of alcohol consumption. The observed level of risk is associated not so much with consuming a particular amount of alcohol, but with the reporting of the consumption of that amount.

Many studies have used drinking status at the start of a prospective study and have used this as an indicator of subsequent exposure to alcohol. Very few studies provide information on drinking at more than one or two points in time. This is not only important when there are changes in the use of alcohol with age but also when they are temporal differences as a population changes its overall consumption. As alcohol consumption tends to decrease with increasing age, epidemiological studies based on the baseline measurement, would tend to lead to an underestimation of risk.

Assumptions about the alcohol content of the reported number of drinks and the need to convert data to grams alcohol/day introduce further areas of difficulty. And lack of information about previous drinking among 'non-drinkers' is of particular importance in relation to discussion of the protective effect of alcohol. This also requires an accurate smoking history, because a non-drinking smoker is much more likely to be an ex-drinker than a lifelong abstainer and a non-drinker who never smoked is much more likely to be a life-long abstainer than an ex-drinker (Kozlowski and Ferrence 1990). There are difficulties in converting data to alcohol consumption per day, since in many studies, drinking patterns or frequencies rarely refer to actual patterns of drinking but to averages of various levels (Knupfer 1987). There is, of course, a huge difference between a pattern of drinking consisting of two drinks every day and one consisting of 14 drinks on one day. Even when good measures of quantity and frequency are obtained, most researchers do not control for body weight and composition, and this could lead to further distortions.

Consumption data require conversion to standard measures of pure ethyl alcohol (ethanol) to facilitate direct comparison between studies because of the wide variety of ways of reporting quantities of alcoholic drinks. Fluid ounces, millilitres, or grams are used to report quantities of either alcohol or of specified beverages; sometimes authors refer to the number of 'drinks' consumed, with differing definitions of a 'drink', or even with no attempt to define a 'drink'. 'Standard drinks' vary in size from country to country, as does average alcohol content (percentage volume) of various beverages. The effect such variations have on the interpretation of data is discussed in full elsewhere (Turner 1990). Anderson *et al.* (1993) converted all data to equivalent grams (g) of alcohol, using the following conversion factors: 1 ml = 0.785 g alcohol; 1 fl oz = 28.41 ml (UK); 1 fl oz = 29.58 ml (USA). If a published paper gave data as a volume of beverage without sufficient information to convert directly to grams of alcohol, the alcohol content was calculated from an assumed average percentage volume, of beer 4 per cent, wine 12 per cent, spirits 40 per cent. If a 'drink' was undefined, the average alcohol content was assumed to be 12 g in the United States, 10 g in Australia/Europe, and 21.2 g in Japan.

For graphical representation of data, the midpoint (in grams of alcohol) of each quoted range of consumption has been calculated. Where the highest consumption category has no upper limit, the lowest value has been used. This tends to overestimate the steepness of the curve at this consumption level.

The epidemiology of risk

A review of published papers may be biased by the greater likelihood of publication of those which demonstrate an association between alcohol and harm (Simes 1986). Comparison between studies is complicated by a number of factors. Most papers reviewed are in the English language but they come from many different countries and involve a variety of racial groups; it is well known, for example, that the Japanese display genetic variations in their ability to metabolize alcohol. Numbers of patients in studies vary, and are often too small to draw definite conclusions; diseases are rarely classified according to International Classification of Diseases (ICD) standards. Studies may be either prospective, case-control, or cross-sectional. Prospective surveys have variable lengths of follow-up and use different end-points, such as death, incidence, prevalence, hospitalization, or a confusing mixture of these. Confounding effects may or may not be controlled for, and different methods are used for doing so. This is particularly important with relation to cigarette smoking, which is so closely interrelated with alcohol consumption. Matching in case-control studies involving both drinking and smoking can be difficult and statistical adjustment for tobacco use could be misleading. It may be better to present results separately for smokers and non-smokers. This is particularly so when smoking rates are declining in many of the countries in which the studies were undertaken.

In some studies, the results of controlling for confounders have provided values of the estimates of the association after adjustment, although this is not always the case (Duffy 1992*a*). Case-control studies vary in the selection of controls; use of hospital controls, for example, may introduce bias because potential alcohol-related disorders are common in such a population. The strength of the approach adopted in existing reviews provides a basis for causal inferences, because of the strength of association, the presence of a dose-response relationship, the temporal relation between risk, and exposure and consistency across different studies. It is often the case that studies relating alcohol consumption to a specific disease are undertaken by different groups of researchers in different countries at different times. When consumption and outcome data are available from relevant studies in similar forms, it is usually quite simple to compare and, if appropriate, combine the results. If, however, there are significant differences in the relationship between consumption and risk in the different studies, it is best not to attempt to provide a combined risk estimate, although for practical purposes it may be necessary to do so. It is, however, possible to conclude that alcohol is associated with a disease if all the odds-ratio estimates of different studies are in the same positive direction. If the interaction between the study and alcohol consumption is not statistically significant, then it can be concluded that all the studies are indicating the same relationship between alcohol consumption and the disease, and it is then legitimate to produce a single estimate.

If not given, relative risk (RR) can be calculated from the crude data (Duffy 1992*a*). In cohort studies, the relative risk can be calculated as the ratio of the rate among those exposed to alcohol to the rate among the unexposed. Relative risk measures how much more or less likely it is that disease occurs among those exposed to the factor in question. The odds ratio is another measure of association. Given the rates of illness, which may be considered as probabilities of illness, the odds for the exposed and unexposed groups can be calculated. The odds ratio may be estimated in situations, such as case-control studies and matched case-control studies where neither the rate difference nor the relative risk can be calculated. The odds ratio approximates the relative risk if the incidence rate of the disease is small. An alternative method of analysing such studies is provided by logistic regression which postulates a linear regression of log-odds of illness risk on values of the exposed variable. Logistic linear models provide an estimate of the regression coefficient relating how the log-odds ratio of a particular condition increases (or decreases) with increasing alcohol consumption. In most papers, non-drinkers are used as a baseline with a relative risk of 1.0; where moderate drinkers are used relative risk can be recalculated using non-drinkers as the baseline where possible.

Cirrhosis of the liver

Men Six studies, which fulfilled the selection criteria of Anderson *et al.* (1993), have shown a significant association between drinking alcohol and cirrhosis (Kagan *et al.* 1981; Péquinot *et al.* 1978; Tuyns and Péquinot 1984; Coates *et al.* 1986; Kono *et al.* 1986; Boffetta and Garfinkel 1990), Fig. 4.1 (the data have been truncated at 70 g per day to enable a clear demonstration of the dose-response relationship at lower levels of consumption). Of these, five showed a dose-response relationship (Kagan *et al.* 1981; Péquinot *et al.* 1978; Tuyns and Péquinot 1984; Coates *et al.* 1986; Boffetta and Garfinkel 1990) which may be log-linear (Péquinot *et al.* 1978; Tuyns and Péquinot 1984; Boffetta and Garfinkel 1990), and one (Kono *et al.* 1986) a significantly increased risk for heavy drinkers only. Three of the studies are prospective (Kagan *et al.* 1981; Kono *et al.* 1986; Boffetta and Garfinkel 1990) and use death from cirrhosis as the end-point of the study. These are the Male Japanese Physicians study of 5477 Japanese doctors, with a 19-year follow-up and data adjusted for the effects of age and smoking (Kono *et al.* 1986), the Honolulu Heart Study of 7591 Japanese men aged 45–69, living in Hawaii, with a 9-year follow-up and data adjusted for age (Kagan *et al.* 1981), and the American Cancer Society Prospective Study of 276 302 men aged 40–59, with a 12-year follow-up and data adjusted for age and smoking (Boffetta and Garfinkel 1990). The three case-control studies review incident cases of cirrhosis (Péquinot *et al.* 1978; Tuyns and Péquinot 1984; Coates *et al.* 1986). Controls used in these studies are from the general population. Current or recent alcohol consumption (Kagan *et*

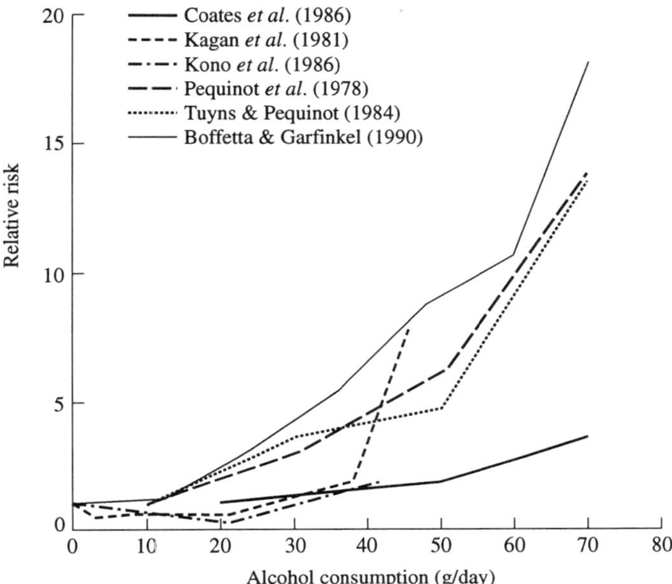

Fig. 4.1 Alcohol consumption and incidence of cirrhosis of the liver in men. Data truncated at 70 g/day.

al. 1981; Péquinot *et al.* 1978; Coates *et al.* 1986; Kono *et al.* 1986; Boffetta and Garfinkel 1990) or an estimate of average daily consumption over a lifetime (Tuyns and Péquinot 1984) were used. Two studies are controlled for both the effects of age and smoking (Kono *et al.* 1986; Boffetta and Garfinkel 1990), whereas other studies are controlled for the effect of age. No study had data on history of hepatitis or on hepatitis serological markers. Studies consider cirrhosis in all adult men except for one study which is limited to those men aged 45–69 (Kagan *et al.* 1981). Using the data from the Péquinot study (Péquinot *et al.* 1978), the estimated regression coefficient from a logistic linear model has been calculated as 0.039, indicating that a man drinking an extra 20 g of alcohol a day multiplies his odds ratio of cirrhosis by approximately 2.2 (Duffy 1992*c*).

Women Two case-control studies considered women (Tuyns and Péquinot 1984; Coates *et al.* 1986) and both demonstrated a dose-response relationship; both found a higher risk for women than men at any given level of alcohol consumption (see Fig. 4.2). It is not possible to calculate the relative risk from a further report (Norton *et al.* 1987).

Men and women A further prospective study of both men and women, using mortality as the end-point, again demonstrated a dose-response relationship (Klatsky *et al.* 1981*a*; Klatsky and Armstrong 1992).

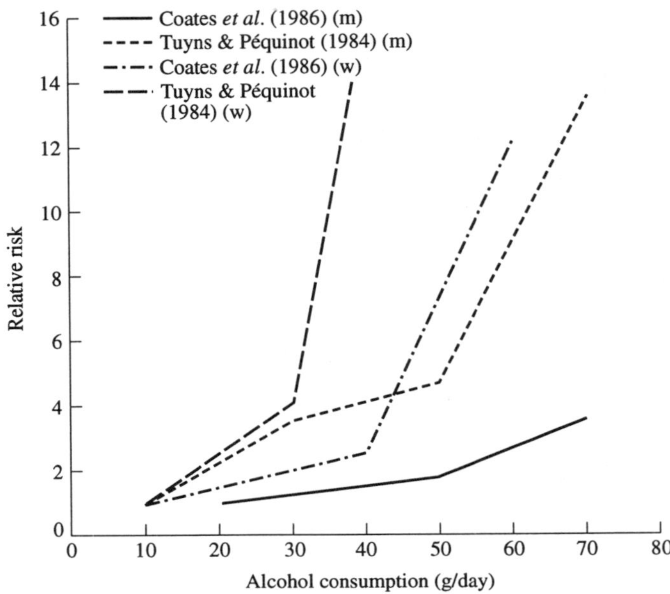

Fig. 4.2 Alcohol consumption and incidence of cirrhosis of the liver in men (m) and women (w). Data truncated at 70 g/day.

Cancers

Alcohol and risk of cancer has been the subject of a number of major and comprehensive reviews (Anderson *et al.* 1993; Holman and Armstrong 1990; Duffy and Sharples 1992; IARC 1988; Doll *et al.* 1993).

The International Agency for Research on Cancer's monograph reviewed cancers across 22 different sites and concluded that alcohol is causally related to cancers of the oral cavity, pharynx, larynx, oesophagus, and liver, independent of cigarette smoking (IARC 1988).

Duffy and Sharples (1992) reviewed cancers across 11 different sites, and concluded that alcohol is causally related to cancers of the oral cavity, pharynx, larynx, oesophagus, and liver. They suggested that breast cancer should probably be added to the list of cancers caused by alcohol drinking and that drinking alcohol may possibly increase the risks of cancers of the large bowel and stomach.

Although there was significant heterogeneity across studies for most of the cancers they reviewed, Duffy and Sharples (1992) calculated pooled relative risks for drinkers compared with non-drinkers and pooled estimates of trends in log-odds ratios with increasing alcohol consumption (ml/day) for cancers, together with a pooled estimate of the increased risk (per cent) at consumption

Table 4.1 Pooled estimate of relative risk in drinkers, compared to non-drinkers, trends in log-odds ratio with increasing alcohol consumption (ml/day) for cancers, and increased risk (%) at consumption levels of, on average, 20 g a day, compared with no consumption

Cancer	Relative risk in drinkers compared to non-drinkers	Trends in log-odds ratio of relative risk	Increased risk (%) with increase in consumption of 20 g
Oral cavity[a]	1.40 (ns)	0.0083 ($P<0.001$)	19
Pharynx[a]	1.49 (ns)	0.010 ($P<0.001$)	24
Larynx[a]	2.20 (ns)	0.013 ($P<0.001$)	31
Oesophagus[a]	1.30 (ns)	0.0049 ($P<0.001$)	10
Stomach	1.17 ($P<0.05$)	0.0025 (ns)	6
Colorectal	1.21 ($P<0.001$)	0.0031 (ns)	7
Lung[a]	0.96 ($P<0.05$)	0.501[b] (ns)	–
Female breast	1.20 ($P<0.001$)	0.59[b] ($P<0.001$)	10
Pancreas	1.03 (ns)	0.0018 (ns)	–
Bladder	1.07 (ns)	0.058[b]	–
Liver	1.56 ($P<0.001$)	0.0066 ($P<0.001$)	14

[a] Adjusted for smoking. [b] Trend in litres of ethanol per week. ns, not significant.

Source: Duffy and Sharples (1992).

levels of an average 20 g a day, compared with no consumption, controlled, where appropriate for cigarette smoking (see Table 4.1).

In their review of cancers across 11 different sites, Holman and Armstrong (1990) identified less heterogeneity between studies for different cancer sites than Duffy and Sharples (1992) and concluded that, with the exception of cancer of the oral cavity, in which women were at lower risk, the magnitude of risk was the same for both men and women.

Doll *et al.* (1993) and colleagues reviewed cancers of the digestive tract (excluding liver) and larynx and concluded that alcohol is causally related to cancers of the mouth (other than salivary glands), pharynx (other than the nasopharynx), larynx, and possibly colorectum.

Anderson *et al.* (1993) reviewed 94 studies of cancers across 11 different sites and summarized data in tabular form. Using data from Anderson *et al.*'s tables, a graphical representation of data for cancer of the oesophagus, and overall cancer mortality are illustrated in Figs 4.3 and 4.4.

Cancer of the female breast

Cancer of the female breast is included for more detailed discussion because of its public health importance.

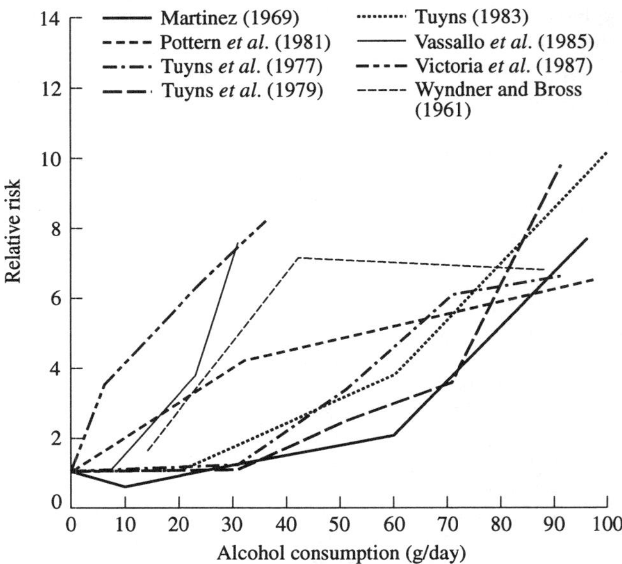

Fig. 4.3 Alcohol consumption and incidence of cancer of the oesophagus in men. *Source:* Anderson *et al.* (1993).

Of the 17 studies of the incidence of breast cancer in women (Schatzkin *et al.* 1987; Willett *et al.* 1987; Hiatt and Bawol 1984; Hiatt *et al.* 1988; Gapstur *et al.* 1992; Lé *et al.* 1984; Rohan and McMichael 1988; Harvey *et al.* 1987; Talamini *et al.* 1984; La Vecchia *et al.* 1985; O'Connell *et al.* 1987; Paganini-Hill and Ross 1983; Harris and Wyndner 1988; Webster *et al.* 1983; Byers and Funch 1982; Miller *et al.* 1987; Begg *et al.* 1983) which fulfil the selection criteria of Anderson *et al.* (1993), 11 show a significant positive association (Schatzkin *et al.* 1987; Willett *et al.* 1987; Hiatt and Bawol 1984; Hiatt *et al.* 1988; Gapstur *et al.* 1992; Lé *et al.* 1984; Rohan and McMichael 1988; Harvey *et al.* 1987; Talamini *et al.* 1984; La Vecchia *et al.* 1985; O'Connell *et al.* 1987). All five cohort studies, four of which are prospective (Schatzkin *et al.* 1987; Willett *et al.* 1987; Hiatt *et al.* 1988; Gapstur *et al.* 1992) and one retrospective (Hiatt and Bawol 1984), show a significant positive dose-response relationship. Six out of 12 case-control studies find a significant positive relationship (Lé *et al.* 1984; Rohan and McMichael 1988; Harvey *et al.* 1987; Talamini *et al.* 1984; La Vecchia *et al.* 1985; O'Connell *et al.* 1987) and in five of these this is a dose-response relationship (Lé *et al.* 1984; Rohan and McMichael 1988; Harvey *et al.* 1987; Talamini *et al.* 1984; La Vecchia *et al.* 1985). The other case-control studies find no significant association (Paganini-Hill and Ross 1983; Harris and Wyndner 1988; Webster *et al.* 1983; Byers and Funch 1982; Miller *et al.* 1987; Begg *et al.* 1983).

The consistency of the findings in the five large cohort studies is convincing

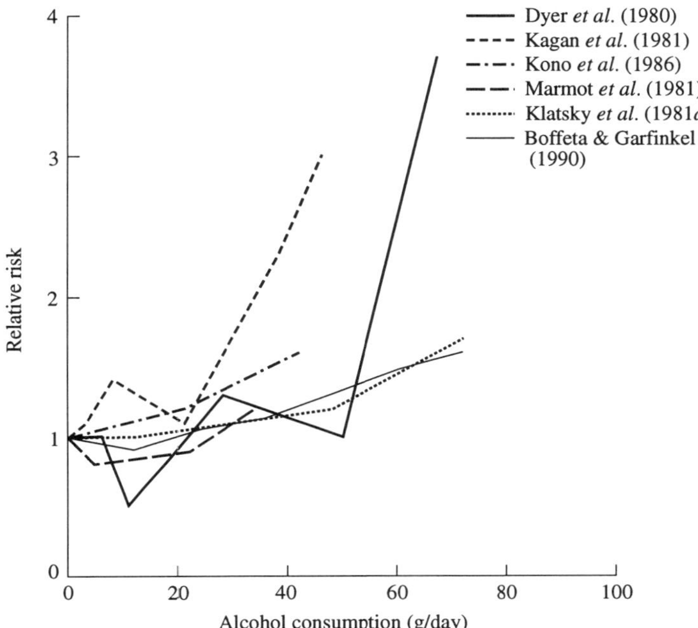

Fig. 4.4 Alcohol consumption and mortality rate from all cancers. (The Klatsky *et al.* (1981*a,b*) data are for both men and women.)
Source: Anderson *et al.* (1993).

(see Fig. 4.5). The 10-year prospective study (from the First National Health and Nutrition Examination Survey: Schatzkin *et al.* 1987) of 7188 women aged 25–74 and the 4-year prospective study (from the Nurses Health Study) of 89 538 women aged 30–55 (Willett *et al.* 1987) are adjusted for other, possibly confounding, breast cancer risk factors (age, diet, smoking, body mass index, family history of breast disease, age at menarche, age at first birth, parity, menopausal status). In addition, one study controls for the effect of education (Schatzkin *et al.* 1987) and the other includes benign breast disease (Willett *et al.* 1987). The remaining two studies are from the Kaiser Permanente group of 88 477 women aged over 15 years, reviewed retrospectively over a period of 13 years (Hiatt *et al.* 1988) and a separate group of 58 347 women followed over 6 years (Hiatt and Bawol 1984). These studies were adjusted for the effects of age, race, smoking, and body mass index in both cases, and, in addition, education, parity, cholesterol level, age at menarche, and menopausal status, in the case of the retrospective study. However, the authors were, unfortunately, unable to control for the effect of diet. The Iowa Women's Health Study followed-up 41 837 postmenopausal women aged 55–69 for 4 years and adjusted for the effects of age, body mass

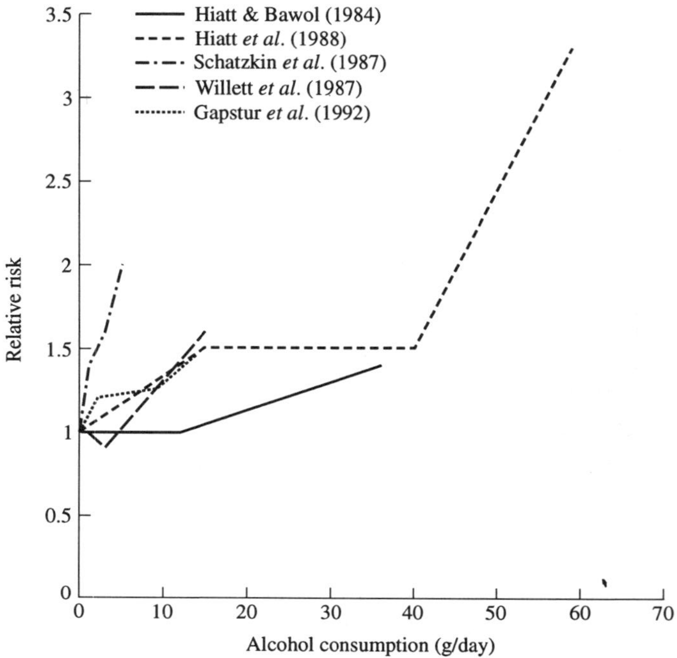

Fig. 4.5 Alcohol consumption and incidence of female breast cancer. Data from five prospective studies.

Source: Anderson *et al.* (1993).

index, age at menarche, age at first live birth, and family history of breast cancer (Gapstur *et al.* 1992).

Of the 12 case-control studies, nine are controlled for the majority of other known risk factors for breast cancer. The three studies which are less well controlled, fail to show a relationship [two control only for age (Byers and Funch 1982; Miller *et al.* 1987), and the other only for age and smoking (Begg *et al.* 1983)]. Diet is controlled for in only three of the case-control studies (Talamini *et al.* 1984; La Vecchia *et al.* 1985; O'Connell *et al.* 1987), all of which show a dose-response relationship. The numbers of cases reviewed in these studies range from 239 to 1799, with a mean of 832 cases. Controls used are from the general population in six studies (Rohan and McMichael 1988; Harvey *et al.* 1987; O'Connell *et al.* 1987; Harris and Wyndner 1988; Webster *et al.* 1983; Miller *et al.* 1987) and from hospitals or clinics in the remainder of the studies. All studies use current or recent consumption in assessing alcohol exposure.

In summary, all five of the cohort studies, and six of the 12 case-control studies show a relationship between level of alcohol consumption and risk of breast cancer. Of these 11 studies, 9 demonstrate a dose-response relationship.

Two papers have presented meta-analyses of individual studies. For case-control studies, Longnecker *et al.* (1988) demonstrated a linear dose-response relationship which increased to a risk of 1.5 at a consumption level of 36 g of alcohol a day or more. For cohort studies, the relationship was steeper with a relative risk of 2.0 at a consumption level of 36 g of alcohol a day or more.

The meta-analysis of Howe *et al.* (1991) represents some of the strongest evidence for a causative association of alcohol with breast cancer because it consists of raw data from studies in which detailed dietary histories were taken and for which dietary adjustments could be made. The adjusted relative risk for alcohol consumption at levels of 40 g or more per day was 1.7.

Although there is discussion on whether the association between alcohol consumption and breast cancer is causal or due to confounding variables (McPherson *et al.* 1993), it can be argued that, until the effect of alcohol consumption can be convincingly accounted for by adjustment of other variables, it should be treated as a predisposing factor.

Cardiovascular disease

Alcohol-related cardiovascular disease includes raised blood pressure, stroke, arrhythmias, cardiomyopathy, and coronary heart disease, including sudden coronary death (Anderson *et al.* 1993).

There is evidence of a dose-response relationship between level of alcoholic beverage consumption and level of blood pressure and stroke, and some evidence of a dose-response relationship for sudden coronary death (Anderson *et al.* 1993). There is also a relationship between heavy alcohol intake and risk of arrythmias and of cardiomyopathy, but there is insufficient evidence to comment on whether or not this is a dose-response relationship.

There appears to be a protective effect of drinking alcoholic beverages on risk of coronary heart disease, excluding sudden coronary deaths, although it is possible that this effect is only apparent in populations with a high risk of coronary heart disease.

There is evidence for a protective effect of alcoholic beverages on risk of total cardiovascular disease mortality, this effect being accounted for by the observed protective effect of alcohol consumption on risk of coronary heart disease.

The following section will focus on the risk of alcohol consumption for stroke and coronary heart disease.

Stroke

Men The results of seven studies of men, two case-control (Gill *et al.* 1986; Shaper *et al.* 1991) and five prospective studies (Kono *et al.* 1986; Boffetta and

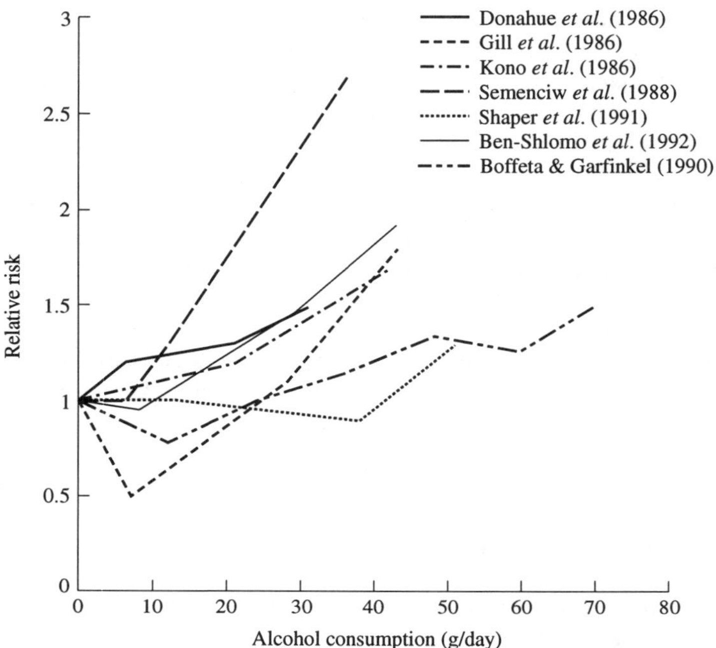

Fig. 4.6 Alcohol consumption and incidence of stroke in men. Data from seven studies.

Garfinkel 1990; Donahue *et al.* 1986; Semenciw *et al.* 1988; Ben-Shlomo *et al.* 1992) are summarized in Fig. 4.6. Four of the prospective studies demonstrate a dose-response relationship (Kono *et al.* 1986; Boffetta and Garfinkel 1990; Donahue *et al.* 1986; Semenciw *et al.* 1988) and one no relationship (Ben-Shlomo *et al.* 1992); one case-control study demonstrates a significant U-shaped curve (Gill *et al.* 1986) and the other a non-significant dose-response relationship (Shaper *et al.* 1991).

The Male Japanese Physicians Study (Kono *et al.* 1986) and the American Cancer Society Prospective Study (Boffetta and Garfinkel 1990) found a significant dose-response relationship between stroke mortality and level of alcohol consumption. Data were adjusted for age and smoking. The Honolulu Heart Study found a dose-response relationship between alcohol consumption levels and incidence of stroke, after a 12-year follow-up (Donahue *et al.* 1986). Data were adjusted for age and smoking, and also for blood pressure, body mass index, serum cholesterol, uric acid, glucose, and haematocrit. In the Nutrition Canada Survey, 3146 men who were free of self-reported heart disease or stroke, aged 35–79, were followed-up for 11 years (Semenciw *et al.* 1988). The data, which were adjusted for age, smoking, diabetes, and diastolic blood pressure showed a dose-response relationship between alcohol consumption and stroke mortality. The British Regional Heart Study found no relationship between alcohol consumption and incidence of stroke in 7735 men with a 7.5-year follow-up (Ben-Shlomo *et al.* 1992). Data were adjusted for age, systolic blood pressure, and smoking. When the total group was subdivided into a group of 5856 'healthy' and 1873 'unhealthy' men, the latter defined as those with any evidence of cardiovascular disease at enrolment (Shaper *et al.* 1988), there was a significant dose-response relationship between alcohol consumption and the risk of stroke among the 'unhealthy' men, after adjustment for age, smoking, and systolic blood pressure, but no relationship was found among the 'healthy' men.

Gill's case-control study of 143 men aged 20–70 also showed a dose-response relationship, but with a U-shaped curve (Gill *et al.* 1986). The data in this study were adjusted for blood pressure, smoking, medication, age, sex, and race. The study, in its first report used hospital controls. The second case-control study showed a non-significant dose-response relationship. Data were adjusted for age, sex, social class, cigarette smoking, and history of hypertension (Shaper *et al.* 1991).

Because there is a linear dose-response relationship between alcohol consumption and blood pressure, controlling for blood pressure will remove some of the alcohol effect for risk of stroke. This was evident for the two studies which demonstrated a significant dose-response relationship when only controlling for age, although failed to demonstrate a dose-response relationship when controlling for age, smoking, and blood pressure (Shaper *et al.* 1991; Ben-Shlomo *et al.* 1992). The stroke studies have also demonstrated how the risk associated with alcohol consumption varies depending on the choice of control group, with different biases associated with selection of different control groups (Ben-Shlomo *et al.* 1992).

Women Two of the above studies are also of women. There was a positive association between stroke mortality and heavy drinking for the 3971 women in one follow-up study, but no dose-response relationship was demonstrated (Semenciw *et al.* 1988). In the case-control study of 87 women, no significant association was found, but there were only three women who usually drank more than one drink a day (Gill *et al.* 1986). A further prospective study, the Nurses Health Study of 87 526 female American nurses, with an 8-year follow-up shows a U-shaped relationship between level of alcohol consumption and combined incidence and mortality from stroke (Stampfer *et al.* 1988). This study adjusts the data for blood pressure, age, family history, obesity, exercise, fat intake, smoking, diabetes, cholesterol, menopausal status, and hormone use.

Men and women Two further studies investigate both men and women. The Kaiser Permanente group followed-up men and women for five years and

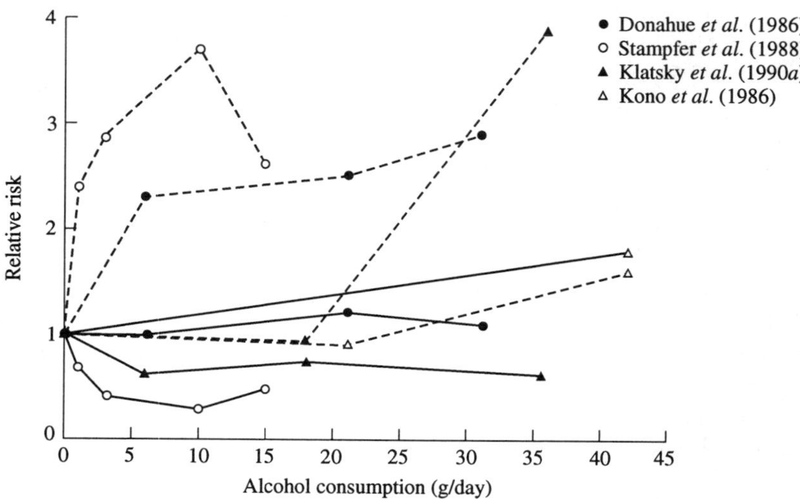

Fig. 4.7 Alcohol consumption and incidence of stroke (– – –, haemorrhagic; ——, non-haemorrhagic). Data from four studies.

found a non-significant dose-response relationship between alcohol consumption and level and risk of hospitalization for stroke (Klatsky *et al.* 1981*b*) and a U-shaped relationship between alcohol consumption and risk of stroke mortality (Klatsky *et al.* 1990*a*). These data are adjusted for age, sex, race, and smoking but not for blood pressure. A case-control study of 209 men and women shows a significant protective effect of drinking for all strokes (Von Arbin *et al.* 1985). The data are adjusted only for age and sex. Four of the above studies subdivide stroke into non-haemorrhagic and haemorrhagic stroke (see Fig. 4.7).

Non-haemorrhagic stroke

A dose relationship was seen for non-haemorrhagic stroke in the Japanese Physicians Study (Kono *et al.* 1986), significant only for heavy drinkers. The Honolulu Heart Study (Donahue *et al.* 1986) showed no significant association, the Nurses' Health Study (Stampfer *et al.* 1988) showed an inverse, U-shaped association, and the Kaiser Permanente study showed a reduced risk among drinkers compared with non-drinkers (Klatsky *et al.* 1990*a*).

The Male Japanese Physicians Study, when analysing data on ex-drinkers, found an overall excessive mortality rate, and this was due in part to a significant excess mortality rate from non-haemorrhagic stroke (Kono *et al.* 1986).

Haemorrhagic stroke

A significant dose-response relationship was found in the Kaiser permanente study for total haemorrhagic stroke (Klatsky *et al.* 1990*a*) and a significant dose-response relationship was found in the Honolulu Heart Study (Donahue *et al.* 1986) for subarachnoid haemorrhage, but not for intracerebral haemorrhage. A dose-response relationship was also seen in the Nurses' Health Study (Stampfer *et al.* 1988) for subarachnoid haemorrhage but this was not significant due to small numbers ($n=28$). The Japanese Physicians Study (Kono *et al.* 1986) showed an increased risk in heavy drinkers, but it was not statistically significant.

In summary, there is evidence of a dose-response relationship between level of alcohol consumption and all strokes in men. There is some evidence of a positive relationship for women, which may be U-shaped. The evidence suggests that drinking alcohol increases the chance of subarachnoid haemorrhage, more than other types of stroke. Further studies should report data both with and without controlling for blood pressure.

Coronary heart disease

Studies vary in their definition of coronary heart disease. Some use death from all 'coronary heart disease' as their definition of the disease studied, others incident myocardial infarction, incident angina, coronary insufficiency, sudden coronary death, or a combination of these (Anderson *et al.* 1993). This makes it difficult to compare data from different studies. Because of these differences in definitions, papers are discussed according to whether they describe coronary heart disease deaths, a combination of incidence and death, or 'sudden coronary death'.

Mortality rates

Men Ten studies of total coronary heart disease (CHD) mortality (Kono *et al.* 1986; Boffetta and Garfinkel 1990; Dyer *et al.* 1980; Yano *et al.* 1977; Hennekens *et al.* 1978; Gordon and Kannel 1983; Suhonen *et al.* 1987; Camacho *et al.* 1987; Gordon and Doyle 1987; Jackson *et al.* 1991) failed to show a significant positive association; five, however, showed a significant negative association (Boffetta and Garfinkel 1990; Hennekens *et al.* 1978; Gordon and Kannel 1983; Gordon and Doyle 1987; Jackson *et al.* 1991) and three of these had a U-shaped curve (Boffetta and Garfinkel 1990; Hennekens *et al.* 1978; Jackson *et al.* 1991).

In the Albany study, Gordon *et al.* followed-up a group of 1910 men aged 38–55 for 18 years (Gordon and Doyle 1987). The study found a non-significant U-shaped association between alcohol use and CHD deaths. They then followed-up 979 of the same men now aged 56–73 for a further 10 years and a significant negative dose-response relationship was shown. This study was controlled for smoking, age, blood pressure, and weight. In the Framingham study, Gordon and Kannel (1983) followed-up a group of 2026 men aged 29–62 for 22 years and found a significant negative response, which was U-shaped. This paper commented that analysis of the various forms of CHD deaths suggested that there may be a positive association for sudden coronary death, and that the negative association was due to acute myocardial infarction and non-sudden CHD deaths. In the American Cancer Society Prospective Study, 276 802 men aged 40–59 were followed-up for 12 years and a significant negative association was found between alcohol consumption and risk of death from coronary heart disease (Boffetta and Garfinkel 1990). Data were adjusted for age and smoking. The protective effect of alcohol remained when excluding subjects with poor health or history of chronic disease at enrolment or excluding subjects who died during the first six years of follow-up. The Auckland Community study is a case-control study of 227 men and demonstrated a significant negative association (Jackson *et al.* 1991). Controls were selected from the community and data were adjusted for age, smoking, hypertension, social class, exercise, and recent change in drinking. Total abstainers had a similar risk of dying from CHD to people who were former drinkers, but who did not currently drink. The final paper suggesting a significant negative relationship (also U-shaped) is a case control study of 568 men aged 30–70 (Hennekens *et al.* 1978). The data are adjusted for smoking, religion, weight, and hospitalization for heart disease. The significance of the protective effect is confined to those drinking less than 46 g/day.

The remaining five papers showing no significant effect can be divided into those with a negative (but non-significant) trend (Kono *et al.* 1986; Yano *et al.* 1977), and those with a non-significant positive trend (Dyer *et al.* 1980; Suhonen *et al.* 1987; Camacho *et al.* 1987). The Honolulu Heart Study showed a non-significant negative trend for all CHD deaths (Yano *et al.* 1977). If the numbers of CHD deaths are added to the numbers of incident cases of myocardial infarction (MI), the trend is of a significant inverse dose-response relationship. The Male Japanese Physicians Study (Kono *et al.* 1986) showed a non-significant negative association for all coronary heart disease deaths. Acute MI deaths show a significant inverse dose-response relationship, whereas other, non-acute MI CHD deaths show a non-significant positive association at high levels of drinking. The Finnish Social Insurance Institute's Mobile Health Clinic Survey (Suhonen *et al.* 1987) followed-up 4532 men for five years and found no significant trend for 40–64-year-olds for all CHD deaths. There was a non-significant positive dose-response relationship, which was strongest in the 60–64-year-old group of men. The Alameda Cohort (Camacho *et al.* 1987) and the Chicago Western Electric Study (Dyer *et al.* 1980) both showed a positive trend in 15- and 17-year prospective studies (respectively). Subsequent analysis of the Alameda Cohort data (Lazarus *et al.*

1991) found no difference in risk of ischaemic heart disease for men who continued to drink and men who gave up drinking during a 10-year period.

Women The Framingham Study (Gordon and Kannel 1983) showed a significant inverse relationship for CHD deaths, and the Alameda Cohort Study (Camacho *et al.* 1987) no significant trend. The Auckland Community Study found a significant negative association with a U-shaped curve (Jackson *et al.* 1991). Additional analysis of the Alameda Cohort data (Lazarus *et al.* 1991), found that there was a significantly higher risk of death from ischaemic heart disease in women who gave up drinking during a 10-year period, compared with women who continued to drink.

Men and women Colditz *et al.* (1985) followed a group of 1184 people aged 66 years or older for an average of 4.75 years and found a significant (U-shaped) protective effect for moderate drinkers, after adjustment for age, sex, smoking, and cholesterol.

Incidence and mortality

Some of the papers mentioned in the preceding section on CHD mortality, also include data about incidence or a combination of incidence and death from CHD. In addition, there are further articles which only give data on incidence or on a combination of incidence and death.

Men In men there are seven such studies (Kagan *et al.* 1981; Suhonen *et al.* 1987; Jackson *et al.* 1991; Shaper *et al.* 1987; Rimm *et al.* 1991; Kittner *et al.* 1983; Scragg *et al.* 1987). Two studies look at a combination of incidence and deaths. An early report from the British Regional Heart Study of 7729 men aged 40–59 followed for 6.2 years (Shaper *et al.* 1987) found a non-significant, U-shaped relationship between consumption and 'major ischaemic heart disease events' (including all CHD deaths and non-fatal myocardial infarction). Data are adjusted for the effects of age, smoking, body mass index, and socio-economic status. Analysis at 9.5-year follow-up found a shallow U-shaped relationship for all CHD events and an inverse association with fatal CHD events. The relationships were strongest in older men and in ex-smokers, current smokers, manual workers, and those with doctor diagnosed cardiovascular disorders or symptomatic coronary heart disease (Shaper *et al.* 1994). The Honolulu Heart Study found that although there was no significant association for CHD deaths alone, if CHD deaths and MI were analysed together there was a significant inverse relationship (Kagan *et al.* 1981), caused by MI alone (Yano *et al.* 1977).

The Auckland Community Study found a negative association with a U-shaped curve for MI incidence (Jackson *et al.* 1991) and the Health Professionals follow-up survey (Rimm *et al.* 1991) found a significant dose-response relationship for coronary heart disease, which remained when excluding current non-drinkers, past heavy drinkers, and men with disorders potentially related to CHD at enrolment. Additional analysis of the Auckland Community data demonstrated a significant negative association between alcohol consumption in the previous 24 hours and risk of MI (Jackson *et al.* 1992).

Three further papers look at the incidence of MI alone. The Finnish Study (Suhonen *et al.* 1987) found a significantly increased risk of MI for abstainers. A non-significant negative association was found in the prospective Puerto Rico Heart Health Programme Study of 8907 men aged 35–79 followed-up for 8 years (data adjusted for age, smoking, exercise, and place of residence) (Kittner *et al.* 1983) and in a case-control study (Scragg *et al.* 1987) of 439 men aged 35–64.

Women In women there are two such studies (Stampfer *et al.* 1988; Jackson *et al.* 1991). The Nurses' Health Study (Stampfer *et al.* 1988) which considered a combination of CHD deaths (including sudden coronary death) and incident cases of MI and angina reported a significant inverse dose-response relationship. Data are adjusted for the effects of menopausal status, family history, hormone use, smoking, blood pressure, diabetes mellitus, serum cholesterol, cholesterol intake, age, body mass index, exercise, and intake of saturated and unsaturated fats. The Auckland Community Study (Jackson *et al.* 1991) found a significant negative association for incidence of MI, without a trend, and as with the men, demonstrated a significant negative association between alcohol consumption in the previous 24 hours and risk of MI (Jackson *et al.* 1992).

Men and women A case-control study of 402 men and women aged 40–69 (Stason *et al.* 1976) showed a significantly lowered risk of non-fatal MI for drinkers of more than about 72 g/day.

Sudden coronary death

Men The Finnish prospective study (Suhonen *et al.* 1987) showed a dose-response relationship which was strongest in older men, for which spirit-drinking was responsible. There were 87 cases of sudden coronary death in this period. Adjustment is made for age, smoking, cholesterol level, and blood pressure. The Puerto Rico prospective study (Kittner *et al.* 1983) showed a non-significant increased relative risk for drinkers compared to non-drinkers for sudden coronary death which contrasted with a non-significant relative risk for other deaths from CHD. This study is adjusted for the effects of age, smoking, exercise, and place of residence, but not for blood pressure. The case-control study of Scragg *et al.* (1987) of 152 men aged 35–64, adjusted for the effects of age, smoking, and blood pressure showed a decreased risk for all drinkers, but numbers were too few for statistical significance.

Women The latter workers found a similar decreased risk in women but numbers were again too small (Scragg *et al.* 1987).

Men and women A cross-sectional study from New Zealand (Fraser and Upsell 1981) of a random sample of 311 men and women with either acute MI or sudden coronary death selected from a community-based register of acute coronary events over a one-year period showed a significant dose-response relationship between alcohol intake and the risk of death from an acute coronary event. Data were adjusted for season, gender, age, prodromal cardiac symptoms, race, smoking, medication, height, weight, ECG features, and autopsy findings.

The authors of the Framingham Study (Gordon and Doyle 1987) comment that 'the indication from several studies that drinking may increase the risk of sudden death is somewhat disquieting. The Framingham study itself, while not conclusive on this point, does raise the possibility that sudden death not preceded by definite clinical evidence of coronary heart disease may occur more frequently than average among heavy drinkers, as well as among non-drinkers'.

Summary

The relationship between level of alcohol consumption and the risk of CHD incidence and death is not consistent. Of 14 reports in men, seven demonstrated a significant negative association (Boffetta and Garfinkel 1990; Hennekens *et al.* 1978; Gordon and Kannel 1983; Gordon and Doyle 1987; Jackson *et al.* 1991; Scragg *et al.* 1987; Rimm *et al.* 1991), Fig 4.8, three a non-significant negative association (Kono *et al.* 1986; Yano *et al.* 1977; Kittner *et al.* 1983), one no relationship (Shaper *et al.* 1987), and three a non-significant positive association (Dyer *et al.* 1980; Suhonen *et al.* 1987; Camacho *et al.* 1987), Fig. 4.9, between alcohol consumption and risk of CHD.

Of four reports in women, three demonstrated a significant negative association (Stampfer *et al.* 1988; Gordon and Kannel 1983; Jackson *et al.* 1991) and one no relationship (Camacho *et al.* 1987), Fig. 4.10.

The effect is present across all age ranges although it appears stronger for older people (Shaper *et al.* 1994) and is present for both men and women. Because CHD is rare in premenopausal women and in men under the age of 35 years, the protective effect cannot be of importance among these groups. In two studies, the negative association appeared to be stronger for CHD incidence, than death (Klatsky *et al.* 1981; Rimm *et al.* 1991), although this was not the case in a third study (Shaper *et al.* 1994). The protective effect is specific to CHD and not to other causes of death apart from non-

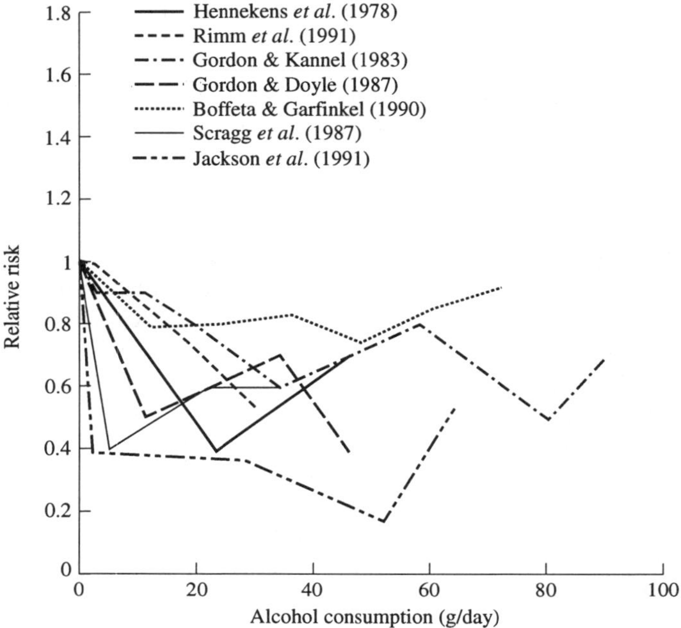

Fig. 4.8 Alcohol consumption and incidence of coronary heart disease in men. Data from seven studies with significant negative association.

haemorrhagic stroke and persists throughout the total length of follow-up periods (Boffetta and Garfinkel 1990; Friedman and Kimball 1986) which has varied from 2 years (Rimm *et al.* 1991) to 22 years (Gordon and Kannel 1983). Although the protective effect is present across populations from many different countries, most studies have been undertaken in populations in economically developed countries, and the effect in lesser developed countries is not known. The protective effect appears to be present for all beverage types (Renaud *et al.* 1993).

The protective effect is greater when alcohol consumption is spread throughout the week on a regular basis than when consumption is concentrated and consumed on one occasion during the week (Rimm *et al.* 1991). The Finnish prospective study showed a dose-response relationship for sudden coronary death and a positive dose-response relationship for CHD in older age groups which resulted from the weekend consumption of spirits (Suhonen *et al.* 1987). The reduced risk is achieved at very low doses of alcohol consumption and is similar for consumption ranging from a few grams of alcohol per day to about 40 g per day (Fig. 4.8) (Maclure 1993).

Some studies have shown an increased risk of CHD at consumption levels of over 60 g a day (Fig. 4.9). Not only former drinkers, but also total abstainers, have a higher incidence of CHD than moderate drinkers (Kono *et al.* 1986;

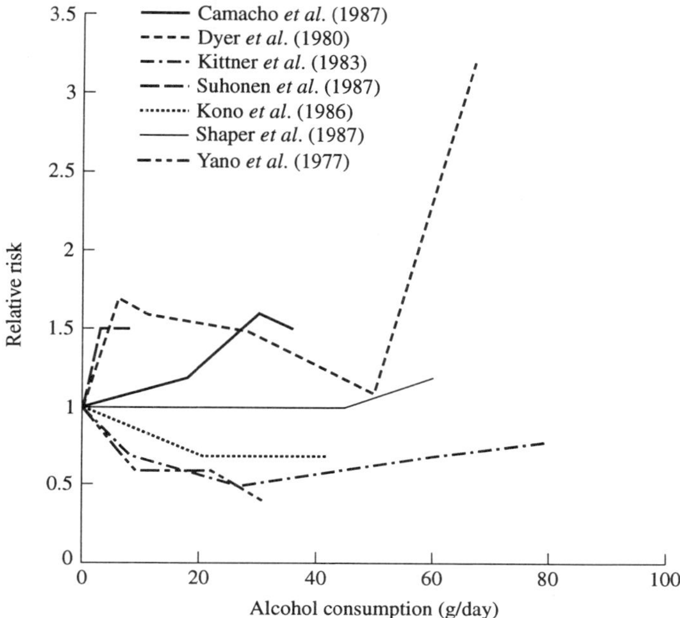

Fig. 4.9 Alcohol consumption and incidence of coronary heart disease in men. Data from seven studies with no significant association.

Yano *et al.* 1977; Jackson *et al.* 1991; Klatsky *et al.* 1989, 1990*b*). However, in one of these studies, former drinkers had a greater incidence of death from CHD than lifetime non-drinkers (Yano *et al.* 1977) and data from the Alameda Cohort study suggested that, at least for women, some of the increased risk of death from ischaemic heart disease associated with not drinking seemed to be accounted for by higher risks among those who gave up drinking (Lazarus *et al.* 1991). A higher risk in non-drinkers has been found in both Japanese Americans of whom 47 per cent of men were non-drinkers (Yano *et al.* 1977) and British civil servants, of whom 6 per cent of men were non-drinkers (Marmot *et al.* 1981).

The reduced risk of CHD from moderate alcohol consumption remains when those with cardiovascular illness or risk factors at enrolment are removed from the analysis (Boffetta and Garfinkel 1990; Klatsky *et al.* 1989), although not all studies have demonstrated this (Shaper *et al.* 1994). The reduced risk of CHD is most pronounced for current cigarette smokers (Shaper *et al.* 1994) and the greatest risk is found amongst non-drinkers who smoke (Klatsky *et al.* 1981*a*,*b*; Friedman and Kimball 1986; Marmot *et al.* 1981; Dyer *et al.* 1977). A smoker who is a non-drinker is likely to be a former drinker and a never drinker who is a non-smoker is likely to be a lifelong

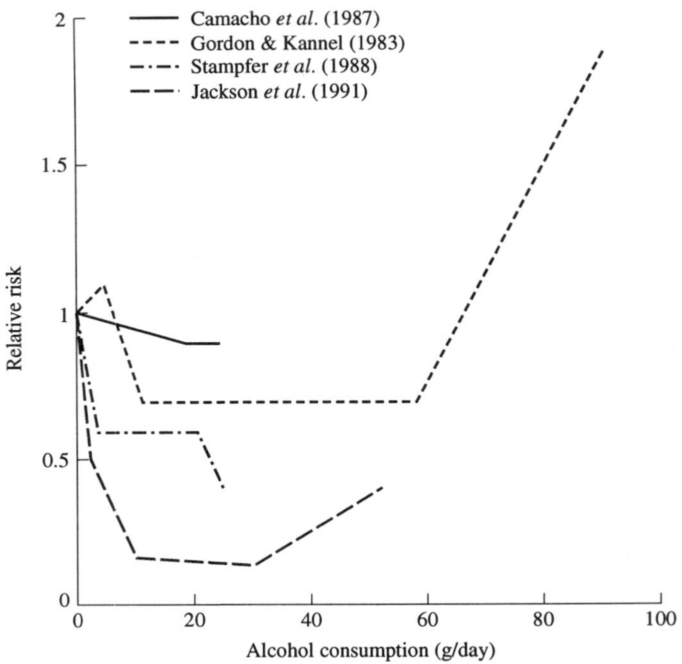

Fig. 4.10 Alcohol consumption and incidence of coronary heart disease in women. Data from four studies.

abstainer (Kozlowski and Ferrence 1990). The reduced risk of CHD is most apparent in manual, as opposed to non-manual workers (Shaper *et al.* 1994).

All cause mortality

Men Of 11 prospective studies of middle-aged men, eight showed a significant association, Fig. 4.11, of which seven showed a J-shaped curve (Kagan *et al.* 1981; Boffetta and Garfinkel 1990, Klatsky *et al.* 1981*a,b*, Shaper *et al.* 1988; Dyer *et al.* 1980; Kittner *et al.* 1983; Marmot *et al.* 1981). These are the Chicago Western Electric Study (Dyer *et al.* 1980) of 1832 American men aged 40–55 followed-up for 17 years, the Honolulu Heart Study (Kagan *et al.* 1981) of 7591 Japanese men aged 45–69 living in Hawaii followed for 9 years, the Whitehall Civil Servants Study (Marmot *et al.* 1981) of 1422 British men aged 40–64 followed-up for 10 years, the Puerto Rico Heart Health Program (Kittner *et al.* 1983) of 8907 Puerto Rican men aged 35–79 followed-up for 12 years, the British Regional Heart Study (Shaper *et al.* 1988) of 7735 British men aged 40–59 followed-up for 7.5 years, the American Cancer Society Prospective Study (Boffetta and Garfinkel 1990) of 276 802 American men aged 40–59 followed-up for 12 years, and the Kaiser Permanente Study

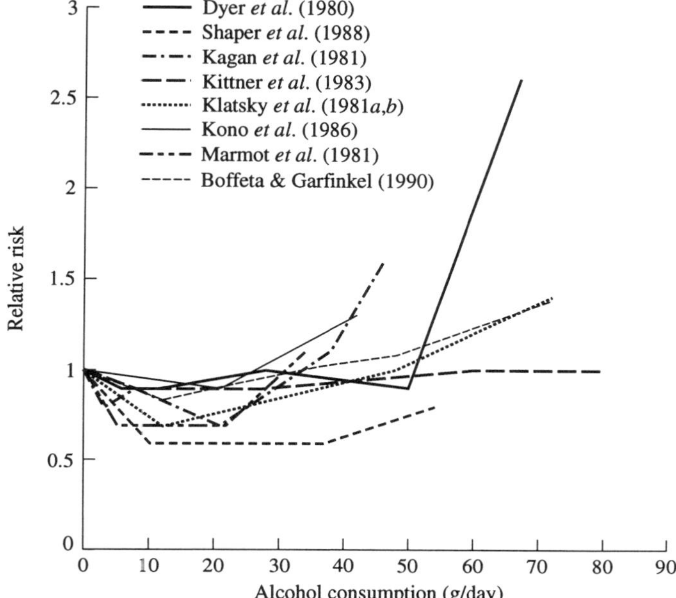

Fig. 4.11 Alcohol consumption and incidence of mortality in men from all causes. Data from eight studies with significant association.

(Klatsky *et al.* 1981*a*,*b*) of 6336 American men aged 15–79 followed-up for 10 years. The eighth study, the Male Japanese Physicians cohort (Kono *et al.* 1986) of 5477 Japanese physicians followed-up for 19 years showed a significantly increased risk for heavy drinkers, but no decreased risk at lower levels.

Further analysis of data from the Chicago Western Electric Study, the Whitehall Civil Servants Study, the British Regional Heart Study, and the Kaiser Permanente Study (Kozlowski and Ferrence 1990) demonstrate that U-shaped relationship is only apparent among current smokers, particularly heavy smokers (Marmot *et al.* 1981) or ex-smokers (Shaper 1990). In the Chicago Western Electric study, the U-shaped curve derives almost completely from the former drinkers who smoke cigarettes (Dyer *et al.* 1977), and in the British Regional Heart Study, shows excess deaths only among non-drinking ex-smokers (Shaper 1990).

The remaining three studies showed a non-significant relationship (Gordon and Kannel 1984; Suhonen *et al.* 1987; Gordon and Doyle 1987), Fig. 4.12. These are the Finnish Social Insurance Institution's Mobile Clinic Health Survey (Suhonen *et al.* 1987) of 4532 Finnish men aged 40–64 followed-up for 5 years, the Framingham Study (Gordon and Kannel 1983) of 2106 American men aged 29–62 followed-up for 22 years, and the Albany study (Gordon and

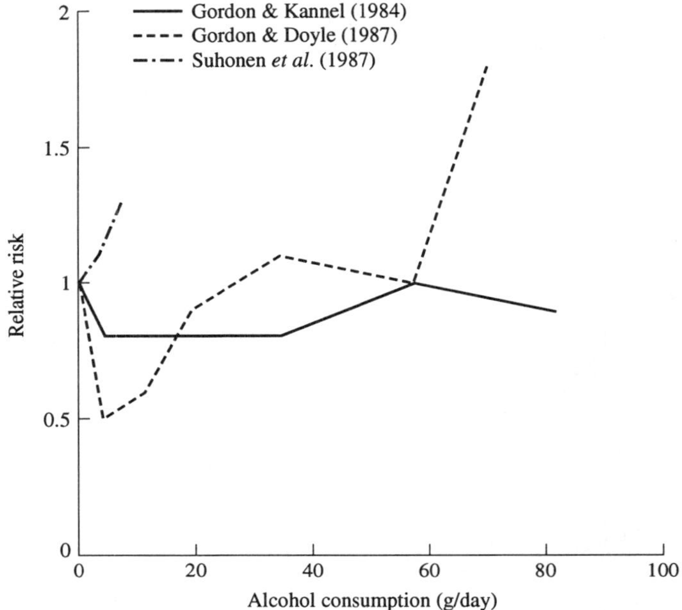

Fig. 4.12 Alcohol consumption and incidence of mortality in men from all causes. Data from three studies with no significant association.

Doyle 1987) of 1910 American men aged 38–55 followed-up for 18 years and 979 men aged 56–73 followed-up for 10 years. In the Finnish study, Suhonen *et al.* (1987) demonstrate a significantly increased risk for coronary death and a significant inverse relationship for MI deaths despite an overall non-significant trend. The Framingham and Albany studies show a significant linear or U-shaped association for non-CHD deaths and a significant inverse association for CHD deaths, despite an overall non-significant relationship.

As with cardiovascular disease mortality, the British Regional Heart data (Shaper *et al.* 1988) demonstrated that the U-shaped curve for total mortality applied only to 'unhealthy' men.

A 15-year follow-up of 11 600 adults drawn from the US National Health and Nutrition Examination study, which controlled for the effects of education, smoking status, BMI, blood pressure, serum cholesterol, and percentage of total calories from fat, demonstrated a significant linear relationship between alcohol consumption and all-cause mortality for females and males under 60 and a non-significant U-shape for older people. The exclusion of persons with heart disease history at baseline led to a more pronounced linear relationship for both females and males under 60 years of age (Rehm and Sempos 1994).

The association between alcohol consumption and 15-year mortality of

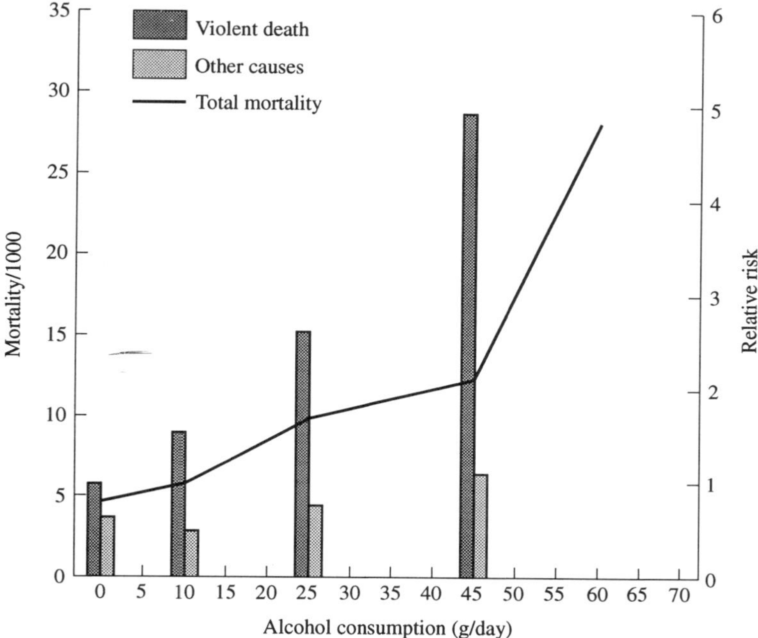

Fig. 4.13 Alcohol consumption and incidence of alcohol-induced mortality in young men aged 18–19.

Source: Andreasson *et al.* (1988).

young men was studied in a cohort of 49 464 Swedish conscripts, mostly aged 18–19 (Andreasson *et al.* 1988), Fig. 4.13. Violent death accounted for three-quarters of all deaths and increased in a linear dose-response relationship with increasing alcohol consumption. A U-shaped curve for total mortality was not confirmed, although when violent deaths were excluded, a U-shaped curve was suggested for other causes of death.

Women The relationship between alcohol consumption and mortality was either not significant in the Framingham Study (Gordon and Kannel 1984) of 2641 women aged 29–62 followed-up for 22 years, or exhibited a U-shaped curve in the Kaiser Permanente Study (Klatsky *et al.* 1981*a,b*) of 1724 women aged 15–79 within a 10-year follow-up.

Men and women Two further surveys showed a significant U-shaped curve (Camacho *et al.* 1987; Colditz *et al.* 1985). The Alameda Cohorts Study of 1845 men and 2225 women aged over 34, with a 15-year follow-up, divides the group into men and women and shows that the significant U-shaped curve is seen in men, but a non-significant relationship is seen in women (Camacho *et al.* 1987). Colditz *et al.* followed-up 1184 American men and women aged over 65 for 4.75 years and showed a U-shaped curve in an elderly cohort, but give no separate data for men and women (Colditz *et al.* 1985).

Discussion

This chapter has focused on the relationship between alcohol consumption and certain forms of physical harm that are of public health importance, including cirrhosis of the liver, cancers, and cardiovascular disease. This review has not considered alcohol-related causes of violent death which is of great concern among the young and forms an important fraction of potential years of life lost.

For many conditions, there is evidence for a dose-response relationship between alcohol consumption and risk, without evidence of a threshold effect (Anderson *et al.* 1993). This applies to cirrhosis of the liver, cancers of the pharynx, larynx, liver, female breast, and possibly colorectum, blood pressure, and stroke. There appears to be a significant negative association, that is not dose-related, between alcohol consumption and risk of coronary heart disease. It appears that much of the protective effect can be achieved at consumption levels of less than 10 g daily and the protective effect cannot be important for men under the age of 35 and premenopausal women. The relationship between alcohol consumption and total mortality appears largely J-shaped.

In general, more data exist for men than for women. Clinical (Turner *et al.* 1984) and biochemical (Hill 1984) data suggests that women may be more susceptible to the toxic effects of alcohol than men. However, the risk function curves for women are, with the exception of cirrhosis of the liver, similar to those for men.

Less data is available concerning age differences. In younger men and women, the dose-response relationship for total mortality appears more linear (Andreasson *et al.* 1988, Rehm and Sempos 1994). Insufficient data exists concerning populations with widely different incidence and prevalence rates of disease. There appears to be no substantial beverage differences in the dose-response relationships.

Little information is available concerning drinking patterns. This is particularly important because the number of drinks per day reported in many studies rarely refers to the actual drinking pattern, but to averages of various other measures of consumption such as usual consumption, very recent consumption or consumption at the beginning of the study. Little information is available concerning social integration and mental health, both of which could be important confounders in the relationship between alcohol consumption and total mortality.

For the adult population, it is possible to give an estimate of risk in relation to alcohol consumption for the conditions reviewed here. At levels of consumption of around 20 g a day, compared with no consumption, it has been estimated that there is a twofold increased risk for cirrhosis of the liver (Duffy 1992*c*), a 20–30 per cent increased risk for cancers of the oral cavity, pharynx, and larynx (Duffy and Sharples 1992), a 10 per cent increased risk for cancer of the oesophagus (Duffy and Sharples 1992), a 14 per cent increased risk for cancer of the liver (Duffy and Sharples 1992), a 10–20 per cent increased risk for cancer of the female breast (Holman and Armstrong 1990; Duffy and Sharples 1992), an increase in blood pressure of between 2 and 4 mmHg (Anderson *et al.* 1993), and possibly a 20 per cent increased risk of stroke (Holman and Armstrong 1990). However, at these levels of consumption, for some segments of the population, the increased risk is balanced by a decreased risk of coronary heart disease of approximately 25–50 per cent (Renaud *et al.* 1993; Marmot and Brunner 1991). Consequently, at levels of intake of around 20 g a day, the relative risk of total mortality is not increased.

Above levels of consumption of 20–30 g a day, compared with abstainers, in terms of mortality, there is a net increase in harm (Anderson 1993).

References

Anderson, P., Cremona, A., Paton, A., Turner, C., and Wallace, P. (1993). The risk of alcohol. *Addiction*, **88**, 1493–1508.

Anderson, P. (1993). Are there net health benefits from moderate drinking? All cause mortality. Paper presented at the *Moderate Drinking and Health Symposium*, 29 April–1 May. Toronto, Canada.

Andreasson, S., Romelsjö, A., and Allbeck, P. (1988). Alcohol and mortality among young men: longitudinal study of Swedish conscripts. *British Medical Journal*, **296**, 1021–5.

Begg, C. B., Walker, A. M., Wessen, B., and Zelen, M. (1983). Alcohol consumption and the risk of breast cancer. *Lancet*, **i**, 293–4.

Ben-Shlomo, Y., Markowe, H., Shipley, M., and Marmot, M. G. (1992). Stroke risk from alcohol consumption using different control groups. *Stroke*, **23**, 1093–8.

Boffetta, P. and Garfinkel, L. (1990). Alcohol drinking and mortality among men enrolled in an American Cancer Society prospective study. *Epidemiology*, **1**, 342–8.

Byers, T. and Funch, D. P. (1982). Alcohol and breast cancer, *Lancet*, **i**, 799–800.

Camacho, T. C., Kaplan, G. A., and Cohen, R. D. (1987). Alcohol consumption and mortality in Alameda County. *Journal of Chronic Disease*, **40**, 229–36.

Coates, R. A. *et al.* (1986). Risk of fatty infiltration or cirrhosis of the liver in relation to ethanol consumption: a case-control study. *Clinical and Investigative Medicine*, **9**, 26–32.

Colditz, G. A. *et al.* (1985). Moderate alcohol and decreased cardiovascular mortality in an elderly cohort. *American Heart Journal*, **109**, 886–9.

Doll, R., Forman, D., La Vecchia, C., and Woutersen, F. (1993). Alcoholic beverages and cancers of the digestive tract. In *Health issues related to alcohol consumption*, (ed. P. M. Verschuren), pp. 125–66. A report for the Amsterdam Group. International Life Sciences Institute (ILSI), Brussels.

Donahue, R. P., Abbott, R. D., Reed, D. M., and Yano, K. (1986). Alcohol and haemorrhagic stroke. The Honolulu Heart Program. *Journal of the American Medical Association*, **255**, 2311–14.

Duffy, J. C. (ed.) (1992*a*). *Alcohol and illness*. Edinburgh University Press.

Duffy, J. C. (ed.) (1992*b*). The measurement of alcohol consumption. In Ed. J. C. Duffy *Alcohol and illness*, pp. 19–25. Edinburgh University Press.

Duffy, J. C. (ed.) (1992*c*). Alcohol consumption and liver cirrhosis. In Ed. J. C. Duffy *Alcohol and illness*, pp. 64–127. Edinburgh University Press.

Duffy, S. W. and Sharples, L. D. (1992). Alcohol and cancer risk. In *Alcohol and illness*, (ed. J. C. Duffy), pp. 1–18. Edinburgh University Press.

Dyer, A. R. *et al.* (1977). Alcohol consumption, cardiovascular risk factors, and mortality in two Chicago epidemiologic studies. *Circulation*, **56**, 1067–74.

Dyer, A. R. *et al.* (1980). Alcohol consumption and 17-year mortality in the Chicago Western Electric Company study. *Preventive Medicine*, **9**, 78–90.

Fraser, G. E. and Upsell, M. (1981). Alcohol and other discriminants between cases of sudden death and myocardial infarction. *American Journal of Epidemiology*, **114**, 462–76.

Friedman, L. A. and Kimball, A. W. (1986). Coronary heart disease moratlity and alcohol consumption in Framingham. *American Journal of Epidemiology*, **124**, 481–9.

Gapstur, S. M., Potter, J. D., Sellers, T. A., and Folsom, A. R. (1992). Increased risk of breast cancer with alcohol consumption in postmenopausal women. *American Journal of Epidemiology*, **136**, 1221–31.

Gill, J. S., Zezulka, A. V., Shipley, M. J., and Beevers, D. G. (1986). Stroke and alcohol consumption, *New England Journal of Medicine*, **315**, 1041–6.

Gordon, T. and Doyle, J. (1987). Drinking and mortality. *American Journal of Epidemiology*, **125**, 263–70.

Gordon, T. and Kannel, W. B. (1983). Drinking habits and cardiovascular disease: The Framingham Study. *American Heart Journal*, **105**, 667–73.

Gordon, T. and Kannel, W. B. (1984). Drinking and mortality. The Framingham Study, *American Journal of Epidemiology*, **120**, 97–107.

Harris, R. E. and Wynder, E. L. (1988). Breast cancer and alcohol consumption. *Journal of the American Medical Association*, **259**, 2867–71.

Harvey, E. B. *et al.* (1987). Alcohol consumption and breast cancer. *International Journal of Cancer*, **78**, 657–61.

Hennekens, C. H., Rosner, B., and Cole, D. S. (1978). Daily alcohol consumption and fatal coronary heart disease. *American Journal of Epidemiology*, **107**, 196–200.

Hiatt, R. A. and Bawol, R. D. (1984). Alcohol beverage consumption and breast cancer incidence. *American Journal of Epidemiology*, **120**, 676–83.

Hiatt, R. A., Klatsky, A. L., and Armstrong, M. A. (1988). Alcohol consumption and the risk of breast cancer in a prepaid health plan. *Cancer Research*, **48**, 2284–7.

Hill, S. Y. (1984). Vulnerability and the biomedical consequence of alcoholism and alcohol related problems among women. In *Alcohol problems in women*, (ed. S. C. Wilsnack and L. Beckman), pp. 120–54. Guilford, New York.

Holman, D'A. J. and Armstrong, B. K. (1990). *The quantification of drug-caused morbidity and mortality in Australia 1988*. Government Printing House, Canberra.

Howe, G. *et al.* (1991). The association between alcohol and breast cancer risk: evidence from the combined analysis of six dietary case control studies. *International Journal of Cancer*, **47**, 707–10.

IARC (International Agency for Research on Cancer) (1988). *IARC monograph on the evaluation of carcinogenic risks to humans: Alcohol drinking*. International Agency for Research on Cancer, Lyon.

Jackson, R., Scragg, R., and Beaglehole, R. (1991). Alcohol consumption and risk of coronary heart disease. *British Medical Journal*, **303**, 21–16.

Jackson, R., Scragg, R., and Beaglehole, R. (1992). Does recent alcohol consumption reduce the risk of acute myocardial infarction and coronary death in regular drinkers? *American Journal of Epidemiology*, **136**, 819–24.

Kagan, A., Yano, K., Rhoads, G., and McGee, D. L. (1981). Alcohol and cardiovascular disease: The Hawaiian experience, *Circulation*, **64**, (suppl. III), 27–31.

Kittner, S. J. *et al.* (1983). Alcohol and coronary heart disease in Puerto Rico. *American Journal of Epidemiology*, **117**, 50.

Klatsky, A. L. and Armstrong, M. A. (1992). Alcohol, smoking, coffee and cirrhosis. *American Journal of Epidemiology*, **136**, 1248–57.

Klatsky, A. L., Friedman, G. D., and Siegelaub, A. B. (1981*a*). Alcohol and mortality. A ten-year Kaiser Permanente experience. *Annals of Internal Medicine*, **95**, 139–45.

Klatsky, A. L., Friedman, G. D., and Siegelaub, A. B. (1981*b*). Alcohol use and cardiovascular disease: the Kaiser-Permanente experience, *Circulation*, **64**, (suppl. III), 32–41.

Klatsky, A. L., Armstrong, M. A., and Friedman, G. D. (1989). Alcohol and cardiovascular deaths. *Circulation*, **80**, 611–14.

Klatsky, A. L., Armstrong, M. A., and Friedman, G. D. (1990*a*). Risk of cardiovascular mortality in alcohol drinkers, ex-drinkers and non-drinkers. *American Journal of Cardiology*, **66**, 1237–42.

Klatsky, A. L., Armstrong, M. A., and Friedman, G. D. (1990*b*). Mortality in ex-drinkers. *Circulation*, **81**, 720.

Knupfer, G. (1987). Drinking for health: the daily light drinker fiction. *British Journal of Addiction*, **82**, 547–55.

Kono, S. *et al.* (1986). Alcohol and morality: a cohort study of male Japanese physicians. *International Journal of Epidemiology*, **15**, 527–32.

Kozlowski, L. T. and Ferrence, R. G. (1990). Statistical control in research on alcohol and tobacco: an example from research on alcohol and mortality. *British Journal of Addiction*, **85**, 271–8.

La Vecchia, C. *et al.* (1985). Alcohol consumption and the risk of breast cancer in women. *Journal of the National Cancer Institute*, **75**, 61–5.

Lazarus, N. B., Kaplan, G. A., Cohen, R. D., and Leu, D-J. (1991). Change in alcohol consumption and risk of death from all causes and from ischaemic heart disease. *British Medical Journal*, **303**, 553–6.

Lé, M. G., Hill, C., Kramar, A., and Flamant, R. (1984). Alcoholic beverage consumption and breast cancer in a French case control study. *American Journal of Epidemiology*, **120**, 350–7.

Longnecker, M. P. *et al.* (1988). A meta-analysis of alcohol consumption in relation to risk of breast cancer. *Journal of the American Medical Association*, **260**, 652–6.

Maclure, M. (1993). Demonstration of deductive meta-analysis: ethanol intake and risk of myocardial infarction. *Epidemiologic Reviews*, **15**, 328–51.

Marmot, M. and Brunner, E. (1991). Alcohol and cardiovascular disease: the status of the U-shaped curve. *British Medical Journal*, **303**, 565–8.

Marmot, M. G., Rose, G., Shipley, M. J., and Thomas, B. J. (1981). Alcohol and mortality: a U-shaped curve. *Lancet*, **i**, 580–3.

Martinez, I. (1969). Factors associated with cancer of the esophagus, mouth and pharynx in Puerto Rico. *Journal of National Cancer Institute*, **42**, 1069–94.

McPherson, K., Engelsman, E., and Conning, D. (1993). Breast cancer. In *Health issues related to alcohol consumption*, (ed. P. M. Verschuren), pp. 221–44. A report for the Amsterdam Group, International Life Sciences Institute (ILSI), Brussels.

Miller, R. D. *et al*. (1987). Breast cancer risk and alcoholic beverage drinking. *American Journal of Epidemiology*, **126**, 736.

Norton, R. *et al*. (1987). Alcohol consumption and the risk of alcohol related cirrhosis in women. *British Medical Journal*, **295**, 80–2.

O'Connel, D. L. *et al*. (1987). Cigarette smoking, alcohol consumption and breast cancer risk. *Journal of the National Cancer Institute*, **78**, 229–34.

Paganini-Hill, A. and Ross, R. K. (1983). Breast cancer and alcohol consumption. *Lancet*, **ii**, 626–7.

Péquinot, G., Tuyns, A. J., and Berta, J. L. (1978). Ascitic cirrhosis in relation to alcohol consumption. *International Journal of Epidemiology*, **7**, 113–20.

Pottern, M. *et al*. (1981). Oesophageal cancer among black men in Washington, DC: Alcohol, tobacco and other risk factors. *Journal of the National Cancer Institute*, **67**, 777–83.

Rehm, J. and Sempos, C. T. (in press). Alcohol consumption and all cause mortality. *Addiction*.

Renaud, S., Criqui, M. H., Farchi, G., and Veenstra, J. (1993). Alcohol drinking and coronary heart disease. In *Health issues related to alcohol consumption*, (ed. P. M. Verschuren), pp. 81–123. A report for the Amsterdam Group International Life Sciences Institute (ILSI), Europe.

Rimm, E. B. *et al*. (1991). Prospective study of alcohol consumption and risk of coronary disease in men. *Lancet*, **338**, 464–8.

Rohan, T. E. and McMichael, A. J. (1988). Alcohol consumption and the risk of breast cancer. *British Journal of Cancer*, **41**, 695–9.

Rydberg, U., Thakker, K. D., and Skerfving, S. (in press). Risk evaluation of alcohol. *International Review of Psychiatry*.

Schatzkin, A. *et al*. (1987). Alcohol consumption and breast cancer in the epidemiological follow-up study of the first national health and nutrition examination survey. *New England Journal of Medicine*, **6**, 1169–73.

Scragg, R., Stewart, A., Jackson, R., and Beaglehole, R. (1987). Alcohol and exercise in myocardial infarction and sudden coronary death in men and women. *American Journal of Epidemiology*, **126**, 77–85.

Semenciw, R. M. *et al*. (1988). Major risk factors for cardiovascular disease moratlity in adults: results from the Nutrition Canada Cohort, *International Journal of Epidemiology*, **17**, 317–24.

Shaper, A. G. (1990). Alcohol and mortality: a review of prospective studies. *British Journal of Addiction*, **85**, 837–47.

Shaper, A. G., Phillips, A. N., Pocock, S. J., and Walker, M. (1987). Alcohol and ischaemic heart disease in middle aged British men. *British Medical Journal*, **284**, 733–7.

Shaper, A. G., Wannamethee, G., and Walker, M. (1988). Alcohol and mortality in British men: explaining the U-shaped curve. *Lancet*, **ii**, 1267–73.

Shaper, A. G., Phillips, A. N., Pocock, S. J., Walker, M., and Macfarlane, P. W. (1991). Risk factors for stroke in middle aged British men. *British Medical Journal*, **302**, 1111–15.

Shaper, A. G., Wannamethee, G., and Walker, M. (1994). Alcohol and coronary heart disease: a perspective from the British Regional Heart Study. *International Journal of Epidemiology*, **23**, 482–94.

Simes, R. J. (1986). Publication bias: the case for an international registry of clinical trials, *Journal of Clinical Oncology*, **4**, 1529–41.

Stampfer, M. J. *et al.* (1988). A prospective study of moderate alcohol consumption and the risk of coronary disease and stroke in women. *New England Journal of Medicine*, **319**, 267–73.

Stason, W. B. *et al.* (1976). Alcohol consumption and nonfatal myocardial infarction. *American Journal of Epidemiology*, **104**, 603–8.

Suhonen, O., Aromaa, A., Reunanen, A., and Knekt, P. (1987). Alcohol consumption and sudden coronary death in middle-aged Finnish men. *Acta Medica Scandinavica*, **221**, 335–41.

Talamini, R. *et al.* (1984). Social factors, diet and breast cancer in a northern Italian population. *British Journal of Cancer*, **49**, 723–9.

Turner, C. (1990). How much alcohol is in a 'standard drink': an analysis of 125 studies, *British Journal of Addiction*, **85**, 1171–6.

Turner, T. B., Mezey, E., and Kimball, A. W. (1984). Measurement of alcohol-related effects in man: chronic effects in relation to levels of alcohol consumption. *Johns Hopkins Medical Journal*, **141**, 235–48; 273–86.

Tuyns, A. J. (1983). Oesophageal cancer in non-smoking drinkers and in non-drinking smokers. *International Journal of Cancer*, **32**, 445–8.

Tuyns, A. J. and Péquinot, G. (1984). Greater risk of ascitic cirrhosis in females in relation to alcohol consumption. *International Journal of Epidemiology*, **14**, 53–7.

Tuyns, A., Péquinot, G., and Jensen, O. (1977). Le cancer de l'oesophage en Ille-et-Vilaine en fonction des niveaux de consommation d'alcool et de tabac. *Bulletin du Cancer*, **64**, 45–60.

Tuyns, A., Péquinot, G., and Abbatucci, J. (1979). Oesophageal cancer and alcohol consumption: importance of beverage. *International Journal of Cancer*, **23**, 443–7.

Vassallo, A. *et al.* (1985). Esophageal cancer in Uruguay: a case control study. *Journal of National Cancer Institute* **75**, 1005–9.

Verschuren, P. M. (ed.) (1993). *Health issues related to alcohol consumption.* A report for the Amsterdam Group International Life Sciences Institute (ILSI), Brussels.

Victoria, C. *et al.* (1987). Hot beverages and oesophageal cancer in southern Brazil: a case control study. *International Journal of Cancer*, **39**, 710–16.

Von Arbin, M. *et al.* (1985). Circulatory manifestations and risk factors in patients with acute cerebrovascular disease and in matched controls. *Acta Medica Scandinavica*, **218**, 373–80.

Webster, L. A. *et al.* (1983). Alcohol consumption and the risk of breast cancer. *Lancet*, **ii**, 724–5.

Willett, W. C. *et al.* (1987). Moderate alcohol consumption and the risk of breast cancer. *New England Journal of Medicine*, **316**, 1174–80.

Wyndner, E. and Bross, I. J. (1961). A study of etiological factors in cancer of the esophagus. *Cancer*, **14**, 389–413.

Yano, K., Rhoads, G. G., and Kagan, A. (1977). Coffee, alcohol and risk of coronary heart disease among Japanese men living in Hawaii. *New England Journal of Medicine*, **297**, 405–9.

5. Alcohol consumption and unintentional injury, suicide, violence, work performance, and inter-generational effects

Anders Romelsjö

Introduction

A variety of consequences of alcohol consumption, including unintentional and intentional trauma, suicide, and various social complications, are reviewed in this chapter. Alcohol-involved problems affect other persons as well as the actual alcohol consumer, such as family members and the victims of traffic accidents and assaults. The figures below illustrate the magnitude of alcohol-involved problems and illustrate variations from study to study, reflecting differences in sample, type of injury, as well as measurement of alcohol involvement.

- Approximately 40–50 per cent of the fatal motor vehicle crashes in the United States (39 800 deaths in 1990) are considered to be alcohol-related, and nearly 560 000 additional people suffer injuries from alcohol-related crashes (NHTSA 1991).
- The risk for a fatal traffic crash, per mile (1.6 km) driven, is increased at least eight times for a driver with a blood alcohol concentration (BAC) of 0.10 per cent or greater than for a driver without any alcohol in the blood (USDHSS 1990).
- Alcohol involvement is more prevalent in serious rather than minor injuries (Roizen 1982).
- Alcohol involvement was noted in 21–77 per cent of fatal falls and in 18–53 per cent of the non-fatal ones (Hingson and Howland 1993) in the United States (12 400 in 1990); in 27–47 per cent of drownings in the United States (5200 in 1990) (Howland and Hingson 1988) and in over 50 per cent of drownings in Sweden (Melinder 1988); in 12–61 per cent of fatal burns in the United States (4300 in 1990) (Hingson and Howland 1993); in 20–36 per cent of suicides in the United States, (USDHHS 1990); in about 50 per cent

of fatally injured adult pedestrians (Baker *et al*. 1984) in the United States; in 53 per cent of deceased accident victims in Lusaka, Zambia during 1958–65 (Haworth 1989); in 66 per cent of murders and victims in Finland (Virkunnen 1974) and in 56 per cent of homicides in Venezuela (Medina-Mora and Gonzales 1989); in 25–50 per cent of cases of wife-beating in the United States (Hamilton and Collins 1981).

- In 1986, 1 800 000 drivers were arrested in the United States for driving while under the influence of alcohol (Greenfield 1988). For 142 000 of 150 000 people who lost their driving licence in West Germany in 1980, the cause was an elevated BAC (Vogt 1989).

This chapter considers causation in alcohol-involved problems, revises methodological issues, such as measurement of alcohol and outcomes, and discusses emergency room studies, and different types of alcohol-involved problems, both presenting empirical data and noting methodological issues.

Causation and alcohol

Many societal, social, and psychological problems which involve alcohol are linked in a causative web. Therefore, understanding alcohol's causal relationship for important and deeply tragic human suffering, such as suicide, violence, and wife battering, could be compared to attempting to catch eels that are escaping out of our grip. As a rule, alcohol consumption is just one of several contributing factors to social and health problems. It is thus necessary to deal briefly with the concept of *causation* (Rothman 1987; Pernanen 1989). For the most part, a disease or a social problem is not caused by one factor, but rather by several factors in combination, and with various time relationships to each other and to the outcome (problem). Alcohol consumption is usually a *contributory* (*component*) *cause*, which, together with other contributory causes, make up a *sufficient cause* for an event. By definition, alcohol consumption is a *necessary cause* for certain alcohol-related problems, such as drunken driving, but neither a sufficient nor a necessary cause for other happenings, such as a fall.

Ten criteria for the establishment of causal associations have been proposed (Rothman 1987; Pernanen 1989; Hill 1965; Honkanen 1988) including:

(1) *strength* (expressed as ratios between incidence rates);
(2) *consistency* of observations on a particular association in different populations under various circumstances;
(3) *specificity*, meaning that a given cause leads to a single effect;
(4) *temporality* (time direction);
(5) *biological gradient* (dose response);
(6) *biological plausibility*;

(7) *coherence* (whether or not the association agrees with other scientific knowledge);
(8) *experimental evidence*; and
(9) *analogy*.

It is possible to find examples which run counter to all these criteria except for temporality. Susser (1991) has recently contended that association, time order, and direction are the essential components of a cause, while Honkanen (1988) proposed temporal sequence, strength, dose-response relationship, consistency, collateral evidence, and biological plausibility. In the end, causal inference is a subjective process and the results are often tentative (Rothman 1987). In this chapter, a cause is pragmatically defined as an event, condition, or characteristic that plays an essential role for the occurrence of the problem (Rothman 1986).

The role of alcohol consumption in unintentional injury

Alcohol has been implicated as one important cause of unintentional injuries, which constitute prominent health problems in many countries (USDHSS 1990). The short-term psychological effects of alcohol include reduced co-ordination and balance, increased reaction time, impaired attention, perception, and judgement, all tending to increase the risk of accidents. Alcohol involvement varies by sex (more common in men); by localization of the injury (more common in head injuries); by severity (more common in fatal than in non-fatal crashes); by age (traffic accidents are more common in young and elderly drivers, and falls in elderly); and by culture. There is evidence that alcohol aggravates the prognosis of a severe trauma. The causes of non-fatal trauma differ considerably from those of fatal trauma (Honkanen and Visuri 1976; Honkanen 1993). The impact of alcohol on injury severity seems to vary with the type of injury. Alcohol involvement in non-vehicular unintentional injuries is less documented for several reasons: a diverse panorama of causes; these injuries are often less dramatic and of less public interest; legislative measures are less applicable. In this review as in others (USDHSS 1990), unintentional injuries refer to motor vehicle injuries, falls, drownings, burns and fires.

The following sections discuss issues of measurement in determining alcohol involvement and the use of the emergency room as a site for measurement.

Measurement of alcohol consumption in conjunction with injury

The information on alcohol consumption in studies of injuries fall into three groups: (1) alcohol use at the time of the event, (2) drinking and a history of problems among those involved, and (3) proportion of heavy drinkers or alcoholics (Roizen 1982, 1989). The first category is the most relevant, and should be the basis for calculations of risk curves and relative risk associated with alcohol use. The estimation of alcohol involvement in the event is usually based on measurement of BAC (recorded as mg per cent) on breathalyser readings, or from self-reports (Roizen 1982, 1989). Each of these have their merits and problems.

Selective measurement may lead to an inflation of alcohol-involved estimates. For example, Williams *et al.* (1988) reported that 70 per cent of all deceased drivers in 1986 had a BAC test, compared to 23 per cent of surviving drivers, while data from a national US survey showed that only 55 per cent of patients admitted to trauma centres were routinely BAC-tested (Söderström and Cowley 1987). In less severe injuries, the subjects involved may not be brought into contact with a hospital or the police, and consequently do not become candidates for testing. Furthermore, the BAC test in most cases probably yields lower values at testing than at the pre-injury and injury phases. This will contribute to an underestimation of the extent of alcohol involvement, but also to overestimation of the relative risk for accidents at various levels of BAC, and consequently to an incorrect dose-response curve. Those who refuse to participate, or are so seriously injured that they cannot be approached, may more frequently be BAC-positive (Cherpitel 1989, 1993*a*). On the other hand, some drivers or victims consume alcohol after the injury. Honkanen (1976) found that 15 per cent of the injury patients had consumed alcohol between the event and the arrival at hospital. Many studies have specified a maximum time lag, often 6 hours (Cherpitel 1993*a*), from the event to the taking of the blood specimen.

Self-reports give information about drinking both prior to and following injury, also stating quantities consumed (Harford 1993). The validity of such self-reports is unreliable, with under-reporting due to denial or forgetting being the foremost problem. In studies with information on both self-reported consumption and BAC, the proportion of persons reporting alcohol consumption within 6 hours prior to the event was greater than the proportion with positive BAC by breathalyser (Cherpitel 1993*a*). In a San Francisco study, 3.6 per cent of the persons who did not report drinking were positive on the breathalyser, while 29 per cent reporting alcohol consumption within a 6-hour period prior to injury were negative on the breathalyser (Cherpitel 1989). Thus, ideally, BACs and breathalyser readings should be supplemented by information about alcohol use from the subjects or witnesses (Harford 1993). BAC estimates with the breathalyser had a correlation coefficient of 0.96 with chemical analysis of the blood in one study (Gibb *et al.* 1984).

The selection of study design and study base (Miettinen 1985) (the study population manifesting the event under study) are fundamental areas. Cohort and case-control studies can enable the estimation of the relative risk of various levels or patterns of alcohol consumption and should ideally include all, or a representative sample of well-defined cases with a given outcome, valid information about alcohol consumption and other relevant risk factors, confounders, and effect modifiers, at time periods in appropriate relation to the outcome in the population (Miettinen 1985; Rothman 1986). Insufficient control groups are common (Roizen 1982, 1989). The selection of controls is a delicate question; hospital controls can be different from the population with respect to alcohol consumption, and perhaps also in other relevant aspects. A control group from the general population, matched by sex, age, site, and time of the day may seem ideal for estimation of relative risk and risk curves, but has rarely been achieved (Cherpitel 1993*a*; Honkanen 1988). Another problem is that all relevant cases are not included. Subjects who die or have minor injuries may not come to the hospital, and will therefore not be included in an emergency room study. Alcohol involvement in these categories can be assumed to be different from those who were included as cases. The role of alcohol can thus only be estimated crudely. However, the data are sufficient to conclude that the involvement is substantial. Both experimental studies and calculations of risk curves from studies with a particularly good methodology show that the risk increases with level of consumption.

Emergency room studies

Emergency room (ER) studies can provide a 'window' for estimation of the association between alcohol consumption and injury and have attracted increasing interest (Cherpitel 1992, 1993*a*). The prevalence of positive BAC or breathalyser readings varies greatly among these studies, partly due to differences in age criteria, variations in length of time for data collection, and seasonal variation (Table 5.1). Probability sampling of patients over the week is important for a correct estimation of the relative risk, as alcohol consumption and causality occurrence vary by day of week and time of day. Most ER studies have recruited controls among non-injured patients in the ER. However, these patients often have higher rates of alcohol use and alcohol-related problems than the general population. Wechsler *et al.* (1969) found that the proportion of persons with a positive BAC was inversely correlated with the length of time between injury and arrival in the ER. One study showed a significantly higher proportion of positive BAC in a non-random sample of persons who refused to participate or were seriously injured, than among those interviewed (Cherpitel 1989). In a unique comparison of ER patients in a health maintenance organization and in the general population, Cherpitel (1992*b*) found a similar association between drinking patterns and problems with causalities. She regarded the findings encouraging in providing support for the generality of ER studies.

Studies find a correlation between persons with a BAC of 0.08 per cent or

Table 5.1 Emergency room (ER) studies measuring BAC[a] among probability samples of patients

Country	Year	Length of collection	Completion rate (%)	Age	Alcohol measure	Injured (% positive BAC) (*n*)	Non-injured (% positive BAC) (*n*)	Source
Boston, MA, USA	1967	1 yr	75	≥16	Breath	23 (2989) 12 ≥0.05	9[b] (2633) 3[b] ≥0.05	Wechsler *et al.* (1969)
Melbourne, Victoria, Australia	1969	7 dys	?	18–65	Breath	31 (246) 19 ≥0.05	–	Gay *et al.* (1970)
Jyväskylä, Finland	1974	?	?	Adults	Blood within 12 h	30 (180) 20 ≥0.10	–	Honkanen and Ottelin (1976)
Exeter, UK	1976–7	4 mths	79	≥15	Blood	11 (700)	10 (240)	Peppiatt *et al.* (1978)
Houston, USA	1980–1	14 mths	100	6 mths–88 yrs	Blood within 1 h	32 (1198) 24 ≥0.10	–	Ward *et al.* (1982)
Broxburn, Scotland, UK	1980	7 wks	99	≥15	Breath	18 (739) 11 ≥0.08	11[b] (301) 3[b] ≥0.08	Walsh and Macleod (1983)
US Army Hospital Nürenburg, Germany	1983	1 mth	75	≥18	Blood and/or breath	34 (356)	19[b] (293)	James *et al.* (1984)
Paris and other towns (21 ERs)	1982–3	6 mths	?	≥15	Blood within 6 h	30 (4796) 21 ≥0.08	–	Papoz *et al.* (1986)
Stockport, UK	1986	2 mths	100	≥17	Breath	10 (126)	–	Redmond *et al.* (1987)
Salford, UK	?	2 wks	74	≥16	Blood or breath	14 (1629) 8 ≥0.08	–	Yates *et al.* (1987)
San Francisco, CA, USA	1984–5	2 mths	75	≥18	Breath	23 (502) 15 ≥0.10	10[b] (1192) 6[b] ≥0.10	Cherpitel (1988*a*)
Contra Costa Co, CA, USA (4 ERs)	1985	3 mths	73	≥18	Breath within 6 h	11 (1026) 4 ≥0.10	5[b] (1306) 3 ≥0.10	Cherpitel (1988*a*)
Acapulco, Mexico (3 ERs)	1987	1 mth	82	≥15	Breath within 6 h	22 (376) 8 ≥0.10	7[b] (308) 1[b] ≥0.10	Rosovsky and Garcia (1988)
Mexico City, Mexico (8 ERs)	1986	1 wk	91	≥18	Breath within 6 h	21 (1644) 11 ≥0.10	3[b] (462) 2[b] ≥0.10	Cherpitel and Rosovsky (1990)
Barcelona, Spain	1987–8	1 yr	80	≥18	Breath within 6 h	10 (1640) 5 ≥0.10	4[b] (657) 1[b] ≥0.10	Cherpitel *et al.* (1991)
Contra Costa Co, CA, USA	1986–7	1 yr	72	≥18	Breath within 6 h	13 (1004) 6 ≥0.10	–	Cherpitel (1992*a*)
Contra Costa Co, CA, USA (3 HMO ERs)	1989	6 wks	76	≥18	Breath within 6 h	6 (452) 1 ≥0.10	3[b] (614) 1 ≥0.10	Cherpitel (1993*b*)

[a] BAC is recorded as mg%: positive is ≥0.01 (10 mg of alcohol per 100 ml of blood), 0.05, 0.08, 0.10 are BACs as indicated. [b] $P<0.05$ comparison of positive breathalyser readings between injured and non-injured in the same sample.
HMO = Health Maintenance Organizations.

Source: Cherpitel *et al.* (1993*a*).

higher and a clinical diagnosis of some degree of intoxication. There is one reporting that 32 per cent of ER patients with a BAC between 0.085 and 0.2 per cent were judged to be clinically sober by medical staff (Yates *et al.* 1987), and that 33 per cent of those with a BAC over 0.2 were diagnosed as either sober or only 'slightly intoxicated'. This means that BAC measurement can complement and assist clinical judgement. Comparative ER studies have shown that the association between alcohol and injury varies with the typical drinking pattern in a given culture (Cherpitel 1993*a*).

Driving while impaired by alcohol

Data from 78 roadside breath-testing surveys in different parts of the United States during 1970–4 showed that 1 per cent of early weekday drivers, 3 per cent of early weekend drivers, and 6 per cent of late weekday and late weekend drivers had a blood alcohol concentration exceeding 0.1 per cent (Lehman *et al.* 1975). The risk of being arrested by the police for drinking and driving has been estimated as 2 per 1000 trips (Ross 1982). There is considerable under-reporting in the official statistics of alcohol involvement in driving.

Unmarried males under the age of 25 in the lower occupational classes is the group most often reported to be driving after drinking heavily (Hingson *et al.* 1982). A follow-up study of 8122 Swedish conscripts showed a significant association between social risk factors and risk of sentence for drinking while intoxicated (DWI), and also that the mortality risk in those convicted of DWI (BAC 0.05 per cent or more) before the age of 27 was elevated 4.9 times (Karlsson *et al.* 1991).

In a study during the 1960s, alcoholics had 10 times as many arrests for DWI as the general population of drivers (Waller 1968). The proportion of alcoholics among DWIs is over 50 per cent in some studies (Waller 1976) and is especially high in those with repeated arrests. A large proportion of DWIs lack a driver's licence. In a study in Norway, which has a low per capita sales of alcohol (4.2 litres of 100 per cent ethanol in 1989, compared to 7.5 litres in the United States and 13.4 litres in France), more than 60 per cent of arrested drunk drivers drank more than 50 g pure alcohol per day (Gjerde and Mörland 1988). In a 2-year prospective study of 293 drunk drivers, 119 (30 per cent) were re-arrested. The re-arrest rate increased with increasing level of BAC and of the alcohol-related enzyme gamma-glutamyltransferase (GGT) at the first arrest, and was especially high in those with more than one previous arrest (Gjerde and Mörland 1988).

Motor vehicle collisions

This type of accident represents a leading cause of fatality in many countries and often involves alcohol. A traffic collision has been defined as alcohol-related when a participant (driver, pedestrian, or bicyclist) has a measured or estimated BAC of 0.01 per cent or above (Waller 1976; NHTSA 1988). Alcohol involvement is more common in fatal than in non-fatal collisions; and fatal collisions are more common during nights and weekends. During heavy daytime traffic, when there is a greater need of concentration, attention, and awareness, a comparatively low blood alcohol concentration (BAC) of 0.01–0.04 per cent can be associated with an increased risk of collision (Waller 1976; Borkenstein *et al.* 1974). Young as well as elderly drivers have been found to be over-represented in both fatal and non-fatal crashes, in addition to drivers cautioned for driving while intoxicated (DWI) (Waller 1976).

Dose-response relationships

Studies have shown that driving performance is reduced for at least three hours after alcohol has been eliminated from the blood and that the impairment is greater for complex driving tasks than for simple ones (Donelson and Beirness 1985). However, the results of experiments do not directly indicate the impairment of driving ability in real life, due to compensatory mechanisms and other factors. In a review, Waller (1976) contended that most of the drivers responsible for accidents had positive BAC—most of them a BAC of 0.1 mg% or more—while about 10 per cent of the 'non-responsible' drivers had a BAC of 0.1 mg% or more, compared to 2–4 per cent of drivers not involved in crashes (Waller 1976). In the Grand Rapids study, the proportion of drivers with a BAC of 0.1 mg% or more in serious non-fatal crashes was 11.3 per cent, while the proportion among drivers with a disabling injury was 6.7 per cent, compared to 0.6 per cent among non-involved drivers (Borkenstein *et al.* 1974).

Laboratory studies show that minimal impairment in performing a simulated driving test can be estimated at BACs of 0.02–0.03 mg%, and that there is a clear risk over 0.05 mg%; the risk of crashing at 0.08 mg% is increased 4 times, at 0.1 mg% 8 times, and at 0.15 mg% 27 times, compared to the risk with no alcohol in the blood (Loomis and West 1958). The most persuasive data, from comparisons of the BACs of drivers in collisions with the BACs of drivers not involved, generate risk curves with double the normal risk at 0.05 per cent BAC and 6 times the normal risk at 0.10 per cent (Voas 1993). The dose-response curves indicate an exponential relationship between blood alcohol concentration, from a BAC of 80–100 mg% and risk of traffic accident (Fig. 5.1) and also interaction with age (Fig. 5.2). In an analysis of data from the US national roadside breath-testing survey conducted in 1986, linked to data on fatal single vehicle collisions, Zador (1991) found that each 0.02 per cent increase in BAC nearly doubles the collision risk of a driver with non-zero BAC, and that the risk in the 0.05–0.09 BAC range was higher in young drivers and in women.

Intoxication among traffic collision victims is also common. Intoxicated

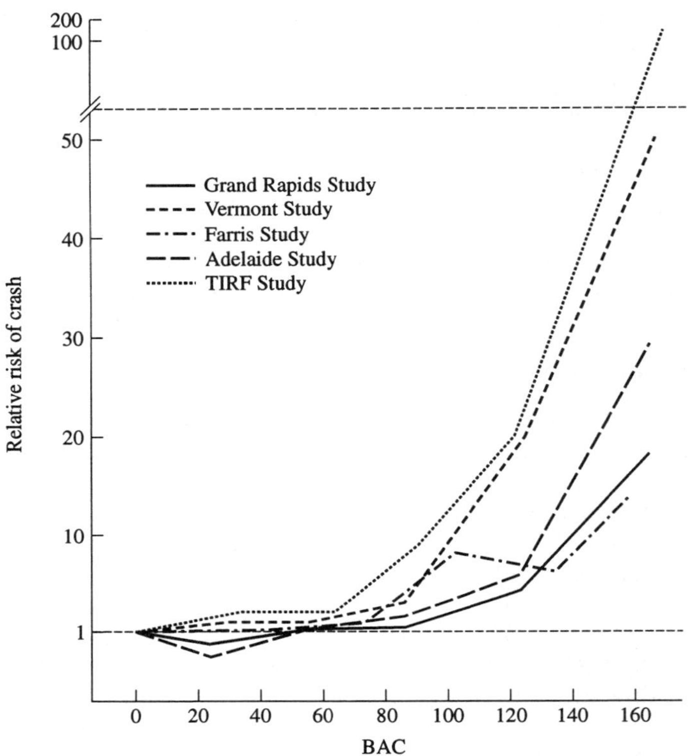

Fig. 5.1 Relative likelihood of a motor vehicle collision as a function of blood alcohol concentration (BAC).

Sources: Donelson and Beirness (1985, p. 48); Mayhew (1983).

pedestrians are 3 to 4 times more likely to be struck by motor vehicles than those who are not intoxicated (USDHSS 1990; Irwin *et al.* 1983). An association between DWI and life style is suggested by data from the United States on reported crashes. The results showed that alcohol intake was more than three times more likely among drivers not using seat belts or having expired licences and five times more likely among drivers with a suspended, revoked licence, or no licence (NHTSA 1988).

Other vehicle accidents

The number of deaths among *motorcyclists* per distance driven has been estimated to be seven times higher than for car occupants. Several studies have demonstrated that alcohol involvement is at least as common in motorcycle fatalities as in other traffic accidents (Roizen 1982; Baker *et al.* 1984). Intoxicated motorcyclists were found to wear helmets one-third less frequently

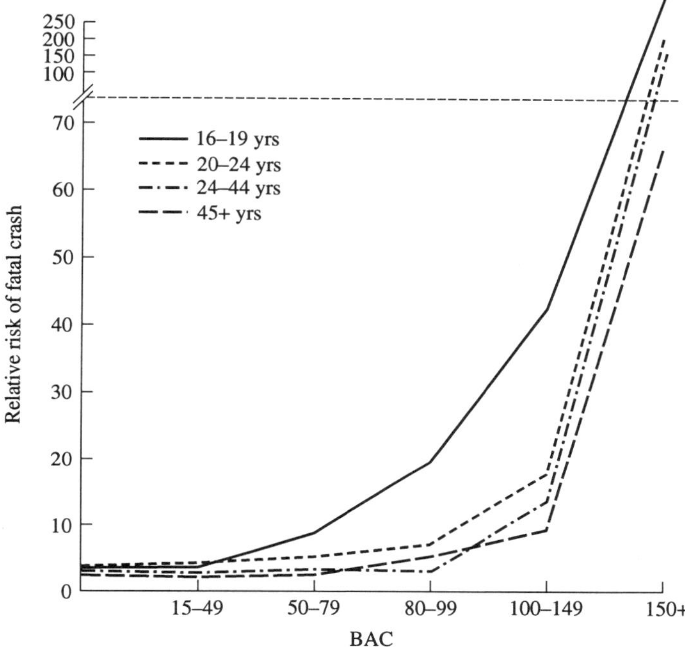

Fig. 5.2 Relative likelihood of a fatal motor vehicle collision as a function of blood alcohol concentration (BAC) and age.

Sources: Donelson and Beirness (1985, p. 64); Mayhew (1983).

than those who were not intoxicated (USDHSS 1990). Alcohol is a frequent contributor to *aviation* crashes (Smith and Kraus 1988) as flying skill is impaired at a blood alcohol concentration of 0.025 per cent (Klein *et al.* 1967). In about 5100 general aviation accidents involving over 10 500 deaths in the United States, during 1963–71, with BAC available on about 53 per cent of the deceased pilots, 18–43 per cent annually had a BAC of 0.15 mg% or more. One study, involving 74 per cent of pilots in non-commercial accidents, showed that 24 per cent had positive BAC (Ryan and Mohler 1979).

Drinking occurred in 40 per cent of *snowmobile* injuries involving adults, which was twice as common as in non-injured snowmobilers (Waller and Lamborn 1975; Smith and Kraus 1988). Thirty per cent of the victims of *moped* accidents had been drinking and about 20 per cent of moped drivers had a recent suspension of their driver's licence (Hunter and Stutts 1979; Roizen 1989). A case-control study in Helsinki comprised 140 adults injured in *bicycle* accidents between 3 p.m. and 10 p.m. and arriving at a hospital within six hours of injury, with 700 bicyclists from the street randomly selected as controls. Twenty-four per cent of the hospitalized persons and 4 per cent of the controls had a positive BAC (Olkkonen and Honkanen 1990).

Other injuries with alcohol involvement

Falls

Falls are also a prominent cause of non-fatal injuries in many countries, especially in the elderly (USDHSS 1990). The risk of falling is related to impairment of balance. Several studies show that individuals with a BAC over 0.1 per cent have an increased risk of swaying, on the Romberg test, which measures the ability to stand upright (Perrine *et al.* 1971; Hingson and Howland 1993). Alcohol was present in 21–77 per cent of fall fatalities and in 17–53 per cent of non-fatal falls in a review of 21 studies published from 1950 to 1985 (Hingson and Howland 1987), and in 18–57 per cent in five more recent studies, encompassing 10 535 subjects (Hingson and Howland 1993). In a case-control study during one summer and one winter week in Helsinki, 60 per cent of the 313 adult emergency room patients who had suffered accidental falls had a positive BAC, and 53 per cent had BAC of 0.2 or more (Honkanen *et al.* 1983). Two controls per case who were at the same site exactly one week later were chosen. The relative risk of falls for individuals with BACs of 0.05–0.10 per cent was three times greater than for individuals with no exposure to alcohol, 10 times greater for individuals with BACs of 0.10–0.15 per cent, and about 60 times greater for individuals with BACs of 0.16 per cent or more.

Drowning

The physiological effects of alcohol intake make it likely that alcohol consumption is a contributory cause of drowning, although the distribution of other contributory causes, such as risk-taking behaviour, may be different between those who drown and those who do not (Hingson and Howland 1993). There are several plausible factors and mechanisms supporting a causal role for alcohol. Alcohol can impair judgement with respect to risk assessment. Intoxicated persons may be more likely to engage in boating without flotation devices, and also in swimming alone at night. Alcohol consumption prior to swimming may lead swimmers to remain in cold water longer than if they were sober, by creating a sense of warmth. In one trial, operators who were both intoxicated and fatigued missed 10 times as many course corrections as tired but sober operators (Wright 1985).

The proportion of alcohol involvement in drowning has also been shown to be high, varying from 27 to 47 per cent with complete ascertainment of a BAC level within a specified time period (important because the decomposition of a submerged body results in fermentation to ethanol) in 36 studies, between 1950 and 1985 (Howland and Hingson 1988). In a study of survivors, a lifesaving association in Australia found that a third of all who came close to death from drowning had been drinking (*BMJ* 1979). In a survey in

Massachusetts in 1990, 36 per cent of the males and 11 per cent of the females reported drinking at the last recreational occasion on or near the water; nearly one-third of the alcohol-consuming males had drunk four or more drinks (Howland and Hingson 1990). In a Finnish study, the breath test was positive for 30 per cent of weekend motorboat drivers tested in a similar way as the roadside test (Penttilä *et al.* 1979).

Burns and fires

In an analysis of 32 studies published between 1947 and 1986, Howland and Hingson (1987) found that alcohol consumption was associated with an increased risk of fires and burns, although these studies were primarily descriptive and did not include control groups. Forty-seven per cent of persons in burn fatalities had been drinking (range: 9–86 per cent). Alcohol involvement in persons with burn injuries requiring emergency room treatment and hospitalization amounted to 17 per cent (median value), with a range of 1–50 per cent. The proportion of cases with alcohol involvement was higher in fatal burns than in non-fatal ones, and especially high in fires ignited by cigarettes. The odds ratio for alcohol involvement in deaths resulting from fires ignited by cigarettes, compared to other fire deaths, ranged between 2.0 and 18.5 in seven studies, and was 0.7 in the eighth study. In a study in California, 64 per cent of the persons whose deaths were attributed to fire, had a BAC of 0.1 per cent or more, while 18 per cent of subjects who died after episodes of acute illness had a similar BAC (Waller 1976).

Hypothermia

Alcohol greatly increases the risk of exposure-related hypothermia and frostbite (Smith and Kraus 1988). Sixty-nine per cent of 63 exposure-related deaths in the District of Columbia had detectable BACs, and 48 per cent had a BAC above 0.15 per cent (Luke and Levy 1982). In five studies of 1195 frostbite patients, alcohol abuse was a predisposing factor in 630 patients (53 per cent) (Urschel 1990).

Occupational injuries

Alcohol consumption has been estimated to have a role in 3–4 per cent of occupational-related injuries (Stallones and Kraus 1993), but higher figures have been reported. In West Germany, alcohol was estimated to be involved in 7–10 per cent of all industrial accidents, while 32 per cent of fatal industrial injury cases in Hamburg had a BAC of at least 0.05 mg% (Shain and Groenveld 1980). In a study from Texas (USA), 13 per cent of the deceased in occupational injuries had a positive BAC (Lewis and Cooper 1989). In 147 occupation-related traffic fatalities, BAC was positive in 20 per cent of the 25 cases and in 7.3 per cent of 122 non-traffic-related occupational injuries (Copeland 1985). Less is known about the role of alcohol in non-fatal occupational injuries. Wechsler *et al.* (1969) found that 16 per cent of emergency room patients injured at work had a positive breathalyser, while only 5 per cent had breathalyser readings greater than 50 mg/100 ml. Maxwell (1959) found that a group of problem drinkers aged below 40 had 3.6 times more accidents than a control group, while there were no differences in these two categories in the ages above 40 years. There is a potential for synergistic, additive, or antagonistic interaction between alcohol and chemical exposure in some work settings, an area which has hardly been studied (Stallones and Kraus 1993).

Alcohol-related casualties outside the United States and Europe

A substantial weakness is that our knowledge is mainly based on research from the United States and some countries in Europe, which together only make up a minority of the world population. The scant available data show, however, an important role for alcohol in other parts of the world. A number of studies conducted in Australia (Norton 1989) conform to the picture given by studies in the United States and Europe. Alcohol involvement in casualties in Latin America has recently been reviewed by Medina-Mora and Gonzáles (1989). High rates have been reported particularly from Chile and Mexico. In a study from Mexico, physicians reported presence of alcohol in 15 per cent of the arrestees at a police station and in 7 per cent in an emergency room, while alcohol involvement in an additional 24 and 10 per cent, respectively, was discovered at an interview (Rosovsky and Lopez 1986). There is very scant information about alcohol use and alcohol-related problems in Africa (Haworth 1989). In Zimbabwe in 1978, 4 per cent of 595 tested drivers had a BAC over 80 mg/100 ml (Kobus 1980). Fifty-three per cent of deceased accident victims in Lusaka, Zambia, during 1958 through 1965 had a BAC over 0.15 mg%, while 14 per cent had BACs between 0.05 and 0.1 mg% (Haworth 1989). Half of 29 dead drivers in fatal accidents in Papua, New Guinea, had a BAC of 80 mg/100 ml or more, the mean level being 212 mg/100 ml (Sinha *et al.* 1981). In a survey of 1710 road casualties in a provincial hospital in New Zealand, 27 per cent had positive BACs and 19 per cent had BACs of 100 mg/100 ml or more (Bailey 1984).

Alcohol and suicide

Many studies have shown that alcohol abuse and alcoholism are associated with increased risk of suicide. In a review, 20–36 per cent of suicide victims had a history of alcohol abuse or had been drinking at the time of the event (USDHSS 1990; Roizen 1982). Between 15 and 64 per cent of suicide attempters and up to 80 per cent of completers had been drinking shortly before their suicide (Roizen 1982). The one year, prevalence rate of drinking problems was significantly greater in suicide attempters, who were also more likely to have been arrested, or to have lost a job, or to have lost a spouse, compared to persons from the general population sample (Roizen 1982). A 16 per cent mortality rate from suicide among alcohol-dependent suicide attempters was noted in a Swedish study, compared to 2.7 per cent among suicide attempters with other diagnoses (Cullberg *et al.* 1988). The risk of suicide varies curvilinearly with age, and linearly with duration and severity of alcohol abuse, depression episodes, social isolation, and loss of emotional support (Murphy and Wetzel 1990).

The Swedish conscript study revealed that the relative risk of suicide death in high consumers of alcohol (250 g of 100 per cent ethanol/week) was 5.1 during a 13-year follow-up, compared with abstainers, while the risk was 9.4 for probable suicide, with a linear risk increase with consumption level for both categories of suicide (Andreasson *et al.* 1988).

Although the lifetime risk of suicide among alcoholics generally has been estimated to be 11–15 per cent (Roizen 1989), Murphy and Wetzel (1990) calculated a much lower risk in untreated or outpatient-treated alcoholics based on data from two studies of 67 male and 9 female active alcoholics, assuming an average abuse period of 19 years. This assumption can be questioned, and further similar analyses based on time at risk are needed.

Murphy and Wetzel (1990) suggest that comorbidity plays an important role in suicide in alcoholics, with depression as the leading complicating factor. They contend that suicide by alcoholics is largely dependent on supervention of a depressive episode, while suicide in personality disorders is conditioned on substance abuse. A depressive episode is found among 50–75 per cent of alcoholic suicides, which is a much higher frequency than in hospitalized alcoholics. Other substance abuse seems to shorten the career from the onset of the substance abuse to suicide. Welte *et al.* (1988) suggested that alcohol intake is associated with impulsive suicides rather than planned ones, and reported that suicides with positive BACs had lower scores for the factors: left a note, diagnosed as depressed, poor health, prior suicide attempt, and being under psychiatric care.

In a 20-year follow-up of 1312 alcoholics in Sweden, 88 (16 per cent) of 537 who died had committed suicide (Berglund 1984). In the evaluation with a multidimensional diagnostic rating scale at first admission, the alcoholics who committed suicide had a higher rate of depressive and dysphoric symptoms and were more brittle and sensitive than others, while the frequency of cognitive impairment and delirium tremens were similar. The rating did not differ between those who committed suicide early or late after admission. Among the 1312 patients, the suicide rate of 257 assaultive alcoholics (having threatened the life of another person) increased 25 times, among the suicidally inclined alcoholics (alcoholics taken in charge by the Temperance Board as dangerous to their lives, or who had tried to commit suicide) the rate increased 21 times, and among the other alcoholics the rate increased 9 times, compared with the general population (Berglund and Tunving 1985). Also, disruption of major personal relationships means increased risk of suicide in alcoholics. Interviews with relatives in the United States showed that almost half of the alcohol abusers who committed suicide had lost their partner or had been in a severe emotional conflict within 6 weeks before the suicide (Murphy and Robins 1967). Thus, there appears to be other important causal factors as well as alcohol consumption for suicide among alcoholics.

The mode of death can also be different in alcohol-involved suicides. One study from the United States found that young suicide victims, with a positive BAC at the time of their death, were almost 5 times more likely to have used firearms than victims with no detectable BAC, while those with a BAC exceeding 0.1 per cent were almost 7.5 times more likely to have used firearms (Brent *et al.* 1987).

There are other, perhaps complementary, perspectives. Menninger (1938) described alcoholism as 'chronic suicide', and Skog (1991), in a similar vein, suggested that suicide is an alternative way of 'solving' problems, and is more common in certain cultures than in others. By this reasoning, social isolation can produce both alcohol abuse and suicide, mainly in people who are poorly integrated from the beginning. Skog (1991) suggests three main mechanisms linking alcohol to suicide: (1) chronic abuse may weaken social integration, (2) weak social integration may increase the risk of both suicide and alcohol abuse, and (3) severe intoxication may produce an anomic state, leading to suicide. Some studies support and others refute this hypothesis.

Alcohol and violence

The association between alcohol consumption and aggression is unclear (Pernanen 1976; Taylor *et al.* 1977; Gustafson 1986*a*,*b*). Experimental research with animals does not provide a clear-cut picture (Chance *et al.* 1973; Yanai and Ginsburg 1977). Different results are obvious in studies of intoxicated behaviour in subcultures. However, most scholars seem to agree that a moderate alcohol intake, with a BAC of at least 0.05 per cent, increases the tendency to aggressive behaviour, provided that the intoxicated person is provoked, for example, by frustration (Gustafson 1986*b*). The results are not homogeneous, the interpretations diverse, and the methodological problems substantial. Neither a simple *disinhibition hypothesis* (suggesting that alcohol causes violence because its psycho-physiological properties releasing violent impulses) nor an *arousal hypothesis* (suggesting that alcohol causes violence by increase in the activity level in the brain) is supported by available studies

(Pernanen 1976; Gustafson 1986*a*). The *attention hypothesis* (suggesting that alcohol causes violence by changes in attention) is supported in several studies with respect to frustration, threat, and social norms (Taylor *et al.* 1976; Gustafson 1986*a*). The central proposition holds that the subjective experience of a salient feature is important. Fewer circumstances and factors in the environment are observed, and if the salient feature is provocative or aggression instigatory this may lead to aggression—aggression inhibitory factors may have the opposite impact. A meta-analysis of 35 studies showed that alcohol can increase social activity, including aggression, especially when the behaviour is influenced by both promoting and inhibitory factors (Steele and Southwick 1985).

There are various limitations in the empirical data: few studies have included females; the alcoholic beverage has usually been strong spirits and the few studies with beer or table wine are not consistent; the outcome generally has been physical aggression, while indirect or verbal aggression was seldom studied; the alcohol dose has generally been rather low in most studies (0.3–1.3 ml pure alcohol/kg).

A high alcohol consumption at a young age carries an increased risk of a violent death, although many people have a peak in consumption when they are young and then consumption is reduced as they grow older (Fillmore 1988). In a 13-year follow-up in a cohort study of 49 464 Swedish military conscripts, the relative risk of violent death increased with reported alcohol consumption at conscription, and was the primary cause of death with 499 cases out of a total of 662 deaths (Andreasson *et al.* 1988) (Fig. 5.3). Similarly, the rate of admissions for accidents increased with the level of self-reported alcohol consumption at conscription.

Alcohol in family violence, marital discord, and child abuse

Most theories on family violence have not included alcohol, but some empirical studies provide information on the relationship between alcohol use and wife-beating. A nation-wide study in the United States with over 2000 couples revealed that the severe violence rate was 2.1 per 100 couples for husbands who were 'never' drunk, but there was an increase in self-reported alcohol consumption during the previous year. For those who were drunk 'very often' the rate of severe violence was 30.8 per 100 couples (Gelles and Straus 1979).

Gerson (1978) analysed police reports on 411 alcohol-related marital assaults. Both persons had been drinking in 43 per cent of cases, while the offender had been drinking in 44 per cent and the victim had been drinking only in 13 per cent. In police reports on 1446 family disputes of which 70 per cent were between the husband and the wife, alcohol or drugs were involved in 46 per cent of all these disputes (Emerson 1979). Fifty-nine per cent of the

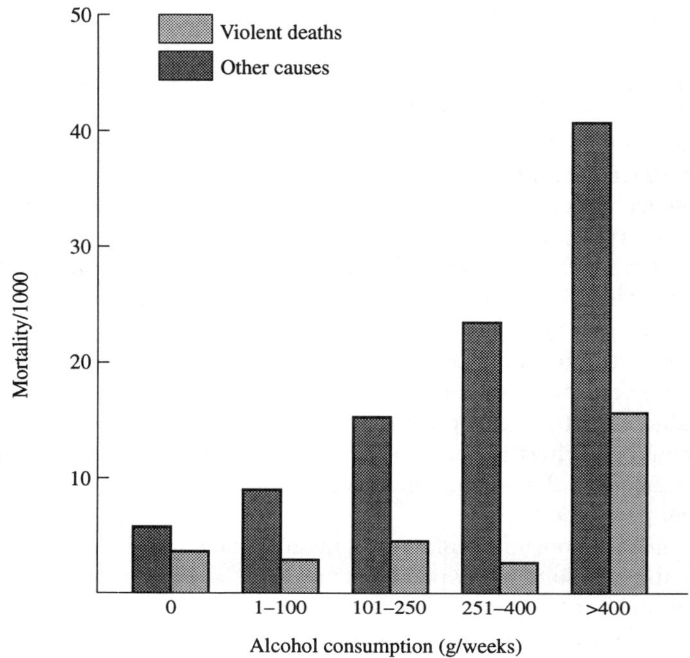

Fig. 5.3 Association between alcohol consumption at conscription, and mortality (violent and other deaths) during follow-up.

Source: Andreasson *et al.* (1988, fig. 1).

disputants under the influence of alcohol were husbands, and 26 per cent were wives. Battered women in clinical facilities report that a very high percentage of the husbands are heavy drinkers, which may partly result from over-reporting. In an interview study of male factory workers, physical conflict with wives were acknowledged by 44 per cent of those who met criteria for alcohol dependence and by 14 per cent of those who did not (Leonard *et al.* 1985). A national US telephone survey of 5000 families showed that the risk of violence increased with alcohol consumption, but also that only 22 per cent of the husbands had been drinking immediately before the event (Kantor and Straus 1987). A combination of alcohol consumption, approval of violence, and blue-collar status was associated with the highest rate of wife-battering.

Some writers assert that there is an association between alcohol use or abuse and child abuse, but not all studies have found this association (Hamilton and Collins 1981). The percentage of alcohol involvement seems to be lower than for wife-beating. Hamilton and Collins (1981) estimated that alcohol was present between 25 to 50 per cent of the cases of wife-beating and in less than 20 per cent in incidents of child abuse.

Homicide and rape

Alcohol is frequently present with perpetrators and victims and considered as a contributory cause in homicide (Pernanen 1976), and was involved in 28–85 per cent of arrested offenders in 11 studies (Roizen 1982). Langevin *et al.* (1982) found that 36 per cent of the murderers had used alcohol or drugs at the time of the offence, compared to 5 per cent among non-violent offenders. Forty per cent of the murderers indicated that they drank too much compared to 15 per cent of non-violent offenders. It can be questioned whether some offenders overstate drunkenness or alcoholism as a means to avoid legal responsibility. In a study of 382 convicted rapists, 81 per cent of those diagnosed as alcoholics and 25 per cent of non-alcoholics at a mental institution had drunk alcohol before the assault (Rada *et al.* 1978). In another study, 33 per cent of 77 rapists had a history of alcoholism, while 27 per cent of 82 rapists in a third study were identified as alcoholics (Rada *et al.* 1978).

Alcohol and working performance and sickness absence

Many studies show that alcohol consumption is associated with increased absenteeism from work (Morawski *et al.* 1991). Jellinek (1947) noted in an early report that a problem drinker lost 24 days per year, on average, because of drinking or alcohol-related diseases. Trice (1962) concluded that 90 per cent of the people in an 'intermediate stage of alcoholism' reported a significant drop in productivity, based on reports from members in Alcoholics Anonymous. In a report from former Yugoslavia, 40 per cent of the registered alcoholics reported a drop of productivity of 25–35 per cent within a year, 3 per cent a complete inability to work due to alcohol, while 21 per cent did not report a productivity decrease (van der Wal 1967; Morawski *et al.* 1991). In Sweden, Kristensen (1982) reported that the total number of sick days, measured retrospectively during 20 years for a group with a high level of the alcohol-related enzyme GGT, was 3.1 times as high as for the group with a GGT-value below the medium. Waern (1977) found that those 12 per cent of men aged 50–60 years who were registered at the Temperance Board in Uppsala, Sweden, for alcohol abuse accounted for 25 per cent of all sick listing and for 45 per cent of all sick listing for psychiatric disorders for men in these ages during a 10-year period. A recent study found that alcohol consumption of over 21 units per week (approximately 210 g of 100 per cent ethanol/week) for male and over 14 units per week (approximately 210 g 100 per cent ethanol/week) for female white-collar workers associated with substantial sickness absence, and lack of promotion in men during a 6-year follow-up (Jenkins *et al.* 1992). Problem drinkers in a large heavy industrial plant in Poland changed work positions within the plant significantly more often than non-problem drinkers (17–12 per cent) (Morawski *et al.* 1991). Many studies have shown that the rates of alcohol problems and mortality in alcohol-related diseases show great differences between different occupational categories (Plant 1977). Brewery workers, seamen, domestic servants, and some other groups have a high level of alcohol problems (Plant 1977). Common explanations of the difference in alcohol-related problems between various occupational categories, generally of *ad hoc* nature, are ready availability of alcohol, social pressure to drink, and separation from ordinary social relationships (Plant 1977; Cooper 1979; Ågren and Romelsjö 1992). Hitz (1973) presented five explanations, Plant (1977) eight, and Whitehead and Simpkins (1976) not less than 39 explanations. Several studies have linked high alcohol consumption to unemployment (Harford 1993).

The inter-generational effects of alcohol problems in families

In a review of 39 studies, Cotton (1979) concluded that male alcoholics were 2.2 times more likely than males in the general population to have an alcoholic father and 1.6 times more likely to have an alcoholic mother. Female alcoholics were 3.3 times more likely to have an alcoholic father and 2.4 times more likely to have an alcoholic mother. Adoption studies have shown that genetic factors can contribute to alcohol abuse, especially in males (Cloninger *et al.* 1981). However, it is not known what percentage of the offspring do well, despite parental heavy drinking or genetic influence.

Studies from Sweden have conveyed interesting information in this difficult area. Nylander (1979) observed 2164 child guidance cases from the age of 9 until they were 29 years old. A total of 123 people (5.7 per cent), of which 99 were males and 24 females, had developed chronic alcohol or drug problems, excluding subjects who had been treated on one or more occasions for their abuse. Ninety-two per cent of the males and 83 per cent of the females showed 'acting-out' behaviour, while 57 and 33 per cent, respectively, showed antisocial behaviour. A large proportion came from homes where parents misused alcohol, were mentally ill, or divorced. Forty-two per cent of the boys and 38 per cent of the girls had fathers who were alcoholics or mentally ill; 29 and 30 per cent, respectively, had mothers who were alcoholics or mentally ill; 61 and 58 per cent, respectively, had parents who were divorced. It was not possible to separate the influence of 'alcoholism' versus 'mental sickness'. This and other studies (McCord *et al.* 1960; Robins 1966) show that anti-social youths often come from homes where parents misuse alcohol or are socially disadvantaged, and that the youths develop alcohol or drug problems to a greater extent than comparison groups. The conclusions must be drawn cautiously, as the study group is highly selected, and the separate influence of alcohol misuse and social and psychological home conditions are difficult to sort out. In another 20-year follow-up register study, sons of treated alcoholics were at increased risk to have been registered due to alcohol and criminal problems, to have needed social service, to have more days of sickness, and to have used more in- and outpatient care, compared with a matched control group (Rydelius 1981). This record was similar, but less pronounced for the daughters. Aggression and signs of neglect in the child correlated best with poor adult adjustment, and these children came from lower social status groups. However, in a third study, Nylander and Rydelius (1982) followed-up the offspring of 40 treated alcoholics from social class I (the highest of three in Sweden) and 50 from the two lower social classes. Social class of origin did not effect the increased level of problems in public records, which was similar to the earlier studies, provided that the father was a 'chronic alcoholic'. One limitation with these studies (Rydelius 1981; Nylander and Rydelius 1982) is that the children were selected because their parents were in treatment, which creates problems in generalizing, as they may have more severe alcohol and/or social problems, or otherwise be different from problem drinkers in general (Velleman 1992*a*,*b*).

Community studies suggest a somewhat different relationship between parental drinking and risk of problems for their children (Velleman 1992*a*,*b*). Vaillant (1983) reported from a 40-year prospective study of working class families in which more than 170 males with one or both parents being alcoholics, were compared with over 230 males without an alcoholic parent. The degree of exposure to alcoholism in childhood was significantly correlated with alcohol use, alcoholism, anti-social behaviour, and death at the 40-year follow-up. Most of this impairment occurred in people who actually developed alcoholism. When these individuals were eliminated from the data analysis, there were no significant differences between the two groups. The interpretation of the result has been challenged by Zucker and Gomberg (1986), who suggest that the importance of social risk factors have been underestimated.

In a recent community study by Velleman and Orford (1990), 170 children (aged 16–35) of problem drinkers and 80 young people in a comparison group were interviewed. They found no group differences in current alcohol use or in illicit drug use, but detrimental effects if both parents had alcohol problems or if one alcohol abusing parent drank at home.

A study of military conscripts in Sweden, where conscription is mandatory, showed that various social factors, including dissatisfaction with the home atmosphere, early maladjustment, and frequent paternal alcohol intake were associated both with high alcohol consumption at conscription and with an increased risk of mortality (Andreasson *et al.* 1988). In those conscripts who did not report high alcohol consumption at conscription, the relative risk of death during a 13-year follow-up increased steeply with a number of social risk factors (Andreasson *et al.* 1991).

Methodological issues in inter-generational studies

The above studies generally show that parental alcohol problems produce an increased risk of alcohol problems in their children, and also a wide variety of emotional and behavioural disorders (poor school performance, learning and reading difficulties, conduct disorder, aggressive behaviour, psychological and emotional problems, and reduction in concentration) (Velleman 1992*a*,*b*). However, a considerable proportion of children seem to do well in spite of poor upbringing conditions. There is also an impact on adulthood adjustment, but studies on community samples and prospective studies of problem-free children suggest that the risk may be exaggerated. There are various possible mechanisms for transmission of alcohol problems from one generation to the next within families. Most researchers seem to favour a *general environmental* mechanism before a *genetic* mechanism or a *specific environmental* mechanism (focusing on what the child learned or failed to learn from parents). The general environmental mechanism stresses that ill-effects are transmitted via disturbed familial relationships or family discord, while parental drinking problems are considered to be of secondary importance (Velleman 1992*a*,*b*). However, alcohol-related parental problems are very likely to be associated with discord—many children will be exposed to both risk factors.

There are many methodological problems in these studies, including: sex bias (most studies concern the relationship between fathers and sons); most studies have not focused on the effects of marital or family disharmony on children, but on effects of parental separation; research has generally not distinguished between father and mother, between a child and each parent independently, and the family group as a whole; different definitions of family disharmony are used; different aspects of family discord have been measured; 'alcoholism' or 'heavy drinking' is defined differently; the offspring is studied at different ages in different studies; and the samples in child guidance studies constitute special groups. Future research must be theory driven and involve an integration of information from many perspectives.

Conclusion

This chapter has covered a variety of consequences of alcohol consumption for the individual—unintentional and intentional trauma, suicide, violence, and various social complications. There is solid empirical support that alcohol consumption is a contributory cause in most kinds of events in these domains. Figures on alcohol involvement in different domains vary with type of injury, sex, culture, environment, and psychological and social factors, but are often high, up to 30–60 per cent of the events. Some of these figures are presented in the introductory section. The cut-off point for increased risk is fairly well known for some of the events, for example, certain accidents, but less well known for others, for example, violence. A minimal deviation in behaviour in a simulated driving test has been estimated at a BAC of 0.02–0.03 mg%, with a clear rise in risk at a BAC of 0.05 mg%. The risk of crashing was estimated to be increased eight times at a BAC of 0.01 mg%. There is substantial evidence that alcoholism and alcohol abuse are linked to a markedly increased risk of suicide. Epidemiological data also show that high alcohol consumption in young men is quite a strong predictor for suicide deaths in the future. Alcohol misuse is associated with violence—several competing or overlapping hypotheses explain this association. A dose-response relationship is well established for most kinds of accidents, while the evidence is lacking or scarce for social complications, violence, and suicide. However, a dose-response relationship was established between self-reported consumption in young men and violent death later in life.

Our chapter confirms that 'alcoholism runs in families'. Alcoholism or alcohol abuse in the family is associated with a definitively increased risk for marital discord, child abuse, and with mental and alcohol problems in the offspring. Many studies from different countries show that alcohol misuse is related to increased absenteeism from work. It is obvious that alcohol is but one of several contributory causes to the reviewed problems. The precise role of alcohol and its often complicated interaction with other factors is difficult to investigate and therefore knowledge is scarce of this complicated process. There are many other, different contributory causes all with different mechanisms. There are several hypotheses and theories which try to explain the interrelationship between alcohol use and other factors in the causation of the problems under review. Often, the methods which are needed to test the various hypotheses abound with severe problems, and there is a real need of methodological development and imagination. Also, a more comprehensive knowledge of the presumptive role of other contributory causes, their possible interaction, confounders, and effect modifiers is necessary for a rational prevention policy.

References

Ågren, G. and Romelsjö, A. (1992). Mortality in alcohol-related diseases in Sweden during 1971–80 in relation to occupation, marital status and citizenship in 1970. *Scandinavian Journal of Social Medicine*, **20**, 134–42.

Andreasson, S., Romelsjö, A., and Allebeck, P. (1988). Alcohol and mortality among young men. Longitudinal study of Swedish conscripts. *British Medical Journal*, **296**, 1021–5.

Andreasson, S., Romelsjö, A., and Allebeck, P. (1991). Alcohol, social factors and mortality among young men. *British Journal of Addiction*, **86**, 877–87.

Bailey, J. P. M. (1984). *The Waikato road accident survey. Analysis and interpretation.* Chemistry Division, Department of Scientific and Industrial Research, Auckland.

Baker, S. P., O'Neill, B., and Karp, R. S. (1984). *The injury fact book*. Lexington and D. C. Heath & Co, Lexington, MA.

Berglund, M. (1984). Suicide in alcoholism. A prospective study of 88 suicides: The multidimensional diagnosis at first admission. *Archives of General Psychiatry*, **41**, 888–91.

Berglund, M. and Tunving, K. (1985). Assaultive alcoholics 20 years later. *Acta Psychiatrica Scandinavia*, **71**, 141–7.

Borkenstein, R. F., Crowther, R. F., Shumate, R. P., Ziel, W. B., and Zylman, R. (1974). The role of the drinking driver in traffic accidents (the Grand Rapids study). *Blutalkohol*, **11**, (suppl. 1), 1–132.

Brent, D. A., Perper, J. A., and Allman, C. J. (1987). Alcohol, firearms, and suicide among youth. *Journal of the American Medical Association*, **257**, 3369–72.

BMJ (*British Medical Journal*) (1979). Drinking and drowning. *British Medical Journal*, **278**, 70–1.

Chance, M. R. A., Mackintosh, J. H., and Doxon, A. K. (1973). The effects of ethyl alcohol on social encounters between mice. *Journal of Alcoholism*, **8**, 90–3.

Cherpitel, C. J. (1988). Alcohol consumption and casualties: a comparison of two emergency room populations, *British Journal of Addiction*, **83**, 1299–1307.

Cherpitel, C. (1989). A study of alcohol use and injuries among emergency room patients. In *Drinking and causalities. Accidents, poisonings and violence in an international perspective*, (eds N. Giesbrecht *et al.*), pp. 288–99. Tavistock/Routledge, London and New York.

Cherpitel, C. J. (1992*a*). Acculturation, alcohol consumption and casualties among US hispanics in the emergency room. *International Journal of Addictions*, **27**, 1067–77.

Cherpitel, C. (1992*b*). Drinking patterns and problems: A comparison of ER patients in an HMO and in the general population. *Alcoholism: Clinical and Experimental Research* **16**, 110–48.

Cherpitel, C. (1993*a*). Alcohol and injuries. A review of international emergency room studies. *Addiction*, **88**, 923–38.

Cherpitel, C. J. (1993*b*). Alcohol consumption among emergency room patients: comparison of county/community hospitals and an HMO. *Journal of Studies on Alcohol*, **54**, 432–40.

Cherpitel, C. J. and Rosovsky, H. (1990). Alcohol consumption and casualties: a comparison of emergency room populations in the United States and in Mexico. *Journal of Studies on Alcohol*, **51**, 319–26.

Cherpitel, C. J., Parès, A., and Rodés, J. (1991). Drinking patterns and populations in the United States and Spain. *Drug and Alcohol Dependence*, **29**, 5–15.

Cloninger, C. R., Bohman, M., and Sigvardsson, S. (1981). Inheritance of alcohol abuse. *Archives of General Psychiatry*, **38**, 861–8.

Cooper, R. (1979). Drinking as conformity. A critique of sociological literature on occupational differences in drinking. *Journal of Studies on Alcohol*, **40**, 868–91.

Copeland, A. R. (1985). Fatal occupational accidents. The five year Metro Dade County experience. *Journal of Forensic Sciences*, **30**, 494–503.

Cotton, N. (1979). The familial incidence of alcoholism: A review. *Journal of Studies on Alcohol*, **40**, 89–116.

Cullberg, J., Wasserman, D., and Stefansson, C. G. (1988). Who commits suicide after a suicide attempt? An 8 to 10 year follow-up in a suburban catchment area. *Acta Psychiatrica Scandinavica*, **77**, 598–603.

Donelson, A. and Beirness, D. (1985). *Impaired drinking. Legislative issues related to drinking and driving*. Traffic Injury Research Foundation of Canada, Ottawa.

Emerson, C. D. (1979). Family violence: A study by the Los Angeles County Sheriff's Department. *The Police Chief*, **46**, 48–50.

Fillmore, K. (1988). *Alcohol use across the life course. A critical review of 70 years of longitudinal research.* Addiction Research Foundation, Toronto.

Gay, T. J., Coates, T. L., Coggins, G. L., Alexander, R. D., and Nayman, J. (1970). Blood alcohol concentrations upon admissions to a hospital based casualty department, *Medical Journal of Australia*, **2**, 778–81.

Gelles, R. and Straus, M. A. (1979). Violence in the American family. *Journal of Social Issues*, **35**, 15–39.

Gerson, L. W. (1978). Alcohol-related acts of violence: Who was drinking and where the acts occurred. *Journal of Studies on Alcohol*, **39**, 1294–6.

Gibb, K., Yee, A., Johnson, C., Martin, S., and Nowak, R. (1984). Accuracy and usefulness of breath alcohol analyzer. *Annals of Emergency Medicine*, **13**, 516–20.

Gjerde, H. and Mörland, J. (1988). A two year prospective study of rearrests for drunken driving. *Scandinavian Journal of Social Medicine*, **16**, 111–13.

Greenfield, L. A. (1988). *Drunk driving* (Special Report, NCJ-109945). US Department of Justice, Bureau of Justice Statistics, Washington, DC.

Gustafson, R. (1986*a*). Alcohol and human physical aggression: The mediating role of frustration. Department of Psychology (thesis), Uppsala.

Gustafson, R. (1986*b*). Threat as a determinant of alcohol-related aggression. *Psychological Reports*, **58**, 287–97.

Hamilton, C. and Collins, J., Jr. (1981). The role of alcohol in wife beating and child: a review of the literature. In *Drinking and crime. Perspectives on the relationships between alcohol consumption and criminal behavior*, (ed. J. Collins Jr.), pp. 253–86. Guilford, New York.

Harford, T. (1993). The measurement of alcohol-related accidents. *Addiction*, **88**, 907–12.

Haworth, A. (1989). Alcohol-related causalities in Africa. In *Drinking and causalities. Accidents, poisonings and violence in an international perspective*, (ed. N. Giesbrecht *et al.*), pp. 83–111. Tavistock/Routledge, London and New York.

Hill, A. B. (1965). The environment and disease: Association or causation? *Proceedings of the Royal Society of Medicine*, **58**, 295–300.

Hingson, R. and Howland, J. (1987). Alcohol as a risk factor for injury or death resulting from accidental falls. A review of the literature. *Journal of Studies on Alcohol*, **48**, 212–19.

Hingson, R. and Howland, J. (1993). Alcohol and non-traffic unintentional death and injuries. *Addiction*, **88**, 877–84.

Hingson, R., Heeren, T., Mangione, T., Morelock, S., and Mucatel, M. (1982). Teenage driving after using marijuana or drinking and traffic accident involvement. *Journal of Safety Research*, **13**, 33–7.

Hitz, D. (1973). Drunken sailors and others. *Quarterly Journal of Studies on Alcohol*, **34**, 496–505.

Honkanen, R. (1976). The effect of time factors on blood alcohol levels in accident victims. *Annales Chirurgiae et Gynaecologiae Fenniae*, **65**, 176–80.

Honkanen, R. (1988). Epidemiological methods in causal accident research. *International Journal of Clinical Psychopharmacology*, **3** (Suppl. 1), 23–33.

Honkanen, R. (1993). Alcohol in home and leisure injuries. *Addiction*, **88**, 939–44.

Honkanen, R. and Ottelin, J. (1976). Blood alcohol levels in injury victims at the emergency station of a rural central hospital. *Annales Chirurgiae et Gynaecologiae*, **65**, 282–6.

Honkanen, R. and Visuri, T. (1976). Blood alcohol levels in a series of injured patients with special reference to accident and type of injury. *Annales Chirurgiae et Gynaecologiae Fenniae*, **65**, 287–94.

Honkanen, R., Ertama, L., Kuosmanen, P., Linnoila, M., Alha, A., and Visuri, T. (1983). The role of alcohol in accidental falls. *Journal of Studies on Alcohol*, **44**, 231–45.

Howland, J. and Hingson, R. (1987). Alcohol as a risk factor for injuries or death due to fires and burns. Review of the literature. *Public Health Reports*, **102**, 475–83.

Howland, J. and Hingson, R. (1988). Alcohol as a risk factor for drownings. A review of the literature (1950–1985). *Accident Analysis and Prevention*, **20**, 19–25.

Howland, J. and Hingson, R. (1990). Alcohol use and aquatic activities in Massachusetts. *Journal of the American Medical Association*, **264**, 9–20.

Hunter, W. W. and Stutts, J. C. (1979). *Mopeds. An analysis of the 1976–1978 North Carolina accidents.* University of Carolina Highway Safety Research Center, Chapel Hill, NC.

Irwin, S. T., Patterson, C. C., and Rutherford, W. H. (1983). Association between alcohol consumption and adult pedestrians who sustain injuries in road traffic accidents. *British Medical Journal*, **286**, 522.

James, J., Dargon, D., and Day, R. (1984). Serum vs breath alcohol levels and accidental injury: analysis among US Army personnel in an emergency room setting. *Military Medicine*, **149**, 369–74.

Jellinek, E. M. (1947). What should we do about alcoholism? *Vital Speeches*, **13**, 252–3.

Jenkins, R., Harvey, S., Butler, T., and Thomas, R. L. (1992). A six year longitudinal study of the occupational consequences of drinking over 'safe limits' of alcohol. *British Journal of Industry Medicine*, **49**, 369–74.

Kantor, G. K. and Straus, M. A. (1987). The 'Drunken Bum' theory of wife beating. *Social Problems*, **34**, 214–30.

Karlsson, G., Romelsjö, A., and Allebeck, P. (1991). Social factors associated with drunken driving and public drunkenness. *36th International Institute on the Prevention and Treatment of Alcoholism*, (Stockholm, Sweden, 2–6 June). (Paper).

Klein, K. E., Breukner, K. L., Brüner, H., and Wegmann, H. M. (1967). Blutalkohol und Fluguntüchtigkeit. Versuch einer Erarbeitung von Richtwerten für die allgemeine Luftfahrt [Blood alcohol and inability to fly (for aviation). Attempts at construction of outlines for general air traffic]. *Internationale Zeitschrift für angewandte Physiologie einschliesslich Arbeitsphysiologie*, **24**, 254–67.

Kobus, H. J. (1980). Breath analysis for control of drunk driving in Zimbabwe, Rhodesia. *Central African Journal of Medicine*, **26**, 21–7.

Kristensen, H. (1982). Studies on alcohol related disabilities in a medical intervention programme in middle-aged males. Thesis, Lund University.

Langevin, R., Paitich, D., and Orchard, B. (1982). The role of alcohol, drugs, suicide attempts, and situational strains in homicide committed by offenders seen for psychiatric assessment: A controlled study. *Acta Psychiatrica Scandinavica*, **66**, 229–42.

Lehman, R. J., Wolfe, A. C., and Kay, R. D. (1975). *A computer archive of ASAP roadside breathtesting surveys, 1970–74* (Technical Report No. DOT HS 801 502). National Highway Traffic Safety Administration, Washington, DC.

Leonard, K. E., Bromet, E., Parkinson, D. K., Day, N. L., and Ryan, C. M. (1985). Patterns of alcohol use and physically aggressive behavior in men. *Journal of Studies on Alcohol*, **46**, 279–82.

Lewis, R. J. and Cooper, S. P. (1989). Alcohol, other drugs and fatal work-related injuries. *Journal of Occupational Medicine*, **31**, 23–7.

Loomis, T. A. and West, T. C. (1958). The influence of alcohol on automobile driving ability. *Quarterly Journal of Studies on Alcohol*, **19**, 30–46.

Luke, L. I. and Levy, M. E. (1982). Exposure-related hypothermia deaths—District of Columbia 1972–1982. *Morbidity and Mortality Weekly Reports*, **31**, 669–71.

Mayhew, D. R. (1982). Age, alcohol and fatal risk. Paper presented at the *19th Annual Meeting of the Traffic Injury Research Foundation of Canada*, pp. 1–21. 27 May 1992. Ottawa, Ontario.

Mayhew, D. R. (1983). Age, alcohol and risk of accident involvement. Paper presented at the *9th International Conference on Alcohol, Drugs and Traffic Safety*. 13–18 November 1983. San Juan, Puerto Rico.

Maxwell, M. A. (1959). A study of abseenteism, accidents and sickness payments in problem drinkers in one industry. *Quarterly Journal of Studies on Alcohol*, **20**, 303–12.

McCord, W., McCord, J., and Gudeman, J. (1960). *The origins of alcoholism*. Stanford University Press, New York.

Medina-Mora, M. and Gonzáles, L. (1989). Alcohol-related causalities in Latin America: A review of the literature. In *Drinking and causalities. Accidents, poisonings and violence in an international perspective* (ed. N. Giesbrecht, *et al.*), pp. 67–82. Tavistock/Routledge, London and New York.

Melinder, K. (1988). *Alkohol och olycksfall*, [*Alcohol and accidents*], Socialstyrelsen, Stockholm.

Menninger, K. A. (1938). *Man against himself*. Harcourt Brace, New York.

Miettinen, O. (1985). *Theoretical epidemiology. Principles of occurrence research in medicine*. Wiley, New York.

Morawski, J., Moskalewicz, J., and Wald, I. (1991). Economic costs of alcohol abuse, with special emphasis on productivity. In *The negative social consequences of alcohol use*, pp. 95–128. Norwegian Ministry of Health and Social Affairs in collaboration with the UN Office at Vienna Centre for Social Development and Humanitarian Affairs, Oslo.

Murphy, G. E. and Robins, E. (1967). Social factors in suicide. *Journal of the American Medical Association*, **199**, 303–8.

Murphy, G. and Wetzel, R. (1990). The lifetime risk of suicide in alcoholism. *Archives of General Psychiatry*, **47**, 383–92.

NHTSA (National Highway Traffic Safety Administration) (1988). *Alcohol involvement in fatal crashes 1986* (Report No. DOT HS 807 268). National Highway Traffic Safety Administration, Washington, DC.

NHTSA (National Highway Traffic Safety Administration) (1991). *Fatal accident reporting system 1990: A review of information on fatal traffic crashes in the United States in 1990* (Report No. DOT HS 807 794). National Highway Traffic Safety Administration, Washington, DC.

Norton, R. (1989). Alcohol-related causality statistics in Australia. (1989). In *Drinking and causalities. Accidents, poisonings and violence in an international perspective*, (ed. N. Giesbrecht *et al.*), pp. 197–214. Tavistock/Routledge, London and New York.

Nylander, I. (1979). A 20-year prospective follow-up study of 2164 cases at the child guidance clinics in Stockholm. *Acta Paediatrica Scandinavica*, (Suppl. 276).

Nylander, I. and Rydelius, P. A. (1982). Comparison between children of alcoholic fathers from excellent versus poor social conditions. *Acta Paediatriatica Scandinavica*, **71**, 809–13.

Olkkonen, S. and Honkanen, R. (1990). The role of alcohol in nonfatal bicycle injuries. *Accident Analysis and Prevention*, **22**, 89–96.

Papoz, L., Weill, J., Gate, C., L'Hoste, J., Chick, J., and Goehrs, Y. (1986). Biological markers of alcohol intake among 4796 subjects injured in accidents. *British Medical Journal*, **292**, 1234–7.

Penttilä, A., Piipponen, S., and Pikkarainen, J. (1979). Drunken driving with motorboats in Finland. *Accident Analysis and Prevention*, **11**, 237–9.

Peppiatt, R., Evans, R., and Jordan, P. (1978). Blood alcohol concentrations of patients attending an accident and emergency department. *Resuscitation*, **6**, 37–43.

Pernanen, K. (1976). Alcohol and crimes of violence. In *The biology of alcoholism: Social aspects of alcoholism*, (ed. B Kissin and H. Begleiter), Vol. 4, pp. 351–444. Plenum, New York.

Pernanen, K. (1989). Causal inferences about the role of alcohol in accidents, poisonings and violence. In *Drinking and causalities. Accidents, poisonings and violence in an international perspective*, (ed. N. Giesbrecht *et al.*), pp. 158–71. Tavistock/Routledge, London and New York.

Perrine, M. W., Waller, J. A., and Harris, S. (1971). *Alcohol and Highway Safety: Behavioral and Medical Aspects*. National Highway Traffic Safety Administration, Washington, DC.

Plant, M. (1977). Alcoholism and occupation: a review. *British Journal of Addiction*, **72**, 309–16.

Rada, R. T., Kellner, R., Laws, D. R., and Winslow, W. W. (1978). Drinking, alcoholism and the mentally disordered sex offender. *Bulletin of the American Academy of Psychiatry and the Law*, **6**, 296–300.

Redmond, A. D., Richards, S., and Plumhett, P. K. (1987). The significance of random breath alcohol sampling in the accident and emergency department. *Alcohol and Alcoholism*, **22**, 341–3.

Robins, L. (1966). *Deviant children grown up*. Williams and Wilkens, Baltimore.

Roizen, J. (1982). Estimating alcohol involvement in serious events. In *Alcohol consumption and related problems* (Alcohol and Health Monograph No. 1), pp. 179–219. National Institute on Alcohol Abuse and Alcoholism, Washington, DC.

Roizen, J. (1989). Alcohol and trauma. In *Drinking and causalities. Accidents, poisonings and violence in an international perspective*, (ed. N. Giesbrecht *et al.*), pp. 158–71. Tavistock/Routledge, London and New York.

Rosovsky, H. and Garcia, G. (1988). *Alcohol-related casualties in Mexico: a comparison between two populations*. Presented at the *Kettil Bruun Society for Social and Epidemiological Studies in Alcohol*, Berkeley, California, USA.

Rosovsky, H. and Lopez, J. L. (1986). Accidentes y violencias relacionidas con el consumo de alcohol revista [Review of accidents and violence resulting from the consumption of alcohol]. *Salud Mental*, **9**, 72–6.

Ross, H. L. (1982). *Deterring the driving drinker. Legal policy and social control*. Lexington Books, Lexington, MA.

Rothman, K. (1986). *Modern epidemiology*. Little, Brown and Company, Boston and Toronto.

Rothman, K. (ed.) (1987). *Causal inference*. Epidemiology Resources, Boston.

Ryan, L. and Mohler, S. (1979). Current role of alcohol as a factor in civil aircraft accidents. *Aviation and Space Environment Medicine*, **50**, 275–9.

Rydelius, P. (1981). Children of alcoholic fathers: Their social adjustment and their health status over 20 years. *Acta Paediatriatica Scandinavica*, (Suppl. 286).

Shain, M. and Groenveld, J. (1980). *Employee assistance programs. Philosophy theory and practice*. D. C. Heath, Lexington, MA.

Sinha, S. N., Sengupta, S. K., and Purohit, R. (1981). A five year review of deaths following trauma. *Papua New Guinea Medical Journal*, **24**, 222–8.

Skog, O. J. (1991). Alcohol and suicide—Durkheim revisited. *Acta Sociologica*, **34**, 193–206.

Smith, G. S. and Kraus, J. F. (1988). Alcohol and residential, recreational and occupational injuries: A review of the epidemiologic evidence. *Annual Review of Public Health*, **9**, 99–121.

Söderstrom, C. A. and Cowley, R. A. (1987). A national alcohol and trauma center survey. *Archives of Surgery*, **122**, 1067–71.

Stallones, L. and Kraus, J. (1993). The occurrence and epidemiologic features of alcohol-related occupational injuries. *Addiction*, **88**, 945–52.

Steele, C. M. and Southwick, L. (1985). Alcohol and social behaviour. *Journal of Personality and Social Psychology*, **48**, 18–34.

Susser, M. (1991). What is a cause and how do we know one? A grammar for pragmatic epidemiology. *American Journal of Epidemiology*, **133**, 635–47.

Taylor, S. P., Gammon, C. B., and Capasso, D. R. (1976). Aggression as a function of alcohol and threat. *Journal of Personality and Social Psychology*, **34**, 938–41.

Taylor, S. P., Schmutte, G. T., and Leonard, K. E. (1977). Physical aggression as a function of alcohol and frustration. *Bulletin of the Psychonomic Society*, **9**, 217–18.

Trice, H. M. (1962). The job behavior of problem drinkers. In *Society, culture and drinking pattern*, (ed. D. J. Pittman and S. Snyder). Wiley and Son, New York.

Urschel, J. D. (1990). Frostbite: predisposing factors and predictors of poor outcome. *Trauma*, **30**, 340–42.

USDHHS (US Department of Health and Human Services) (1990). *Alcohol and health*. National Institute on Alcohol Abuse and Alcoholism, Rockville, MD.

Vaillant, G. (1983). *The natural history of alcoholism*. Harvard University Press, Cambridge, MA.

van der Wal, H. J. (1967). Work absenteeism and alcohol consumption. *Alcoholism* (Zagreb), **III**, 95–103.

Velleman, R. (1992*a*). A review of environmentally oriented studies concerning the relationship between parental alcohol problems and family disharmony in the genesis of alcohol and other problems. I. The intergenerational effects of alcohol problems. *International Journal of Addictions*, **27**, 253–80.

Velleman, R. (1992*b*). A review of environmentally oriented studies concerning the relationship between parental alcohol problems and family disharmony in the genesis of alcohol and other problems. II. The intergenerational effects of family problems. *International Journal of Addictions*, **27**, 367–89.

Velleman, R. and Orford, J. (1990). Young adult offspring of parents with drinking problems: Recollections of parents' drinking and its immediate effects. *British Journal of Clinical Psychology*, **29**, 297–317.

Virkunnen, M. (1974). Alcohol as a factor precipating to aggression and conflict behaviour leading to homicide. *British Journal of Addiction*, **69**, 149–54.

Voas, R. (1993). Cross-national comparisons of crash data. *Addiction*, **88**, 959–67.

Vogt, I. (1989). Federal Republic of Germany. In *Alcohol-related problems in high-risk groups*, (ed. M.A. Plant), pp. 64–80. WHO, Regional Office for Europe, Copenhagen.

Waern, U. (1977). Findings at a health survey of 60-year old men and recorded disease during their proceeding 10 years of life. Acta Universitatis Upsaliensis (thesis), Uppsala.

Waller, J. and Lamborn, K. (1975). Snowmobiling. Characteristics of owners, patterns of use and injuries. *Accident Analysis and Prevention*, **7**, 213–23.

Waller, J. A. (1976). Alcohol and unintentional injury. In *The biology of alcoholism. Social aspects of alcoholism*, (ed. B. Kissin and H. Begleiter), pp. 307–49. Plenum, New York.

Waller, J. A. (1968). Patterns of traffic accidents and violations related to drinking and to socio-medical conditions. *Quarterly Journal of Studies on Alcohol*, **29** (Suppl. 4), 118–37.

Walsh, M. E. and Macleod, D. (1983). Breath alcohol analysis in the accident and emergency department, *Injury*, **15**, 62–6.

Wechsler, H., Kasey, E., Thum, D., and Demone, H. W. (1969). Alcohol level and home accidents. *Public Health Reports*, **84**, 1043–50.

Welte, J. W., Abel, E. L., and Wieczorek, W. (1988). The role of alcohol in suicides in Erie County, NY, 1972–84. *Public Health Reports*, **103**, 648–52.

Whitehead, P. and Simpkins, J. (1976). Occupational factors in alcoholism. In *The biology of alcoholism: The pathogenesis of alcoholism*, (ed. B. Kissin and H. Begleiter), Vol. 6, pp. 405–96. Plenum, New York.

Williams, G. D., Grant, B., Stinson, F. S., Zobeck, T., Aitken, S., and Noble, J. (1988). Trends in alcohol related morbidity and mortality. *Public Health Reports*, **103**, 592–7.

Wright, S. I. (1985). SOS, alcohol, drugs, and boating. *Alcohol Health and Research World*, **9**, 28–33.

Yanai, J. and Ginsburg, B. E. (1977). Long term reduction of male agonistic behaviour in mice following early exposure to ethanol. *Psychopharmacology*, **52**, 31–4.

Yates, D., Hafield, J., and Peters, K. (1987). The detection of problem drinkers in the accident and emergency department. *British Journal of Addiction*, **82**, 163–7.

Zador, P. (1991). Alcohol-related relative risk of fatal drivers injuries in relation to driver age and sex. *Journal of Studies on Alcohol*, **52**, 302–10.

Zucker, R. and Gomberg, L. (1986). Etiology of alcoholism reconsidered: The case for a biopsychosocial process. *American Psychologist*, **41**, 783–93.

Part II

Strategies with potential to reduce harm

6. Do alcohol prices affect consumption and related problems?

Esa Österberg

Introduction

In many countries, public emphasis regarding responses to the alcohol question has come to be laid more and more on education, information, and treatment, in recent decades. In addition, market forces and economic considerations have increasingly overshadowed preventive policies, and in some countries a strengthening of liberal attitudes has led to a stress on individual responsibility and a denial of the justification of any control measure. Accordingly, limiting the physical availability of alcoholic beverages or imposing high taxation as a means to control consumption and related harmful effects, are nowadays regarded by an increasing number of people as an archaic patchwork of laws and as irrelevant to contemporary life.

The real price of alcoholic beverages has decreased in many countries during the last decades at the same time as many other alcohol control measures have been liberalized or abandoned completely. The fact that the pricing instrument has not been used actively as an alcohol control measure does not, however, by any means prove that an increase in alcohol prices would not be an effective measure to curb alcohol consumption and alcohol-related problems. Indeed, it is of some importance to re-investigate the empirical evidence on the effects of changing alcohol prices on alcohol consumption and related problems.

This chapter begins by considering the relationship between the price and the consumption of alcoholic beverages, and different lines of research, mainly econometric studies, will be discussed. In addition, the cross-elasticities between different types of alcoholic beverages are discussed and studies based on individual data are reviewed. This chapter will also investigate those studies which try to explore the relationship between alcohol prices and different kinds of alcohol-related problems. Alcohol taxation is also discussed.

Econometric models

The effect of changing prices of alcoholic beverages on alcohol consumption has been more extensively investigated than any other potential alcohol control measure, and the most common way to study these effects has been to rely on econometric methods. For example, according to different reviews, there are currently econometric studies dealing with all alcoholic beverages or a certain category of these available in at least the following countries: Australia, Belgium, Canada, Denmark, Germany, Finland, France, Ireland, Italy, Kenya, the Netherlands, New Zealand, Norway, Poland, Portugal, Spain, Sweden, the United Kingdom, and the United States (see Huitfeldt and Jorner 1972; Lau 1975; Bruun *et al.* 1975; Ornstein 1980; Ornstein and Levy 1983; Godfrey 1986; Olsson 1991; Clements and Selvanathan 1991; Yen 1994). This list of countries also shows that our knowledge of the effects of changing alcohol prices on alcohol consumption chiefly derives from Western industrialized nations.

In econometric studies, the responsiveness or sensitivity of quantity demanded to the determinants of demand is measured by elasticity. The sensitivity of the quantity demanded to changes in prices, when other determinants of the demand remain unchanged, is called the price-elasticity of demand, or own-price elasticity. In a similar manner we may speak about income-elasticity, that is, the response of the quantity demanded to changes in consumer income, or elasticities for changing the number of liquor stores or restaurants, or for changes in advertising expenditure.

The values of price-elasticities for alcoholic beverages estimated in different studies have consistently shown that when other factors remain unchanged, a rise in the price of alcohol has generally led to a drop in consumption, and that a decrease in price has usually led to a rise in consumption. In the same manner, income-elasticities estimated in different studies have shown that when other factors remain unchanged, a rise in consumer disposable income has generally led to a rise in alcohol consumption and a decrease in income has generally led to a decrease in alcohol consumption. In other words, alcoholic beverages appear to behave on the market like most other commodities and in the way presupposed by the theory of consumer demand. On the other hand, in studies dealing with different geographical regions and periods, different values of income- and price-elasticities have been found with respect to both total alcohol consumption and the consumption of different types of alcoholic beverages. These variations are partly due to the methods applied, the accuracy of the basic data, and the statistical factors of uncertainty relating to the elasticities. However, disparities in elasticity values also stem from differing social, cultural, and economic circumstances prevailing in different regions and in different periods. Therefore, when looking at the results of different studies, it is not very sensible to seek for any general, typical, or mean elasticity value for all alcoholic beverages, or even for beer, wines or spirits separately, because elasticities describing the reactions of the consumers to price increases are not inherent attributes of alcoholic beverages, but rather reflections of the prevailing drinking habits and culture.

On a very general level, we may say that consumer preferences are linked to the benefits consumers derive from using different commodities, in our case, drinking alcoholic beverages, and consumer preferences are therefore indicated by elasticity values; or to put it another way, consumer preferences are reflected in elasticity values. When taking into account the many different uses of alcoholic beverages—they can be used as an intoxicant, a thirst quencher, a drink with meals, medicine, or as means of recreation and enjoyment—it is not surprising that the demand for alcoholic beverages or a certain category of these may respond very differently to a certain change in price in different countries and in different periods. The interpretation of elasticity values—and changes in elasticity values—therefore calls for a close examination of drinking habits and the uses alcoholic beverages are put in a certain society at a certain point of time.

Effects of price changes on consumption

The values of price elasticities given in Table 6.1 all have an absolute value greater than zero and they are all negative, indicating that changes in prices affect consumption and that the effects of price changes are in the direction consistent with economic theory, that is, if prices go up consumption goes down, and if prices go down consumption goes up. However, the values of price elasticities for different beverages are not the same, indicating that the effects of price changes were quite different in different countries.

If the demand for a given category of alcoholic beverages is price-elastic, that is, relatively sensitive to price changes, a rise in price will have a strong diminishing effect on consumption, and decreases the share of personal disposable income allocated to that beverage. Consequently, a decline in price will have a strong increasing effect on consumption, and raise the share of personal disposable income allocated to that beverage. According to Table 6.1, this was the case with spirits in Canada in 1949–69, wine in Norway in 1960–74, and with strong beer in Sweden in 1956–68.

Alcoholic beverages can also be price-inelastic, that is, relatively insensitive to price changes. In this case, a price increase would have only a small impact on alcohol consumption, and increase the share of personal disposable income allocated to alcohol. A decline in price will have a relative slight positive effect on consumption and decrease the share of personal disposable income allocated to that beverage. According to Table 6.1, this was the case with wine in France in 1954–71, with beer in Ireland in 1953–67, and with spirits in Australia in 1956–77.

Table 6.1 Values of price-elasticities for beer, wine, and distilled spirits in different econometric studies

Country	Period	Beer	Wine	Distilled spirits	Source
UK	1870–1938	−0.66	NA	−0.57	Prest (1949)
UK	1920–48	−0.69	−1.17	−0.57	Stone (1951)
Finland	1949–62	−0.49	−0.83	−0.13[b] −0.95[c]	Nyberg (1967)
Ireland	1953–67	−0.17	NA	−0.64	B. Walsh and D. Walsh (1970)
Sweden	1956–68	−3.0[a]	−0.7	−1.2	Huitfeldt and Jorner (1972)
Canada	1949–69	−0.03	−1.65	−1.45	Lau (1975)
France	1954–71	NA	−0.06	NA	Labys (1976)
Norway	1960–74	NA	−1.5	−1.2	Horverak (1979)
Australia	1956–77	−0.11	−0.40	−0.53	Clements and Johnson (1983)
Finland	1969–86	−0.6	−1.3	−1.0	Salo (1990)
New Zealand	1983–91	−1.1	−1.1	−0.5	Wette *et al.* (1993)

[a] Strong beer. [b] Vodka. [c] Other distilled spirits. NA, figures not available.

If the demand for alcoholic beverages is unit price-elastic, a rise in price will have a diminishing effect on consumption of equal proportion and keep the share of personal disposable income allocated to alcohol about equal. Consequently, lower prices will increase consumption and keep the share of personal disposable income allocated to that beverage equal. According to Table 6.1, this was what almost happened with distilled spirits in Finland in 1969–86, and with wine in the United Kingdom in 1920–48 as well as with beer in New Zealand in 1983–91.

As Table 6.1 indicates, there are great differences between countries in the way the consumers have reacted to price changes. This is something we expected because of the differences in drinking habits between countries. But to make it more difficult, even the results of econometric studies dealing with one and the same country do not present a very clear picture. For instance, in his review of price-elasticities, Ornstein (1980) wanted to see whether the weight of the evidence indicates that beer, wine, and spirits are price-elastic, -inelastic, or unit-elastic, and whether they are substitutes, complements, or unrelated in consumption. He also discussed the possibility of identifying a range of 'true' elasticities for the United States (and Canada) by a comparison of diverse studies which according to him 'is clearly risky if not outright erroneous' (Ornstein 1980, p. 810).

For beer, the studied price-elasticities in the United States range from an estimate of approximately zero by I. Horowitz and A. Horowitz in the 1950s to Comanor and Wilson's long-term estimate of −1.39 (Table 6.2). As these two studies show serious econometric problems, they are dismissed by Ornstein (see also Ornstein and Levy 1983). The remaining estimates available ranged from

Table 6.2 Values of price-elasticities for beer, wine, and distilled spirits in the United States and Canada

Country	Period	Beer	Wine	Distilled spirits	Source
USA	1934–60	−0.50 −0.33	−1.59 −0.35	−2.03 −0.93	Niskanen (1962)
USA	1949–61	0.00	NA	NA	I. Horowitz and A. Horowitz (1965)
USA	1956–9	−0.89	NA	NA	Hogarty and Elzinga (1972)
USA	1955–61	NA	NA	−0.79	Simon (1966)
USA	1947–64	−0.56[a] −1.39[b]	−0.68[a] −0.84[b]	−0.25[a] −0.30[b]	Comanor and Wilson (1974)
USA	1946–70	−0.87	NA	NA	Norman (1975)
Canada	1949–69	−0.03	−1.65	−1.45	Lau (1975)
Canada	1955–71	−0.22[a] −0.38[b]	−0.50[a] −1.30[b]	−0.91[a] −1.60[b]	Johnson and Oksanen (1974)
Canada	1955–71	−0.27[a] −0.33[b]	−0.67[a] −1.78[b]	−1.14[a] −1.77[b]	Johnson and Oksanen (1977)
USA	1954–71	NA	−0.44[c] −1.65[d]	NA	Labys (1976)
USA	1960	NA	NA	0.08	Wales (1968)
USA	1970	NA	NA	−1.95	Smith (1976)
California, USA	1953–75	NA	NA	0.02	Lidman (1976)
USA	1970–5	NA	NA	−1.06	Barsby and Marshall (1977)
USA	1949–82	−0.09	−0.22	−0.10	Clements and Selvanathan (1987)
USA	1945–82	−0.11	−0.05	−0.11	Selvanathan (1991)
Canada	1953–82	−0.28	−0.58	−0.30	Quek (1988)
Canada	1956–83	−0.26 to −0.31[a] −0.14[b]	−0.70 to −0.88[a] −1.17[b]	−0.45 to −0.82[a] NA	Johnson *et al.* (1992)

[a] Short term. [b] Long term. [c] Domestic. [d] Imported. NA, figures not available.

−0.33 to −0.89. Comparing the US results with those of Canada and other countries, Ornstein suggests that beer price-elasticity in the United States is about −0.3 to −0.4 (Ornstein 1980, p. 811).

The price-elasticities for distilled spirits in the United States range from 0.08 to −2.03 (Table 6.2). According to Ornstein, none of the studies (done before 1980) finding low elasticity values are econometrically convincing (see also Ornstein and Levy 1983). Therefore, the data suggest a price-elasticity for distilled spirits between −1.0 and −2.0 for the United States (Ornstein 1980, p. 815).

The US estimates of wine price-elasticities available ranged from −0.44 to −1.78 (Table 6.2). According to Ornstein, no consensus on wine price-elasticity is possible. However, in a later review, Ornstein and Levy (1983), using the same data as Ornstein (1980), make a reconsideration of the range of price-elasticity

Table 6.3 Values of price-elasticities for beer, wine, and distilled spirits in the United Kingdom

Period	Beer	Wine	Distilled spirits	Source
1920–38	−0.25	−0.99	−0.51	Wong (1988)
1955–75	−0.19	−0.23	−0.29	Clements and Selvanathan (1987)
1955–75	−0.13	−0.28	−0.47	Walsh (1982)
1956–79	−0.30	−0.17	−0.38	McGuinness (1983)
1963–78	NA	−1.00	−0.77	Duffy (1983)
1956–80	NA	−0.76 to −1.14	−0.56 to −0.99	Godfrey (1988, 1989, 1990)
	−0.50	−1.3[a] −1.6[b] −0.5[c]	−1.30	Treasury
1963–83	−0.29	−0.77	−0.51	Duffy (1987)
1963–83	−0.09	−0.75	−0.86	Duffy (1991)
1967–83	−0.27	−0.77	−0.95	Jones (1989)
	−0.40	−0.94	−0.79	
1955–85	−0.13	−0.37	−0.32	Selvanathan (1988)
1955–85	−0.13	−0.40	−0.31	Selvanathan (1991)
1970–86	−0.88	−1.37	−0.94	Baker and McKay (1990)

[a] Light wine. [b] Other wine. [c] Cider. NA figures not available.

estimates in the United States. After a detailed description, comparison, evaluation, and discussion of 20 studies, they report that their 'summary estimates of own-price elasticities for beer, wine, and distilled spirits were −0.3, −1.0 and −1.5, respectively. These are crude at best, particularly for wines, but seem the best available' (Ornstein and Levy 1983, p. 343).

In her review of demand models, Godfrey (1986) puts more weight on the underlying demand theory and the methodology employed in econometric studies than on presenting results of many empirical studies (see also Maynard 1983; Godfrey and Maynard 1988). In her reviews from 1989 and 1990, Godfrey discusses three alcohol demand studies in the United Kingdom as well as her own estimates and the estimated elasticities used by the Treasury in revenue calculations (Godfrey 1989, 1990). These figures, which are presented in Table 6.3, show that the demand for beer has generally been price-inelastic, that is, a rise in beer prices results in a less than proportionate fall in beer consumption and a decrease in prices results in a less than proportionate increase in consumption. On the other hand, demand for wines and spirits has been found to be more price-responsive than beer (Godfrey 1989). Later studies accord this interpretation (see Table 6.3).

Partanen (1991) has estimated price- and income-elasticities for beer in Kenya for the 1963–85 period. His first crude estimates had negative signs and they were quite large; the value of price-elasticity was −1.5. Partanen, however,

Table 6.4 Values of price-elasticities of beer, wine, and spirits in Sweden

Period	Beer	Wine	Distilled spirits	Source
1923–39	NA	−0.9	−0.3	Malmqvist (1948)
1920–51	−1.2	−1.6	−0.5	Bryding and Rosén (1969)
1931–54	NA	−1.6	−0.3	Sundström and Ekström (1962)
1956–68	−3.0[a]	−0.7	−1.2	Huitfeldt and Jorner (1972)
1970–88	−1.3	−0.9	−0.9	Assarsson (1991)

[a] Strong beer.

deemed the simple model unsatisfactory. In a more sophisticated model, he then estimated both short- and long-term price- and income-elasticities, the short-term price-elasticity estimate for beer (−0.3) being one-third of the corresponding long-term estimate (−1.0). This suggests that Kenyan beer drinkers are not, in the short-term, very sensitive to price increases. Sooner or later, however, they must face economic realities and the growth of the beer market is effectively constrained by price development (Partanen 1991).

According to Partanen, a comparison of the Kenyan results, with the elasticities found in Europe and North America, is hardly justified in view of the differences in variables and model specifications. However, the general observation is that, on the whole, the price-elasticity for beer in Kenya is greater than the elasticities obtained for beer in North America and Europe. There is no special reason to doubt that this indicates a real difference in the social position of beer (Partanen 1991).

Changes in price-elasticity values

Malmqvist (1948), studying the price-elasticities for distilled spirits and wine in Sweden, argued that alcohol control measures other than prices affect the values of price-elasticities. This argument seems to be reasonable, since lifting of other alcohol control measures gives alcohol prices more regulative power. As Table 6.4 shows, lifting the '*motbok*' connected with the Bratt rationing system (where the possibility to buy distilled spirits in Sweden was individually regulated until 1955) in fact led to a rise in the value of the price-elasticity for distilled spirits. It can, therefore, be argued that the more restricted the availability of alcohol—apart from prices and other factors affecting alcohol consumption being the same—the smaller is the influence of changing prices on consumption (Huitfeldt and Jorner 1972).

In Table 6.5, a set of price-elasticities is presented for Finland for the period 1955–80. The decrease in the value of price-elasticities is interpreted to show that alcoholic beverages have come to be seen more and more as an everyday

Table 6.5 Values of price-elasticities for total alcohol consumption in Finland; 1955–80

Period	Price-elasticity
1955–6	−0.93
1957–8	−0.95
1959–60	−0.92
1961–2	−0.89
1963–4	−0.86
1965–6	−0.82
1967–8	−0.79
1969–70	−0.75
1971–2	−0.72
1973–4	−0.69
1975–6	−0.68
1977–8	−0.67
1979–80	−0.70

Source: Ahtola *et al.* (1986).

commodity; in the mid-1950s, the total alcohol consumption per capita was under 2 litres in terms of 100 per cent alcohol, while in the beginning of the 1980s it was over 6 litres. These figures could also be interpreted to show that the value of price-elasticity has a tendency to decrease as incomes and the standard of living are rising.

Econometric studies use as their material factual changes in alcohol prices which are normally relatively small. It can, therefore, be asked if they have any predicting value in cases where changes in alcohol prices are dramatic. An unusual example of the effects of radical price changes on consumption comes from Denmark. Due to food shortage during World War I, the price of Danish *akvavit* was raised more than 10 times and the price of beer was almost doubled. These drastic price increases reduced per capita consumption of alcohol by 75 per cent within two years. The decrease was mostly due to the diminished consumption of *akvavit* and only later did the consumption of beer increase to change Denmark from a spirit-drinking country to a beer-drinking country. Not only was the total alcohol consumption affected, but also the rate of registered cases of delirium tremens declined to one-thirteenth, and deaths due to chronic alcoholism to one-sixth of their previous rates (Bruun *et al.* 1975).

Other examples of great price changes are not as dramatic as the Danish one. They have, however, taken place more recently. For instance, a 10 per cent increase in real alcohol prices in Finland in 1975 put an end to the increase in alcohol consumption that had continued in the country since the early 1960s (Salo 1987). In Sweden, the marked increase in consumption which followed the abolition of the Bratt system in 1955 was halted and eventually reversed by radical increases in prices. In 1957 and 1958, for instance, the real price of distilled spirits went up by more than 30 per cent. This contributed to a decline in spirits consumption from 0.8 litres per capita per month in 1956 to 0.6 litres in 1958, that is, a decrease of one-quarter (Huitfeldt and Jorner 1972).

The value of price-elasticity denotes the way consumers have reacted to changes in prices during the study period. If alcohol prices have, for instance, fallen steadily during that period, the estimated price-elasticity may not necessarily apply to a situation of increasing alcohol prices because the assumption that elasticities are symmetrical may not be valid as far as alcoholic drinks are concerned. A symmetrical elasticity would mean that a given rise or fall in alcohol prices produces an equivalent effect in the opposite direction on consumption. However, since some people may become addicted to alcohol, it is quite possible that a rise in alcohol consumption introduced by a cut in prices would not be checked by an equivalent increase in alcohol prices (Bruun *et al.* 1975). At the moment we do not, however, have any empirical evidence to support this hypothesis.

In the long term, elasticity values may change markedly along with changes in social, cultural, and economic conditions. It has already been pointed out that this may apply to changes in alcohol control policy and changes in the standard of living. In this context the extent to which social change creates new opportunities for using alcohol and the extent to which the suppliers of alcohol strive to create new markets for their products are also important considerations (Bruun *et al.* 1975).

Cross-elasticities

In econometric analyses of demand, the estimation of cross-elasticities—that is, of the change in demand for one type of alcoholic beverage caused by a change in the price of some other type of alcoholic beverage—has proved to be an extremely difficult task. Although the price changes in the cases studied in the Nordic countries have mostly been within a modest range, they, nevertheless, seem to result in the substitution of one type of beverage for another (Nyberg 1967; Huitfeldt and Jorner 1972).

When discussing cross-price elasticities in North America, Ornstein (1980) regards the studies by Johnson and Oksanen (1974) and Niskanen (1962) as being the most comprehensive. The results, however, show that elasticities are inconsistent both within and across the two studies: 'For example, Johnson and Oksanen found that beer was a substitute for wine, but wine was not a substitute for beer. . . . Johnson and Oksanen found that beer and spirits are complements, whereas Niskanen found that they are substitutes' (Ornstein 1980, pp. 815–16). Niskanen's own conclusion was that consumption of each beverage class is significantly related to its own-price and little affected by changes in the price of substitute alcoholic beverages (Niskanen 1962).

In the survey by Ornstein and Levy (1983), no summary estimates are given for cross-price elasticities. According to Godfrey (1989, p. 9), 'estimates of demand models based upon time series data have in general been unsuccessful in identifying the cross-substitution effects with accuracy, even for the case of close substitutes', and, for instance, 'Duffy's analysis of U.K. annual data from 1963 to 1983 found all cross-price elasticities to be very small and insignificant, (p. 16).

The cross-elasticities estimated in econometric studies may also be of little use in actual alcohol policy-making. The estimated elasticities are derived from aggregate data using average price rates. However, it has been observed in many studies that heavy consumers usually prefer the cheaper beverages in each type of alcoholic beverage. Under such circumstances, the substitution between different types of alcoholic beverage is perhaps not so much determined by changes in the average price of each type as by changes in prices of the cheapest brands in each type (Bruun *et al.* 1975).

Alcoholic beverages, because they all include ethyl alcohol, are potential substitutes for each other. A substitution between different classes of alcoholic beverages means that alcohol is substituted by alcohol, that is, with the same substance from the public health point of view. Alcoholic beverages also serve as substitutes for other commodities and thus they can be replaced by other commodities. This means that the level of alcohol consumption is related to the prices of alcoholic beverages relative to other commodities. When discussing other commodities as substitutes for alcoholic beverages, it should be noted that the substitution process may equally well lead to either unhealthier or healthier drinking habits. A rise in wine prices may result in a substitution of commercially produced wine by soft drinks, by self-produced wine, by 'moonshine', or even by drugs. Although a rise in alcohol prices can lead to a shift in consumption to illegal alcohol or drugs, it should be remembered that these types of substitution processes are affected by restrictions and limitations of those beverages or drugs to which consumers are apt to move. In all probability, the more decisive factors in these substitutions are the control measures that bear upon the availability of those substitutes, and it is scarcely conceivable that illicit traffic of alcohol could be altogether eliminated by cutting the prices of legally produced alcohol. Furthermore, if prices of legally produced alcohol are kept constant or lowered because of the possible undesirable substitution for illegal alcoholic beverages, the harmful effects of the legitimate alcohol may exceed the socially acceptable level of alcohol problems.

Studies based on individual data

In econometric studies based on time series, the values of price-elasticities reflect in many ways the average reactions of consumers to changes in prices. It is particularly the treatment of consumers as one group that has raised doubts about the validity of elasticity values. Although it can be inferred from econometric studies that a rise in alcohol prices has the effect of reducing consumption, it cannot be determined who the people are that have cut down on their consumption and by how much.

All the studies mentioned in the previous sections are based on aggregate data. During the last decade, the proliferation of economic work based on individual data and the development of econometric techniques of these data have also begun to exert their influence on research dealing with the price-sensitivity of alcohol consumption. The availability and the use of individual data can shed light on debates that cannot be solved by using aggregate data. One good example is the debate on whether heavy drinkers are responsive to price changes. This is important because alcohol literature frequently asserts that increases in prices of alcoholic beverages will only affect moderate and problem-free drinkers and will have no effect on heavy drinkers and problem drinkers because they are either addicted to or physically dependent on alcohol. Consequently, unwillingness to raise prices is likely to be provoked if the effect on pricing policy is felt mainly by moderate drinkers and leaves the heavy drinkers to carry out as before.

In the United States, Grossman *et al.* (1987) studied the price-sensitivity of young people's demand for alcohol. The result provides weak evidence that heavy drinkers are more sensitive to price changes than moderate drinkers. A similar study by Coate and Grossman (1988) also found that heavy drinkers were more sensitive to price changes than moderate drinkers. In Heien and Pompelli's (1989) study data was obtained from a household food consumption survey. They attempted to estimate a complete demand system for beer, distilled spirits, wine, and non-alcoholic beverages. According to their analysis, the three types of alcoholic beverages are weak complements to each other. The own-price elasticities are all negative, the demand for spirits being the most inelastic and the demand for beer being almost unitary elastic (Heien and Pompelli 1989).

The first work on the effect of price on consumption at an individual level was the study by Kendell *et al.* (1983). They studied the effect of price on consumption in Scotland, 1981, with two surveys, the second survey being conducted after a rise in price of alcohol. According to this study, the impact of the price increase is strongest among the heaviest drinkers, for both men and women (Kendell *et al.* 1983). Heavy drinkers also experienced the largest reduction in the number of adverse effects related to alcohol consumption. There are, however, several shortcomings in Kendell *et al.*'s analysis.

In the early 1970s many bars, taverns, and restaurants initiated a variety of sales programmes to attract more customers. These programmes, called 'happy hours' included some kind of price reduction; it might be two beverages for the price of one, a 25 per cent reduction for all beverages, free beverages for a particular type of patron, or all 'you can drink' specials. Happy hours offer one possibility to study the effect of decreasing prices on consumption, but only one experimental study seems to have been made. Babor *et al.* (1980) studied 34 men who were admitted to McLean Hospital in Boston for 30 days. Those 34 men consisted of 14 heavy drinkers and 20 fairly light drinkers. Their patterns of drinking were tested under happy hour or non-happy-hour conditions. As expected, both light and heavy drinkers drank more when drinks were less expensive: light drinkers drank about twice as much and heavy drinkers drank about 2.4 times as much as those drinking in the non-happy-hour conditions. Both light and heavy drinkers had longer episodes of drinking under happy hour conditions, but heavy drinkers also increased their short drinking episodes.

Babor *et al.* (1978) supplemented the experimental happy hour study with observations of the drinking habits of 16 regular bar patrons, in happy hour and non-happy-hour times. Happy hour patrons drank 9.56 drinks per day while non-happy-hour patrons drank only 3.73 drinks, despite the fairly small reduction in drink prices during the happy hour. Happy hour patrons engaged in more drinking sessions which also lasted longer.

Price changes and alcohol-related problems

One development in the field has been to link price changes directly to alcohol-related problems. This is, on one hand, one way to get indirect evidence of the effects of price policy on heavy consumers. On the other hand, this kind of study design takes care of the problems caused by possible substitution of recorded and unrecorded alcohol consumption.

Schweitzer *et al.* (1983) developed an econometric model of alcoholism which could incorporate its causes, its effects, and its possible control. According to them, such a model should give more complete and more direct insights into the problems of alcoholism than previous demand studies. They used cross-sectional data on 35 US states in 1975 to estimate a simultaneous model of beer and spirits consumption, alcoholism, and alcohol-related mortality. According to the results, a rise in the price of spirits lowers alcoholism, but a rise in the price of beer appears to increase it.

Cook (1981) adopted Simon's (1966) approach, using as a quasi-experiment the changes in state liquor excise-tax rates legislated between 1960 and 1975 in licence states. A follow-up study by Cook and Tauchen (1982) sought to improve this method while still taking advantage of the underlying quasi-experiment. They did not only consider the relationship between spirits consumption and tax changes, but also cirrhosis and car accidents in relation to tax changes. In the study by Cook and Tauchen, the median price elasticity for liquor was −1.8. The 1981 study discovered that the states that raised their liquor tax had a greater reduction or smaller increase in cirrhosis mortality than other states in the corresponding year (Cook 1981). In the 1982 study, Cook and Tauchen concluded that liquor consumption, including that of heavy drinkers (as indicated by cirrhosis mortality), is quite responsive to price and that a liquor tax increase tends to reduce car accidents' fatality rate (Cook and Tauchen 1982; Cook 1987).

Alcohol taxation

In the past, before the introduction of income and sales taxes, governments were heavily dependent on foreign trade duties and excise taxes for the bulk of their revenues. Special alcohol duties and taxes have been and are still an established means of raising government revenue. In some countries, alcoholic beverages have been susceptible to such taxation because of their characterization as luxury commodities. In other countries, in turn, special taxes have been levied on alcoholic beverages because they have formed a wide tax basis as everyday necessities. In the past, many other necessities, such as salt and matches, have also been specially taxed or priced.

Alcoholic beverages are especially suitable for special taxation because of their detrimental social and health consequences. In some countries, where the basic aim of alcohol consumption control is of social or public health origin, raising alcohol prices higher than the production costs has often been the result of granting monopoly rights to state-owned companies. This occurs in the Nordic countries and North America, in particular.

The rationale for levying a special tax on alcoholic beverages is seldom questioned, and the potential discussions on the subject are usually concerned with such questions as how the alcohol taxes should be formed, for example, should special alcohol taxes be based on the value of the product or the amount of ethyl alcohol in the product, how expensive alcoholic beverages should or could be relative to other commodities, and whether prices should vary according to the beverage category—distilled spirits, wine, and beer—and according to the type of outlet or to the category of the restaurant (see Crooks 1989; Baker and McKay 1990; Cook and Moore 1993). In addition, the impact of alcohol taxation on the distribution of consumer disposable incomes has been discussed because it is often felt that alcohol taxation is repressive by nature, that is, the percentage of total personal income that the state collects by means of alcohol taxes is higher in the low income groups than among the affluent members of the society (see, for example, Ashton *et al.* 1989).

A highly restrictive pricing policy is not always feasible, especially in the cases where alcoholic beverages are a substantial part of the daily diet of the population. Many consumers are naturally affected and very likely opposed to high alcohol taxation or to any increase in the price of alcoholic beverages. On the other hand, if alcoholic beverages are essential commodities for the population, alcohol consumption would be price-inelastic and quite resistant to price increases. Therefore, any increase in alcohol tax rates would collect a larger amount of tax revenues for the public treasury.

Tax increases, either motivated by social and public health or state finance considerations, may also have an adverse effect on the prospects of the alcoholic beverage industry and alcohol trade. The effects of tax-induced price increases on the volume of production and sales would be smaller if alcoholic beverages are used rather as everyday necessities than as luxury commodities when they are price-elastic as opposed to price-inelastic.

From the point of view of collecting tax revenues, the most important information regarding the effects of changing alcohol prices is how sensitive alcohol consumption is in relation to changing alcohol prices. From the point of view of the alcohol industry and trade, this knowledge may be sufficient because it does not matter where the demand for their products and their profits comes from as long as it occurs. Even from the point of view of public health considerations, the overall sensitivity of demand is most crucial if increases or decreases in the mean alcohol consumption are very likely to be accompanied by increases or decreases in alcohol-related problems or increased or decreased prevalence of heavy alcohol consumers.

Discussion

The evidence examined above suggests that alcohol price levels do have an independent effect on the level of alcohol consumption. More specifically, recent evidence has supported rather than weakened the conclusions reached by Bruun and his colleagues in 1975. They noted (p. 83) that 'in many respects, alcoholic beverages behave like other commodities on the market, so that their consumption is affected by their price level', and that 'the availability of alcohol is an important factor in the general level of consumption'.

One clear limitation of price policy is its concentration in societies that have been very concerned about drinking. In other words, available evaluation studies mostly originate from northern Europe and North America, and recently also from Australia and New Zealand (for example, Clements and Johnson 1983; Pearce 1986; Clements and Selvanathan 1987; Selvanathan 1991; Clements and Selvanathan 1991; Wette *et al.* 1993). Even though the basis of relevant evidence has broadened geographically, we still know too little about the effects of changes in alcohol prices in wine-growing countries of southern Europe, or in Moslem societies, for instance.

When looking at the results of different studies, it is easy to find a wide variety of elasticity values. Many variations may and can be explained by problems in study designs or basic data, by methodological problems, and by misinterpretations. For instance, Ornstein (1980, p. 817) concluded his review by stating that 'the main lesson to be learned from this survey is that demand estimation is a difficult and inexact business. The results are strongly affected by the data and econometric technique used. One should be cautious before adopting the results of any given study, and especially cautious if such results are to be used as a basis for public policy'. This pessimism is partly exaggerated because of the fact that Ornstein was seeking 'true' elasticity values for different types of alcoholic beverages.

One should remember that even similar alcohol policies yield different results in different societies because of the different economic, cultural, political, and social circumstances. We may of course speculate, referring to econometric studies presented above, that, the demand for beer is, particularly, inelastic with respect to its price. This may even be true in the countries studied—Western industrialized nations. But as soon as we are able to get similar analyses from wine-growing countries, this generalization may not apply any longer.

Bruun *et al.* (1975) concluded that although the price changes in the cases studied were mainly within a modest range, they nevertheless seem to result in the substitution of one type of beverage for another. On the basis of research presented above, it is difficult to add much more to this. One could, perhaps, conclude that there appear to be no studies indicating that consumption of a certain type of alcoholic beverage would be greatly affected by changes in the price of a substitute alcoholic beverage. Furthermore, there seems to be hardly any studies of the substitutive process between alcoholic beverages and other commodities, whether they are non-alcohol drinks, drugs, or leisure activities.

Since the mid 1970s, some empirical evidence has appeared on the effects of changing prices on different population groups. These studies seem to indicate that price policy affects both moderate drinkers and heavy consumers. In this sense, the legitimacy of pricing policy as a means to affect alcohol-related problems has increased.

References

Ahtola, J., Ekholm, A., and Somervuori, A. (1986). Bayes estimates for the price and income elasticities of alcoholic beverages in Finland from 1955 to 1980. *Journal of Business and Economic Statistics*, **4**, 199–208.

Ashton, T., Casswell, S., and Gilmore, L. (1989). Alcohol taxes: do the poor pay more than the rich? *British Journal of Addiction*, **84**, 759–66.

Assarsson, B. (1991). Efterfrågan på alkohol i Sverige 1970–1988 [Demand of alcoholic beverages in Sweden in 1970–1988]. In *Alkoholbeskattningen. Betänkade av alkoholskatteutredningen* [*Alcohol taxation. A report from the alcohol tax committee*]. Government Official Reports, Stockholm.

Babor, T. F., Mendelson, H., Greenberg, I., and Kuehnle, J. (1978). Experimental analysis of the 'happy hour': effects of purchase price on alcohol consumption. *Psychopharmacology*, **58**, 34–41.

Babor, T. F., Mendelson, J. H., Uhly, B., and Souza, E. (1981). Drinking patterns in experimental and bar-room settings. *Journal of Studies on Alcohol*, **41**, 635–51.

Baker, P. and McKay, S. (1990). *The structure of alcohol taxes: A hangover from the past?* Institute for Fiscal Studies, London.

Barsby, S. L. and Marshall, G. L. (1977). Short term consumption effects of a lower minimum alcohol-purchasing age. *Journal of Studies on Alcohol*, **38**, 1665–79.

Bruun, K., *et al.* (1975). *Alcohol control policies in public health perspective*, Vol. 25. Finnish Foundation for Alcohol Studies, Helsinki.

Bryding, G. and Rosén, U. (1969). Konsumtionen av alkoholhaltiga drycker 1920–1951, en efterfrågeanalytisk studie [Consumption of alcoholic beverages in Sweden 1920–1951, an econometric study], (stencil). University Statistics Institute, Uppsala.

Clements, K. W. and Johnson, L. W. (1983). The demand for beer, wine and spirits: a system-wide approach. *Journal of Business*, **56**, 273–304.

Clements, K. W. and Selvanathan, E. A. (1987). Alcohol consumption. In *Applied demand analysis: Results from system-wide approaches* (ed. H. Thiel and K. W. Clements), pp. 185–264. Ballinger Publishing Company, Cambridge, MA.

Clements, K. W. and Selvanathan, S. (1991). The economic determinants of alcohol consumption. *Australian Journal of Agricultural Economics*, **35**, 209–31.

Coate, D. and Grossman, M. (1988). Effects of alcoholic beverage prices and legal drinking ages on youth alcohol use. *Journal of Law and Economics*, **31**, 145–71.

Comanor, W. S. and Wilson, T. A. (1974). *Advertising and market power*. Harvard University Press, Cambridge, MA.

Cook, P. J. (1981). The effect of liquor taxes on drinking, cirrhosis and auto accidents. In *Alcohol and public policy: Beyond the shadow of prohibition*, (ed. M. H. Moore and D. Gerstein), pp. 255–85. National Academy Press, Washington, DC.

Cook, P. J. (1987). The impact of distilled-spirits taxes on consumption, auto fatalities, and cirrhosis mortality. In *Advances in substance abuse: Behavioral and biological research. Control issues in alcohol abuse prevention: Strategies for states and communities*, (ed. H. D. Holder), pp. 159–67. JAI, Greenwich, CT.

Cook, P. J. and Moore, M. J. (1993). Taxation of alcoholic beverages. *Economics and the Prevention of Alcohol-Related Problems*. National Institute on Alcohol Abuse and Alcoholism, Rockville, Maryland.

Cook, P. J. and Tauchen, G. (1982). The effect of liquor taxes on heavy drinking. *Bell Journal of Economics*, **13**, 379–90.

Crooks, E. (1989). *Alcohol consumption and taxation*. Institute for Fiscal Studies, London.

Duffy, M. (1983). The demand for alcoholic drink in the United Kingdom, 1963–78. *Applied Economics*, **15**, 125–40.

Duffy, M. (1987). Advertising and the inter-product distribution of demand: a Rotterdam model approach. *European Economic Review*, **31**, 1051–70.

Duffy, M. (1991). Advertising and the consumption of tobacco and alcoholic drink: a system-wide analysis. *Scottish Journal of Political Economy*, **38**, 369–85.

Godfrey, C. (1986). *Factors influencing the consumption of alcohol and tobacco—A review of demand models*. Addiction Research Centre for Health Economics, York, UK.

Godfrey, C. (1988). Licensing and the demand for alcohol. *Applied Economics*, **20**, 1541–58.

Godfrey, C. (1989). Factors influencing the consumption of alcohol and tobacco: the use and abuse of economic models. *British Journal of Addiction*, **84**, 1123–38.

Godfrey, C. (1990). Modelling demand. In *Preventing alcohol and tobacco problems*, (ed. A. Maynard and P. Tether), Vol. 1, pp. 35–53. Avebury, Aldershot.

Godfrey, C. and Maynard, A. (1988). An economic theory of alcohol consumption and abuse. In *Theories on alcoholism*, (ed. C. D. Chaudron and D. A. Wilkinson), pp. 411–35. Addiction Research Foundation, Toronto.

Grossman, M., Coate, D., and Arluck, G. M. (1987). Price sensitivity of alcoholic beverages in the United States: Youth alcohol consumption. In *Advances in substance abuse: Behavioral and biological research. Control issues in alcohol abuse prevention: Strategies for states and communities*, (ed. H. D. Holder), pp. 169–98. JAI, Greenwich, CT.

Heien, D. and Pompelli, G. (1989). The demand for alcoholic beverages: Economic and demographic effects. *Southern Economic Journal*, **55**, 759–70.

Hogarty, T. F. and Elzinga, K. G. (1972). The demand for beer. *The Review of Economics and Statistics*, **54**, 195–8.

Horowitz, I. and Horowitz, A. (1965). Firms in a declining market; the brewing case. *Journal of Industrial Economics*, **13**, 129–53.

Horverak, Ø. (1979). *Norsk alkoholpolitikk 1960–1975. En analyse av alkoholpolitiske virkemidler og deres virkninger*. [Norwegian alcohol policy 1960–1975. An analysis of alcohol political means and their effects]. National Institute for Alcohol Research (SIFA), Oslo.

Huitfeldt, B. and Jorner, U. (1972). *Efterfrågan på rusdrycker i Sverige* [The demand for alcoholic beverages in Sweden]. Rapport från Alkoholpolitiska utredningen [Report from the Alcohol Policy Commission]. Government Official Reports, Stockholm.

Johnson, J. A. and Oksanen, E. H. (1974). Socio-economic determinants of the consumption of alcoholic beverages. *Applied Economics*, **6**, 293–301.

Johnson, J. A. and Oksanen, E. H. (1977). Estimation of demand for alcoholic beverages in Canada from pooled time series and cross sections. *Review of Economics and Statistics*, **59**, 113–18.

Johnson, J. A., Oksanen, E. H., Veall, M. R., and Fretz, D. (1992). Short run and long run elasticities for Canadian consumption of alcoholic beverages: an error-correction mechanism/cointegration approach. *The Review of Economics and Statistics*, **74**, 64–74.

Jones, A. M. (1989). A system approach to the demand for alcohol and tobacco. *Bulletin of Economic Research*, **41**, 3307–78.

Kendell, R. E., de Roumanie, M., and Ritson, E. B. (1983). Effect of economic changes on Scottish drinking habits 1978–82. *British Journal of Addiction*, **78**, 365–79.

Labys, W. C. (1976). An international comparison of price and income elasticities for wine consumption. *Australian Journal of Agricultural Economics*, **20**, 33–6.

Lau, H.-H. (1975). Cost of alcoholic beverages as a determinant of alcohol consumption. In *Research advances in alcohol and drug problems*, (ed. R. J. Gibbins, Y. Isreal, and H. Kalant), Vol. 22, pp. 211–45. Wiley, New York.

Lidman, R. M. (1976). *Economic issues in alcohol control*. Social Research Group, School of Public Health, University of California, Berkeley.

Malmqvist, S. (1948). *A statistical analysis of demand for liquor in Sweden*. A study of the demand for a rationed commodity. Uppsala, Appelbergs Boktryckeri AB.

Maynard, A. (1983). Modelling alcohol consumption and abuse: The powers and pitfalls of economic techniques. In *Economics and alcohol*, (ed. M. Grant, M. Plant, and A. Williams), pp. 128–39. Croom Helm, London.

McGuinness, T. (1983). The demand for beer, spirits and wine in the UK, 1956–1979. In *Economics and alcohol*, (ed. M. Grant, M. Plant, and A. Williams), pp. 238–42. Croom Helm, London.

Niskanen, W. A. (1962). *The demand for alcoholic beverages*. University of Chicago Press.

Norman, D. (1975). *Structural change and performance in the US brewing industry*. Unpublished dissertation. University of California, Los Angeles.

Nyberg, A. (1967). *Alkoholijuomien kulutus ja hinnat* [Consumption and prices of alcoholic beverages], Vol. 15. Finnish Foundation for Alcohol Studies, Helsinki.

Olsson, O. (1991). *Prisets och inkomstens betydelse för alkoholbruk, missbruk och skador* [The effect of prices and income on alcohol consumption and related problems]. The Swedish Council for Information on Alcohol and other Drugs (CAN), Shockholm.

Ornstein, S. I. (1980). Control of alcohol consumption through price increases. *Journal of Studies on Alcohol*, **41**, 807–18.

Ornstein, S. I. and Levy, D. (1983). Price and income elasticities and the demand for alcoholic beverages. In *Recent developments in alcoholism* Vol. 1, (ed. M. Galanter), pp. 303–45. Plenum, New York.

Partanen, J. (1991). *Sociability and intoxication. Alcohol and drinking in Kenya, Africa and the modern world*, Vol. 39. Finnish Foundation for Alcohol Studies, Helsinki.

Prest, A. R. (1949). Some experiments in demand analysis. *Review of Economics and Statistics*, **21**, 33–49.

Quek, K. E. (1988). *The demand for alcohol in Canada: an econometric study*. Discussion paper No. 88.08, Department of Economics, The University of Western Australia.

Salo, M. (1987). *Alkoholijuomien anniskelukulutuksen määrän kehitys vuosina 1969–1986 ja eräitä anniskelua koskevia kysyntämalleja* [Developments of on-premise retail sales of alcoholic beverages, 1969–1986, and some demand models for on-premise retail sales], Research Report No. 9. Economic Research and Planning Department, Finnish Alcohol Company, Helsinki.

Salo, M. (1990). *Alkoholijuomien vähittäiskulutuksen analyysi vuosilta 1969–1988* [An analysis of off-premises retail sales of alcoholic beverages, 1969–1988], Research Report No. 9. Economic Research and Planning Department, Finnish Alcohol Company, Helsinki.

Schweitzer, S. O., Intriligator, M. D., and Salehi, J. (1983). Alcoholism: An econometric model of its causes, its effects and its control. In *Economics and alcohol*, (ed. M. Grant, M. Plant, and A. Williams), pp. 107–27. Croom Helm, London.

Selvanathan, E. A. (1988). Alcohol consumption in the UK, 1955–85: a system-wide analysis.

Selvanathan, E. A. (1991). Cross-country consumption comparison: an application of the Rotterdam demand system. *Applied Economics*, **20**, 1071–86.

Simon, J. L. (1966). The price elasticity of liquor in the US and a simple method of determination. *Econometrica*, **34**, 193–205.

Smith, R. T. (1976). The legal and illegal markets for taxed goods: Pure theory and an application to state government taxation of distilled spirits. *Journal of Law and Economics*, **19**, 393–432.

Stone, R. (1945). The analysis of market demand. *Journal of the Royal Statistical Society*, **108**, 286–382.

Stone, R. (1951). *The role of measurement in economics*. Cambridge University Press.

Sundström, Å. and Ekström, J. (1962). Dryckeskonsumtionen i Sverige [Beverage consumption in Sweden], Report No. 22. Industrins utredningsinstitut [Research Institute of the Industry], Stockhom.

Wales, T. J. (1968). Distilled spirits and interstate consumption effects. *American Economic Review*, **58**, 853–63.

Walsh, B. M. (1982). The demand for alcohol in the UK: a comment. *Journal of Industrial Economics*, **30**, 439–46.

Walsh, B. and Walsh, D. (1970). Economic aspects of alcohol consumption in the Republic of Ireland. *Economic and Social Review*, **12**, 115–38.

Wette, H. C., Zhang, J.-F., Berg, R. J., and Casswell, S. (1993). The effect of prices on alcohol consumption in New Zealand 1983–1991. *Drug and Alcohol Review*, **12**, 151–8.

Wong, A. Y.-T. (1988). *The demand for alcohol in the UK 1920–1938: An econometric study*. Discussion Paper No. 88.13, Department of Economics, The University of Western Australia.

Yen, S. T. (1994). Cross-section estimation of US demand for alcoholic beverage. *Applied Economics*, **26**, 381–92.

7. The social and public health significance of individually directed interventions

Thomas F. Babor

Introduction

Since the end of World War II, a wide variety of individually directed interventions have been developed to deal with alcohol-related problems (Klingemann *et al.* 1992; Mäkelä *et al.* 1981; Babor *et al.* 1986; Roman and Gilbert 1979), in both the developing and developed countries. These interventions can be classified into three general categories: (1) early intervention, (2) specialized treatment programmes, and (3) mutual help groups. Early detection is directed at the reduction of alcohol-related harm and the prevention of alcohol dependence through screening and brief interventions. Specialized treatment is designed to treat the medical complications of drinking and to assist the problem drinker with social and psychological rehabilitation. Mutual help programmes are concerned with the long-term rehabilitation of problem drinkers, many of whom require continuing care and support over the course of years. Alcoholics Anonymous is a prime example of this approach.

This chapter considers the aggregate-level significance of individually directed interventions, which have been developed primarily to ameliorate the health and social consequences of problematic drinking. It begins with a discussion of the information requirements for estimating the impact of individually directed interventions. After defining important terms and concepts, selected interventions that have been applied to alcohol problems are reviewed. In the final section, the chapter discusses where most effectively in the public health interest interventions directed at the individual drinker should be mounted. Implicit in this review is the notion that in addition to their public health functions, individually directed interventions serve a variety of humanitarian purposes such as providing shelter to the homeless drinker and long-term domiciliary care for the chronic inebriate.

Ideally, the following kinds of information should be available to understand the impact of individual-level programmes on public health and social welfare:

the prevalence of the disorder, condition or problem; the efficacy of intervention programmes; the cost of identification and intervention; the reduction in morbidity and mortality due to treatment of identified cases; and the potential barriers to successful implementation of cost-effective measures. By combining these kinds of information, it is possible to estimate the gap or difference between the current 'burden' of an illness (the combined health, economic, and social impact of a health problem) and the lesser burden that is achievable through the application of present knowledge. For example, Stoudemire *et al.* (1987) attempted to estimate the gap between current efforts and the preventable burden of alcohol abuse in the United States by reviewing evidence about the aetiology of alcohol problems; estimating the morbidity, mortality and disability attributable to alcohol; evaluating the costs of alcohol problems; identifying populations at risk; and summarizing information about the effectiveness of primary prevention measures. They did not evaluate the actual or potential contributions of individual level interventions, presumably because they considered these efforts insignificant in relation to interventions directed at the general population. They conclude that 'for society to adequately address alcohol-related problems, it is necessary to shift attention away from the individual and focus on the system in which the individual acts'.

This conclusion in part reflects the difficulty involved in estimating how individual treatment interventions can affect aggregate-level mortality, morbidity, disability, social problems, and health care costs attributable to alcohol misuse. Evaluating the success of alcohol intervention programmes depends on clinical, epidemiological, and economic information that is unavailable in most countries. In addition, cultural and national differences in health beliefs, health resources, and drinking patterns make research findings from one country inappropriate or ungeneralizable to another country. Nevertheless, a first approximation can be made by reviewing the available evidence pertaining to early intervention programmes, specialized treatment programmes, and mutual help organizations. In the following sections, individual-level interventions are reviewed in relation to their potential impact on the prevalence of alcohol problems. The sections are organized according to the following format. First, an attempt is made to review the history of the intervention and the types of alcohol-related problems it is most likely to affect. Next, causal evidence for the effectiveness of the intervention is discussed. Third, evidence for its aggregate-level impact is presented, when available. Finally, the feasibility of the intervention and its cross-national generalizability are considered.

Early intervention and secondary prevention programmes

Early intervention means that a therapeutic or preventive activity is initiated before the onset of severe alcohol dependence or serious alcohol-related problems. Its purpose is to prevent alcohol-related disabilities in persons at risk. Early intervention as a public health strategy is likely to be most effective when there is a clear consensus about aetiology and risk factors, as when an infectious or toxic agent is identified as the cause of an illnes. Because alcohol dependence and other addictive disorders appear to result from complex interaction of biogenetic and psychosocial factors, it is difficult to identify specific causes and vulnerability factors. As a result, true early intervention programmes have been rare and are unlikely to be feasible for alcohol problems.

In contrast to the pro-active nature of early intervention, secondary prevention is directed at persons *after* the onset of alcohol-related problems. Secondary prevention is the provision of therapeutic or remedial interventions to persons who have already manifested alcohol-related problems, but who have not developed severe alcohol dependence. Secondary prevention involves the early treatment of a disorder or condition to decrease the length of the illness or prevent the further development of symptoms, with the intent of reducing prevalence.

This section discusses the evidence for the effectiveness of measures based on research on primary care interventions as well as screening and referral programmes. These measures have been developed in part because a substantial proportion of a country's alcohol problems are experienced by people unlikely to meet diagnostic criteria for alcohol dependence (Moore and Gerstein 1981; Krietman 1986). Drinking problems are directly related to the quantity and the frequency of alcohol consumed, and they manifest themselves in terms of biological, social, and psychological consequences. Drinking patterns and alcohol-related consequences vary considerably from one country to another. Acute consequences tend to vary with the amount consumed per occasion, while many of the medical consequences, such as liver cirrhosis, vary with chronic alcohol use (Babor *et al.* 1987). Although heavy and frequent drinking are not necessarily indicative of alcoholism, they are important risk factors and can lead to health problems in the absence of alcohol dependence.

Primary care and other health settings

The prevalence of problem drinking in patients seeking treatment for other health problems ranges from 15 to 20 per cent of males and from 4 to 10 per cent of females in general hospital settings of many of the developed countries (McIntosh 1982). In many parts of the world, health workers encounter heavy drinkers routinely in primary care clinics, educational settings, and general practitioners' offices. In an effort to evaluate a public health approach to the secondary prevention of alcohol-related problems, randomized studies have been conducted in more than 13 countries to evaluate the efficacy of screening technologies and low-cost intervention strategies (Bein *et al.* 1993; Babor 1994). Because life style risk factors, such as alcohol intoxication and frequent drinking, are often amenable to behavioural interventions, increasing attention has been devoted to the development of educational and motivational interventions designed to preclude the need for costly medical care. An underlying assumption of this approach is that regular drinking and frequent alcohol intoxication increase substantially the risk of social, medical, and psychological problems.

Evidence for causal effects During the 1970s there were a number of research reports evaluating the effectiveness of broad-spectrum behavioural treatment techniques with problem drinkers. Although the early studies were encouraging (Miller and Hester 1980), the multimodal approaches used in these studies were time-consuming. Later studies have used a less time-consuming approach, referred to as behavioural self-control training (Miller and Munoz 1976). One unanticipated finding that emerged from these studies (Miller and Taylor 1980) is that a self-help manual may be as effective as self-control training provided by a therapist. This suggests that interventions utilizing a manual or brief counselling are appropriate as the first attempt to intervene with people who drink heavily, but who are not dependent on alcohol. Other studies support this conclusion.

In one investigation in Malmö, Sweden, Kristenson and colleagues studied a group of 529 middle-aged men who had been identified as 'heavy drinkers' as part of a community-wide health screening project (Kristenson *et al.* 1982, 1983). Men having an abnormal liver enzyme, gamma-glutamyltranspeptidase (GGT), were randomly assigned to either a counselling group or a control group. Over a six-year period, the intervention group improved more in terms of absenteeism, sick days, and days hospitalized. There were also small but significant differences in mortality. The study showed that a simple intervention based on regular feedback about a biochemical marker had a beneficial effect on the drinking habits and physical health of a population at risk.

A related study was conducted in Scotland to assess the effectiveness of brief counselling and a self-help manual with non-alcoholic, socially stable problem drinkers identified in a general hospital (Chick *et al.* 1985). Screening was conducted by a nurse using a 10-minute interview covering drinking habits, medical history, and social background. Both the counselling and control groups reported significantly less alcohol consumption at the one-year follow-up evaluation. However, the counselling group indicated fewer alcohol-related problems, greater reduction in GGT values, and better performance on a global measure of improvement.

These studies inspired further research to investigate the effectiveness of minimal interventions using self-help manuals, simple advice, and brief, time-limited counselling. Common features of these interventions are their low cost, ease of implementation, and minimal involvement of professional service providers.

Wallace and colleagues (1988) studied 47 group practices in England to determine the effectiveness of advice given to heavy drinkers by general practitioners. Patients in the intervention condition received one session of advice to reduce their alcohol consumption, and the opportunity to participate in additional sessions. The control group received no advice about drinking. Follow-up assessments of drinking at 6 and 12 months revealed a twofold reduction in the intervention group compared with controls.

Anderson and Scott (1992) conducted a randomized trial of brief interventions with heavy drinkers identified at eight group primary care practices in the United Kingdom. The intervention consisted of 10 minutes of advice about drinking, feedback concerning the results of a liver enzyme test (GGT), and information about the risks of heavy drinking. In comparison with an untreated control group, the intervention group at one-year follow-up showed a small but statistically significant reduction in the quantity consumed and the proportion of heavy drinking days, as well as a 13 per cent reduction in the proportion of hazardous drinkers. A parallel study was conducted in a sample of 72 women (Scott and Anderson 1990). At one-year follow-up there was a significant reduction in the alcohol consumption of both the intervention and the control groups. The authors suggest that many women in the control group may have received advice from other sources to reduce their drinking.

Antti-Poika *et al.* (1988) randomly assigned 120 male patients with alcohol-related injuries to a control group or an intervention group that received between three and five counselling sessions with a nurse and a doctor. At six-months follow-up evaluation significantly more patients in the intervention group (45 per cent) were considered improved than in the control group (20 per cent). Patients considered to be alcoholics had worse outcomes than those who did not demonstrate signs of chronic alcoholism.

Nilssen (1991) randomly assigned 338 at-risk drinkers to a control group or to two intervention conditions: (1) a single consultation devoted to a discussion of laboratory test results (GGT) and a pamphlet giving advice about drinking habits; (2) an extensive diagnostic evaluation followed by several follow-up meetings and repeated laboratory tests. At the one-year follow-up evaluation significant reductions in both self-reported alcohol consumption and GGT levels were found in both of the intervention groups but not in the control group.

A major cross-national study sponsored by the World Health Organization was conducted at collaborating centres in Costa Rica, Australia, the United Kingdom, Norway, Mexico, Kenya, Bulgaria, the former Soviet Union, Zimbabwe, and the United States (Babor and Grant 1992). Non-alcoholic heavy drinkers ($N = 1490$), recruited from a combination of hospital settings, primary care clinics, and work sites, were randomly assigned to a control group, a simple advice group, or a group receiving brief counselling. The results of a nine-month follow-up evaluation of 75 per cent of the intake sample showed a significant effect of the interventions on both average alcohol consumption and intensity of drinking in the male samples, even after controlling for demographic factors and sociocultural influences. For females, significant reductions were observed in both the control and the intervention groups. The results also showed that the intensity of the intervention was not related to the amount of change in drinking behaviour, with 5 minutes of simple advice as effective as 20 minutes of brief counselling.

Evidence of aggregate effects This review of controlled trials indicates that modest but reliable effects on drinking behaviour and related problems can follow from brief interventions, especially with the less serious type of problem drinkers. To date, there has been little effort to apply these findings to general health care systems in a way that might have an impact on prevalence rates in the general population. One exception is the French secondary prevention programme. Beginning in 1970, the French Health Ministry established a system of outpatient clinics as part of a national programme to prevent alcoholism. These clinics respond to the needs of habitual excessive drinkers who do not have serious psychological problems (LeGo 1977). More than 150 'Centres of Nutritional Hygiene' have now been established in France, with at least one to be found in every major city. Although systematic evaluation research has not been conducted, two critical reviews (Babor *et al.* 1983; Chick 1984) concur that the programme merits careful attention because of its low cost (compared to inpatient treatment), widespread accessibility throughout France, and apparent effectiveness in treating large numbers of problem drinkers.

Lacking clear evidence of the aggregate level impact of screening programmes, few studies can be cited to estimate even the potential effects of brief interventions in primary care. The Wallace *et al.* (1988) study suggests that if sufficient numbers of general practitioners can be trained and mobilized, the effect could be significant. Kristensen *et al.* (1983) showed that population screening for risk factors can have a beneficial impact on alcohol-related morbidity and mortality. Nilssen (1991) found a significant reduction in drinking following a brief intervention directed at heavy drinkers in a small Norwegian community. Babor and Grant (1992) found that approximately 20 per cent of male patients respond in a clinically meaningful way to simple advice, and that these effects are consistent across different cultures. These studies suggest that the effects of brief interventions on heavy drinkers are consistent, robust, and could have a significant impact on the heavy drinking population of a community if they were employed routinely in primary care and other health settings.

Feasibility Despite the relative complexity of alcohol-related problems, secondary prevention strategies directed at individuals are feasible, in part because the toxic agent, alcohol, is easily identifiable. Almost all alcohol-related health and social consequences can be minimized by reducing the frequency and quantity of alcohol consumed. There is, however, considerable evidence that physicians often fail to provide preventive services to their patients, particularly with regard to alcohol abuse. The reasons for this are complex and not clearly understood. Cost, time constraints, limited resources, lack of organizational support, and insufficient training are possible explanations. Despite the promising results of controlled trials, there is little information to estimate the feasibility of screening and brief intervention programmes, except for the community-wide research programmes tested successfully in Norway (Nilssen 1991) and Sweden (Kristenson *et al.* 1983).

Fetal alcohol effects

Concern about the effects of alcohol on the fetus has increased interest in how brief intervention techniques might be employed with pregnant women who drink. Research on the prevention of fetal alcohol effects has developed during the last 15 years following reports of children born to alcoholic mothers with craniofacial, limb, and cardiovascular defects. This constellation of abnormalities, called the fetal alcohol syndrome (FAS), is thought to be an extreme manifestation of less serious but possibly more prevalent fetal alcohol effects (FAE) of maternal alcohol intake. The scientific evidence for FAE has focused attention on the need to monitor alcohol intake by pregnant women, at least in the industrialized countries where a significant proportion of women drink.

Evidence for causal effects There is some evidence that early intervention can reduce the risk of adverse effects of alcohol on the fetus, although there are methodological limitations with the existing studies (Schorling 1993). In the United States, Rosett *et al.* (1983) systematically evaluated all pregnant women attending the prenatal clinic for excessive alcohol intake. Among 791 women evaluated, 11 per cent were heavy drinkers. They were told that they had a better chance of having a healthy baby if they abstained from alcohol use during pregnancy. Supportive therapy with a psychiatrist and/or counsellor was provided one to four times a month in conjunction with the prenatal visit. Approximately two-thirds of women who participated in at least three counselling sessions stopped heavy drinking before the third trimester. The five cases of FAS diagnosed in this study all occurred in women who continued to drink heavily.

Larsson (1983) implemented a similar programme among 464 women at four maternal health centres in Stockholm. Four per cent of the population were identified as alcohol abusers. Women were given counselling similar to that provided in the Boston study. There was a reduction in alcohol use by all of the women classified as excessive drinkers, and by 78 per cent of those considered to be abusers. More infants from mothers classified as excessive drinkers or abusers (33 per cent) were placed in the intensive care nursery than were those born to social drinkers (12 per cent). The two babies born to mothers who continued to drink heavily exhibited significant growth retardation, and one was diagnosed as having FAS.

Evidence for aggregate effects and feasibility In a review of these and three other studies, Schorling (1993) concluded that a simple message may be sufficient to lead to behaviour change for a majority of women. Nevertheless, there is no evidence to estimate the aggregate level impact of fetal alcohol programmes. If prenatal screening and intervention programmes could be instituted throughout the health delivery system in countries where women drink frequently, it is likely that there would be a substantial reduction in fetal alcohol effects. Because a large percentage of women in all nations see a physician during their pregnancy, it is likely that alcohol screening, brief intervention or referral to more intensive treatment could be made a routine part of prenatal care. Unfortunately, not all women would receive screening early enough in their pregnancy to prevent all fetal alcohol effects, and screening would not be an economic investment of resources in countries with low prevalence rates.

Occupational programmes

Industry-based programmes designed to identify and manage problem drinkers have expanded dramatically in North America since the early 1940s (Roman 1981; Walker and Shain 1983). Parallel developments have occurred in France, (LeGo 1968), the Soviet Union (Roman and Gilbert 1979), and other countries. The following ingredients are characteristic of these programmes: identification of problem drinkers through impaired work performance rather than medical signs and symptoms, although in some countries (for example, France) industrial screening is conducted using physical exams and laboratory tests (LeGo 1968); confrontation of the problem-drinking employee by the work supervisor; referral to an agency external to or associated with the work organization for appropriate counselling or treatment; the threat of disciplinary action or dismissal in cases where there has been a breach of discipline if the employee fails to accept help or improve job performance. Despite these common ingredients, there is no single, generally accepted method for conducting an occupational programme. Programmes differ widely in nature and scope, some focusing specifically on problem drinking, others on a broader range of psychosocial problems. Programmes also differ in the use of coercion, the types and intensity of treatment made available to the employee, and the degree of supervisory follow-up aimed at maintaining compliance with treatment.

Evidence for causal effects While there is general agreement that industry based programmes have great potential for secondary prevention, there has been very little systematic research conducted on the effectiveness of these programmes. Nor have there been attempts to determine how various programme procedures or components affect outcome. It is conceivable, for example, that the process of identification and confrontation, rather than counselling or treatment, are responsible for the general impression that employee programmes are cost-effective, relative to dismissal or demotion.

Evidence for aggregate level effects and feasibility Occupationally based programmes vary widely in their nature and purpose. There has been little systematic evaluation of their effectiveness, in part because they often serve as referral agencies without providing direct intervention services, and in part because of the variability among programmes in the use of job sanctions. Nevertheless, the use of coercion and employment-related sanctions is likely to affect both compliance with treatment and relapse rates after treatment (Weisner 1990). The fact that occupationally based programmes have been established in large enterprises in many countries indicates that such programmes are feasible.

Specialized treatment

Specialized treatment, sometimes referred to as tertiary prevention, refers to interventions directed at the limitation of disability or fatal complications, generally through optimal clinical management. Specialized treatment is directed primarily at the management of alcohol withdrawal, the social and psychological rehabilitation of the problem drinker, the prevention of relapse to alcohol dependence, and the management of alcohol-related medical conditions. Tertiary prevention is accomplished if the patient does not relapse and progress to a more serious level of alcohol problems.

Specialized treatment for the management of alcohol-related problems began with the establishment of inebriate asylums in the United States and England during the late 19th century. The network of specialized residential facilities that grew up prior to World War I virtually ceased to exist as a result of national prohibition laws, the two world wars, and the global depression. It was only in the late 1940s that the modern approach to alcoholism treatment emerged. The treatment paradigm for the new alcoholism movement in North America was established on a professional level in the form of the 'Yale Plan Clinics', and on the non-professional level in the form of Alcoholics Anonymous (Keller 1986). The Yale clinics were specialized outpatient programmes that experimented with a variety of medical, psychological, and social interventions considered appropriate for the complex task of rehabilitating alcohol-dependent people. These methods included group therapy, aversive conditioning, individual psychotherapy, vocational counselling, alcohol education, as well as using disulfiram and other pharmacotherapies when these became available.

With these modest beginnings in the English-speaking, industrialized countries, the management of alcohol problems also took on a special identity within the health care systems of many other nations. Several international surveys (Moser 1974; Mäkelä *et al.* 1981; Klingemann *et al.* 1992) have shown that during the post-war period national policy shifted away from legal and repressive measures toward medico-social approaches to the management of alcohol problems. In countries with an organized system of health services, treatment for the medical complications of alcohol use most often became the concern of general hospitals, while alcohol-related psychological disabilities were treated in psychiatric facilities. Increasingly, however, specialized facilities became available for the rehabilitation and re-socialization of alcoholics. What has emerged in most of these countries is a network of treatment facilities and other supportive services. These services include counselling and outpatient treatment in both general and mental hospitals, specialized detoxification centres and sobering-up stations, half-way houses and hostels, and programmes within industry and the penal system. In some countries, responsibility for treatment and rehabilitation has been assumed by special governmental administrative bodies (for example, Norway and the former Soviet Union). In other countries, there is a close link between the health and social service system, as in Finland and Scotland. In most countries, however, there is little integration of the various components of alcoholism treatment on a national level (Moser 1985).

In addition to the expansion of residential rehabilitation programmes, the management of acute alcohol intoxication and the alcohol withdrawal syndrome (commonly referred to as detoxification) was improved by the development of specialized detoxification facilities in North America and Europe (DenHartog 1982). These facilities expanded rapidly following widespread adoption of laws decriminalizing public intoxication.

Evidence of efficacy The specialized treatment system that emerged following World War II is varied, complex, and still in the process of development. Many of its components (for example, detoxification facilities, inpatient residential programmes, outpatient clinics), and the therapeutic approaches used in these components (for example, the Twelve Steps of AA, chemical aversion therapy, relapse prevention), have only recently begun to receive systematic research attention. Listed below are a series of summary statements that borrow heavily from recent literature reviews (Holder *et al.* 1991; Institute of Medicine 1990; Miller and Hester 1986) focusing on the effectiveness of alcoholism treatment.

1. Despite its methodological limitations, the available evidence suggests that any treatment for alcoholism is better than no treatment. Although as many as two-thirds of those treated demonstrate improvement, perhaps one-third would have improved without treatment or with minimal intervention.

2. Although many of the studies of alcoholics' utilization of health services are limited, the evidence suggests that: (a) alcoholics and their families demand more health care services than non-alcoholics; (b) this elevated demand can be reduced substantially by treatment for alcoholism; and (c) the benefits of alcoholism treatment clearly outweigh its costs.

3. There is little evidence that any one treatment approach is better than any other. There is some support for certain kinds of behaviour therapy, but the effectiveness of chemical aversion therapy and disulfiram seem to depend on patient characteristics and compliance. Several kinds of carefully specified and theoretically derived therapeutic approaches show promise as a basis for a new generation of ambulatory treatments. These include the Community Reinforcement Technique that attempts to create an environment conducive to abstinence; relapse prevention strategies that teach the alcoholic how to avoid high-risk relapse situations; and new pharmacological agents that appear to dampen the alcoholic's craving for alcohol.

4. Controlled studies have not found pronounced differences in outcome according to intensity or duration of treatment. Nevertheless, most of these studies have been conducted in the United States, where long-term institutionalization (for example, 3–36 months) typical of other countries has not been evaluated.

5. There is little support for the superiority of either inpatient or outpatient care alone. Some evidence indicates that continuing aftercare helps to maintain abstinence following short-term intensive rehabilitation in inpatient settings. Medically based inpatient rehabilitation services are far more costly than non-medical residential or outpatient treatment, but not necessarily more effective.

Evidence for aggregate-level effects Given the increasing number of problem drinkers involved in specialized treatment in many countries, it is reasonable to expect that these programmes may have a significant impact on aggregate level indicators of alcohol-related harm. For example, a recent review of specialized treatment programmes in the United States (Weisner and Morgan 1992) reported that in 1987 there were approximately 6000 identifiable units, with approximately 350 000 patients in treatment on a given day. In the former Soviet Union, where alcoholism treatment also expanded rapidly in the past two decades (Ivanets *et al.* 1992) it is estimated that more than 4.5 million alcoholics are under medical observation throughout the nation's system of outpatient dispensaries, general health clinics, and compulsory treatment facilities.

Unfortunately, there is little evidence of an aggregate-level impact of treating such large numbers of problem drinkers, in part because of the lack of reliable statistical data. Nevertheless, several researchers have identified relationships between declining liver cirrhosis rates and the growth of specialized treatment. Mann *et al.* (1988) found that decreased hospital discharges for liver cirrhosis were associated with increased treatment for alcoholism in Ontario, Canada. Similarly, research by Romelsjö (1987) suggests that in addition to decreased per capita consumption, outpatient treatment of alcoholics may have accounted for the reduction in liver cirrhosis rates in Stockholm, Sweden. In a qualitative description of aggregate statistics, Ivanets *et al.* (1992) report that as the numbers of alcoholics registered for medical observation achieved asymptote in the mid 1980s, the annual incidence of alcoholism and alcoholic psychosis declined in the former Soviet Union. The evidence from these studies is correlational and not particularly compelling in terms of the magnitude of the effects. But they do suggest that aggregate-level effects may be detectable with better reporting statistics and systematic monitoring of trends in specialized treatment. This is confirmed by a 20-year time series analysis of data from the US State of North Carolina pertaining to cirrhosis deaths, alcohol treatment, and per capita alcohol consumption (Holder and Parker 1992). The results showed that the increasing availability of alcoholism treatment over a large geographical area was associated with significant reductions in liver cirrhosis mortality. The authors suggest that: 'even if alcoholics are not cured and/or continue to relapse, the provision of treatment can produce sufficient disruption in the natural progression of the disease cirrhosis such as to delay deaths'.

Feasibility The implications of these findings for estimating the potential aggregate-level effects of treatment services in countries without a significant investment in specialized treatment are not clear. Despite the amount of treatment evaluation research conducted during the past 20 years, many of the conclusions regarding treatment efficacy must be considered tentative. Furthermore, there is little basis for determining whether treatment approaches shown to be effective in one culture will be equally effective in another. The indiscriminate transfer to health technologies and treatment concepts from one country to another may not be appropriate for several reasons. First, there may be pronounced differences in the mix of patient characteristics such as the proportion of treatment-seeking drinkers with severe psychopathology. Different services may be required for different types of patients. Secondly, culturally learned patterns of drinking, culturally mediated drinking customs, and culturally sanctioned alcohol availability, all may demand special intervention strategies and different approaches to clinical management. For these reasons, extreme caution should be exercised in any attempt to adopt or adapt treatment approaches considered effective in some of the developed countries.

The same caveat applies to the example provided by developed countries for the expansion of alcoholism treatment services. Despite the dramatic and costly expansion of the specialized treatment system, the demand for treatment services has still not been satisfied. As Hawks (1980) has suggested, this implies that even in industrialized countries the provision of adequate resources for treatment may be an unrealistic possibility. The virtual non-existence of specialized treatment facilities in developing countries makes it unlikely that investment in expensive tertiary care facilities will be an effective way to manage alcohol-related problems on an aggregate level.

Impaired driver rehabilitation programmes

The use of coercive measures to restrict access to alcohol, to punish the drinker, and to motivate sobriety has been a standard part of alcohol control policies since the 19th century. Coercion is any form of institutionalized pressure that influences a person to enter treatment involuntarily (Weisner 1990). Coercion usually involves the use of negative consequences as an alternative to treatment, and includes civil commitments by the criminal justice system, family interventions guided by a treatment provider, and workplace referrals with the threat of job sanctions. Curren *et al.* (1987) reported that 20 of 43 countries surveyed in a World Health Organization study had some type of legislation that allowed for the diversion of criminal justice offenders to some form of treatment. The most common offences are connected with driving under the influence of alcohol (DUI).

The use of education and rehabilitation as alternatives to court-imposed legal sanctions has increased steadily in many countries since the 1970s (Mäkelä *et al.* 1981). In some nations, these programmes are used in lieu of traditional punitive sanctions such as jail, fines or licence revocation. In France for example, the Centres d'Hygiène Alimentaire (CHA) receive a large proportion of their referrals from the traffic courts (Bernadou *et al.* 1981).

Evidence for causal effects In the United States, a concerted effort has been made by the National Highway Traffic Safety Administration (NHTSA) to evaluate the effectiveness of programatic sentencing alternatives. Between 1970 and 1977 the NHTSA evaluated the impact of 35 Alcohol Safety Action Projects (ASAPs) on subsequent drinking behaviour, drunken driving, and fatal crash involvement (Nichols *et al.* 1978). The ASAP programmes consisted primarily of didactic driver education classes. One-half of the sites reported positive results in terms of overall rehabilitation effectiveness. However, there was a tendency for poorly controlled evaluations to report more optimistic results than better controlled studies. In those studies examining the effects of alcohol education schools, positive outcome was reported most frequently in the participant's knowledge and attitudes. Fewer than 25 per cent of the studies found reductions in impaired driver re-arrest statistics. Social drinkers exposed to treatment had lower re-arrest rates than social drinkers not so exposed. The nature of the school programme did not seem to make a difference. Problem drinkers, on the other hand, gave no evidence of being responsive to any type of programme.

A related series of studies was conducted in California to evaluate a treatment demonstration project designed to compare the effects of several educational and counselling programmes (Reis 1983). One type of programme consisted of short-term alcohol safety education. First offenders were randomly assigned to a four-session education programme, a home study programme, or a no-treatment control group. Both the home study and the in-class education programmes were associated with lower re-arrest rates relative to the control group during the three-year period after the programme. No differences were noted in self-reported alcohol consumption and other alcohol-related indicators. These findings replicate those reported in a related study (Swenson and Clay 1980) that found no difference between the home study and in-class education methods in their ability to reduce recidivism.

Hoffmann *et al.* (1987) compared DUI arrestees who were court referred for substance abuse treatment with non-DUI and non-court-referred patients attending the same 'Minnesota Modal' outpatient treatment programmes. DUI arrestees were more likely to complete treatment and showed as much general improvement as non-DUI patients.

In general, the research indicates at best a small effect of some interventions on DUI recidivism and drinking behaviour (Wells-Parker *et al.* 1989). Recent efforts to increase the effectiveness of remedial programmes with DUI offenders have focused on better matching of clients with interventions. There is some evidence that education programmes benefit offenders with less severe alcohol problems but not offenders with more severe problems. Given these modest effects, some have argued that the use of education and rehabilitation as a DUI sanction option, while probably better than doing nothing at all, is not a suitable replacement for licensing sanctions (Hagen 1985). Nevertheless, these may be used effectively in conjunction with licensing sanctions.

Evidence for aggregate effects and feasibility There is virtually no data from any nation that suggests that individual level interventions that combine coercion, education, and treatment have a significant effect on aggregate-level prevalence. Although there has been a decline in alcohol-related traffic accidents in some countries following the implementation of impaired driver programmes, these effects cannot be separated from other measures, such as direct licence sanctions, that are likely to exert a strong influence on both driving and drinking behaviour.

Mutual help societies

The fellowship of Alcoholics Anonymous (AA) was established in 1935 in the north-eastern region of the United States. Almost 60 years later, AA has evolved into a world-wide mutual help movement with groups established in 132 countries and an estimated membership of two million recovering alcoholics (Mäkelä 1991; AA 1990). In addition to the AA, two related 'fellowships' have been developed to facilitate the involvement of the alcoholic's family and friends in the recovery process. The first is Al-Anon Family Groups, a fellowship of relatives and friends of alcoholics who provide mutual support and practical advice to families affected by another person's drinking. The second is Alateen, which sponsors weekly meetings for adolescents who consider themselves to be alcoholics. These complementary organizations have established groups in 102 countries, 70 per cent of these in the United States and Canada. Mutual help societies not affiliated with the AA have developed in France, Finland, the former Soviet Union, and a number of other countries (Klingemann *et al.* 1992). Unfortunately, these societies have not been studied to the same degree as AA.

Evidence of efficacy Sociological and psychological analyses have identified a number of ingredients that may contribute to the popularity of AA as a social movement and its apparent success as a method of maintaining sobriety (Ludwig 1988; Mäkelä 1991). For example, AA engenders crucial attitude changes and teaches effective behavioural techniques that seem to be particularly effective during the early stages of recovery. Nevertheless, there is surprisingly little scientific information about the effectiveness of AA. Baekeland (1977) reported an improvement rate of 35 per cent among members who attended at least 10 AA meetings. Smart *et al.* (1989) assumed that AA is as effective as formal treatment for alcoholics, which was estimated to be successful for 35 per cent of alcoholics.

Even with controlled studies using random assigned procedures, it is difficult to estimate the direct and unique effects of AA because of sampling problems (for example, obtaining a sample representative of the general population of alcoholics), confounding with other treatment interventions (AA members often receive conventional treatments in conjunction with AA), and difficulty in measuring the amount of 'treatment' AA members receive. AA functions not only as a unique source of recovery for an alcoholic, it also can be used as part of a formal treatment plan or as an aid in sustaining the recovery achieved through formal treatment. While AA does not consider itself to be a formal treatment modality, in the United States it plays a prominent role in the design and delivery of residential treatment programmes. This is achieved through the sponsorship of AA meetings within programmes, the arrangement of referrals to AA following discharge from treatment, the use of AA members as alcoholism counsellors, and the incorporation of the Twleve-Step philosophy, methods, and materials into the daily routine of treatment programmes (Institute of Medicine 1990).

Evidence of aggregate effects Given the ability of AA to involve large numbers of problem drinkers and their family members in its group meetings, it is reasonable to ask about its impact on the prevalence of heavy drinking and alcohol-related problems in communities and nations. As with other individual-level interventions, the impact of AA is difficult to estimate. Reliable data on the medical problems and drinking habits of AA affiliates are lacking and there is a dearth of systematic evaluation research concerning its efficacy in promoting sobriety among alcohol-dependent persons. Furthermore, the AA philosophy and fellowship activities have become closely linked to the specialized treatment system in countries like the United States and Canada (Weisner and Morgan 1992). It is likely that if AA is as effective as other forms of intervention for alcoholics, then its impact on morbidity and mortality would depend on the number of alcoholics actively involved in its programmes. According to AA Headquarters, there were 46 400 groups in the United States in 1990. Membership is estimated to be approximately one million. Active members attend meetings with equal or greater frequency than standard outpatient treatment (once per week). In Canada, AA membership in 1983 was estimated to be 75 per cent of the number of patients treated for alcohol problems in health care facilities. To the extent that AA groups are more numerous than outpatient treatment, they may constitute a significant resource for drinkers who are attempting to stop drinking.

According to the most recent survey of US and Canadian affiliates (AA 1990), the majority of members (66 per cent) are men between 31 and 50 years of age, and most (60 per cent) have had prior counselling. This demographic profile is consistent with that of alcoholics involved in specialized treatment.

Smart and colleagues (Smart *et al.* 1989; Smart and Mann 1990; Mann *et al.* 1991) studied longitudinal trends as well as geographical differences in AA membership in relation to cirrhosis rates and alcohol-related problems in Canada. Increased AA membership was not associated with decreases in cirrhosis rates, nor was there a simple relationship with drinking-driving offences and Liquor Act offences. A decline in drinking-driving convictions was associated with increased AA membership, but this occurred only at higher levels of per capita consumption increases. The data suggest that the impact of AA on morbidity and mortality may be affected by the type of drinker typically attracted to AA in a given country, as well as the kinds of drinkers who are coerced to attend. To the extent that AA attracts socially stable binge drinkers in the Anglo-Saxon countries, it may not influence cirrhosis rates. In addition, when large numbers of drinking-driver offenders are referred to AA, increased membership may be related to reduced recidivism and lower conviction rates.

Although there was no clear evidence for an association between AA membership and cirrhosis rates in the Canadian data, a subsequent study using US data (Mann *et al.* 1991) showed that changes in cirrhosis mortality rates were positively associated with changes in per capita consumption and negatively associated with AA membership.

In a study undertaken primarily for heuristic purposes, Smart and Mann (1990) attempted to account for recent declines in cirrhosis mortality in the United States and Canada. Based on estimates of the effectiveness of formal treatment and AA, as well as the likelihood of alcoholics developing cirrhosis, they concluded that increased treatment and AA membership could have accounted for a substantial proportion of the reductions in cirrhosis deaths and hospital discharges in Ontario and the United States between 1975 and 1982. Although it cannot be assumed that these relationships are causal, the implication is that with greater availability of treatment and AA, alcoholic cirrhosis could be reduced significantly.

Feasibility What are the potential contributions of AA to the reduction of morbidity and mortality in relation to the barriers that must be overcome to achieve maximum impact of its services? Mann *et al.* (1991) estimate that a 1 per cent increase in AA membership could result in a 0.06 per cent decrease in cirrhosis mortality. They conclude (p. 364) that 'large increases in AA membership would be necessary to justify an expectation of substantially reduced cirrhosis deaths'. Nevertheless, the impact of AA is not likely to be limited to cirrhosis mortality. Small reductions in cirrhosis mortality may be accompanied by comparable or greater changes in other alcohol-related problems, and this additive effect may well justify policies that encourage AA membership.

It must be emphasized that without a clear estimate of its total and specific impact in countries like the United States and Canada where AA is well established, it is virtually impossible to estimate its potential influence elsewhere in the world. Indeed, as Mäkelä (1991) had found, AA typically emerges in non-socialist, non-Islamic countries that have relatively high standards of living. The growth and strength of AA vary with socio-economic factors, per capita alcohol consumption, and religious beliefs. AA has grown faster in Catholic countries in recent years. Beer consumption is positively correlated with the strength of AA while wine consumption is negatively correlated. The strength of AA is greatest in the United States, Canada, Finland, Germany, Costa Rica, El Salvador, Honduras, Mexico, and Nicaragua. The movement has shown considerable growth in Eastern Europe and the former Soviet Union since the dissolution of communist governments in those countries.

Summing the evidence

Marked changes have occurred during the past century in life-expectancy as well as the disease patterns affecting the populations of both the industrialized and developing nations. Substantial improvements in life-expectancy have resulted primarily from achievements in infectious disease prevention and general improvements in public health (Amler and Dull 1987). The major causes of death in most Western and industrialized countries are no longer infectious diseases like tuberculosis, dysentery, smallpox, and diphtheria, but chronic diseases and violent deaths. An important lesson for the present analysis of alcohol problems is that the control of infectious diseases has resulted less from breakthrough cures than from intervention against precursors of fatal disease that could be eliminated or reduced with existing technology (Amler and Eddins 1987).

This chapter has reviewed a variety of individual level interventions designed to provide humane care, medical/psychiatric treatment, secondary prevention, and long-term rehabilitation to persons with alcohol-related problems. During the 20th century, and particularly in the last two decades, various combinations of these interventions have developed into service networks, called treatment systems, in a large number of countries (Klingemann *et al.* 1992). As summarized in Table 7.1, the interventions range from brief counselling in primary care settings to specialized treatment in hospitals and clinics. Each intervention tends to have a particular target group and a specific alcohol-related problem as its primary focus, although some interventions, like occupational programmes, are addressed at several types of alcohol problems.

The research findings indicate mixed evidence for efficacy of these interventions. Efficacy has not been defined consistently across studies. At times, it refers to abstinence, at times to reduced alcohol consumption, at other times to reduced alcohol-related problems. This lack of consistency reflects the different functions of these interventions, which cannot be evaluated against a common criterion of effectiveness. As Hunt *et al.* (1992) have noted, some programmes are designed to cure alcoholics, others to care for them, and still others to control their behaviour. Not all interventions would therefore be expected to have a direct impact on morbidity and mortality. Despite this diversity of purpose, it is nevertheless possible to provide an admittedly crude estimate of the extent to which these interventions are capable of achieving their objectives. As shown in Table 7.1, brief counselling with heavy drinkers shows the most evidence of efficacy, while mutual help programmes have the least empirical support. It should be noted that the lack of causal evidence may be attributable as much to the difficulty of conducting well-controlled evaluation studies as to the inconclusiveness of existing research.

Assuming that most of these interventions have at least some evidence of efficacy, there is considerably less evidence about the aggregate level impact of these programmes. Ironically, interventions directed at the treatment of alcohol dependence and chronic alcoholism (specialized treatment and AA) are the only programmes that have demonstrated an impact at the aggregate level. This may be due to the low density of other interventions in most countries, and to the lack of systematic research.

The final column in Table 7.1 describes the feasibility of these interventions

Table 7.1 Causal evidence, aggregate-level evidence, and potential feasibility regarding individual-level interventions

Intervention	Target group	Problem	Causal evidence	Aggregate evidence	Potential feasibility
Brief counselling	Primary care patients	Hazardous drinking	++	?	++
Prenatal counselling	Pregnant women who drink heavily	Fetal alcohol effects	+/?	?	+
Drinking-driver programmes	Impaired drivers	Accidents, injuries	+/?	?	+
Server intervention	Heavy drinkers	Acute intoxication	+/?	?	+
Occupational programmes	Problem drinking employees	Impaired work performance	?	?	+
Specialized treatment	Alcoholics, problem drinkers	Alcohol dependence, Alcoholm problems	+	+	+/?
Mutual help	Alcoholics	Chronic alcoholism	?	+	+

++, good; +, minimal; ?, questionable or not known.

as methods for reducing the prevalence of alcohol-related morbidity and mortality. As with the ratings of evidence, these ratings must be qualified in relation to their cross-national generalizability. For example, the feasibility of many of these interventions depends on the economic development of the country, the organization of health care, the type of alcohol problems, the cost of delivering the intervention to the target group, and the nation's political commitment to treatment interventions. Applying these criteria, most nations, particularly developing countries, could support screening and brief interventions in primary care and occupational settings. In addition, most governments could facilitate the development of mutual help societies, which may influence the prevalence of liver cirrhosis and other consequences of chronic drinking. Although specialized treatment demonstrates evidence of efficacy and is feasible in developed countries, it may not be the best way to allocate scarce resources unless the ingredients of a public health approach have first been put into place.

As a general policy recommendation, this review supports the development of strategies that take into account the traditional public health model of disease prevention. An important ingredient of that model consists of individual level interventions based on population screening for disease detection and risk factors (Safer 1986; Amler and Eddins 1987). It has been estimated that early detection, immunization, and other health promotion efforts in the United States could prevent or delay the onset of 23 per cent of cancer cases, 45 per cent of cardiovascular deaths, and 50 per cent of the complications of diabetes (Amler and Dull 1987). Although the benefits of immunization and screening tests are widely accepted, the potential advantages of applying behavioural change efforts to the reduction of alcohol problems are less clear.

Screening programmes are likely to be successful when the risk factors for an illness are well understood, its aetiology has been precisely identified, screening tests are accurate and available, and treatment interventions are effective. Estimating the relevance of a public health approach is much more difficult when the concepts of preventive medicine are applied to the broad range of diseases, disorders, and social problems that are associated with the misuse of beverage alcohol. Nevertheless, the number of health and social problems connected with drinking, and the concentration of multiple problems in the same drinker, may make individual-level interventions cost-effective. But without clear evidence of a direct relationship between the cost, intensity, and effectiveness of services, it would seem inadvisable to recommend specialized and labour-intensive interventions when scarce resources might be allocated to less expensive alternatives.

One approach that is supported by a growing amount of research evidence is to emphasize secondary prevention and early intervention where some investment in health services is indicated. As recommended in a WHO Expert Committee report (WHO 1980), 'further investment in treatment should be concentrated on developing inexpensive and cost-effective services'. These services should be targeted at high-risk groups and designated to fit the specific needs of these populations (Hawks 1980). For example, the concentration of heavy drinking within the shanty towns surrounding large urban centres in developing countries suggests that alcohol treatment resources might be focused on emergency services and primary care clinics where large numbers of problem drinkers are likely to be encountered. Another area for the expansion of services is the development of low-cost social support networks that rely on volunteer help using trained para-professionals or recovering patients who are motivated to help others. AA stands as the model for such services, but other examples of effective self-help techniques should be considered.

Because of the competition for health resources and the shortage of trained professional staff, emphasis might be given to the integration of treatment interventions with the existing primary care systems in both developed and developing countries. According to Hawks (1980), the planning of treatment in developing countries must be relevant to the setting in which it is carried out. It must acknowledge the constraints of the situation, especially the absence of specialized staff and in-patient facilities. Treatment cannot be highly technical, sophisticated, or time-consuming. A nucleus of alcoholism specialists may be needed, however, if only to supervise the training of primary health care workers.

In summary, creation of a separate health care delivery system for the management of alcohol-related problems is neither feasible nor practical for most countries. A highly structured, geographically oriented public health, and primary care delivery system is often in place in these countries. By integrating brief intervention and specialized treatment into these existing structures, large numbers of problem drinkers may be identified and treated without placing serious demands on resources and personnel.

This approach may also be relevant to the developed nations that have already established a specialized treatment system. A study by Drummond *et al.* (1990) found that after an initial detailed assessment and advice session, the treatment provided by general practitioners is at least as effective as that from a specialist clinic with respect to improvements in drinking behaviour and alcohol-related problems.

Future directions

There is a pervasive tendency to make global distinctions that limit the purview of certain kinds of policy analyses. The distinction between alcoholism and social drinking limits the analysis of treatment policy to considerations of extreme cases. The distinction between treatment and prevention limits the analysis of prevention policy to discussions of population-level interventions that are implemented through structural and normative changes rather than programmes directed at individuals. And distinctions between public health, clinical medicine, and legal coercion limit the consideration of common pathways to improve the health of the general population.

Although the evidence is far from compelling, studies conducted in Sweden (Romelsjö 1987), Canada, and the United States (Mann *et al.* 1988; Smart *et al.* 1989) suggest that the combination of population-based policies (for example, reduced per capita consumption through increased taxes) and individual-based interventions (for example, AA, formal treatment) can each make significant contributions to reduced morbidity and mortality. The potential benefit of this approach is in synergistic effects: changes made by individuals are supported by concomitant changes in the social and physical environment. This is based on the recognition that most risk factors for alcohol problems are linked to life style behaviours that are supported by the general culture.

Beyond the integration of individual-level interventions within a broader preventive strategy, there is a critical need for a greater investment in evaluation research. Although evidence for causal and aggregate level effects is inadequate, this review has shown that existing research technologies are capable of providing policy-relevant information. Without a greater investment in demonstration programmes and well-controlled evaluations, policy-makers will continue to allocate scarce resources without a sound scientific basis.

Acknowledgements

The writing of this paper was supported in part by a grant from the US National Institute on Alcohol Abuse and Alcoholism (2 P50 AA03510).

References

AA (Alcoholic Anonymous World Headquarters) (1990). *1989 membership survey*. AA World Services, New York.

Amler, R. W. and Dull, H. B. (eds) (1987). *Closing the gap: The burden of unnecessary illness*. Oxford University Press.

Amler, R. W. and Eddins, D. L. (1987). Cross-sectional analysis: Precursors of premature death in the United States. In *Closing the gap: The burden of unnecessary illness*, (eds R. W. Amler and H. B. Dull), pp. 181–7. Oxford University Press.

Anderson, P. and Scott, E. (1992). Randomized controlled trial of general practitioner intervention in men with excessive alcohol consumption. *British Journal of Addiction*, **87**, 891–900.

Antti-Pika, I., Karaharju, E., Roine, R., and Salaspuro, M. (1988). Intervention of heavy drinking—A prospective and controlled study of 438 consecutive injured male patients. *Alcohol and Alcoholism*, **23**, 115–21.

Babor, T. F. (1994) Avoiding the horrid and beastley sin of drunkeness: Does dissuasion make a difference? *Journal of Consulting and Clinical Psychology*, **62**(6), 1127–40.

Babor, T. F. and Grant, M. (1992). *Project on identification and management of alcohol-related problems. Report on Phase II: A randomized clinical trial of brief interventions in primary health care.* World Health Organization, Geneva.

Babor, T. F., Treffardier, M., Weill, J., Fegueur, L., and Ferrant, J. P. (1983). The early detection and secondary prevention of alcoholism in France. *Journal of Studies on Alcohol*, **44**, 600–16.

Babor, T. F., Ritson, E. B., and Hodgson, R. J. (1986). Alcohol-related problems in the primary health care setting: A review of early intervention strategies. *British Journal of Addiction*, **81**, 23–46.

Babor, T. F., Kranzler, H. R., Lauerman, R. J. (1987). Social drinking as a health and psychosocial risk factor, Anstie's limited revisited. *Recent developments in alcoholism*, (ed. M. Galanter), Vol. 5, pp. 373–402. Plenum, New York.

Baekeland, F. (1977). Evaluation of treatment methods in chronic alcoholism. In *Treatment and rehabilitation of the chronic alcoholic*, (ed. B. Kissen and H. Begleiter), pp. 385–440. Plenum, New York.

Bernadou, M., *et al.* (1981). Enquête sur les CHA. *Alcool ou Santé*, **157**, 21–4.

Bien, T. H., William, R., and Tonigan, S. (1993). Brief interventions for alcohol problems: a review. *Addiction*, **88**, 315–36.

Chick, J. (1984). Secondary prevention of alcoholism and the Centres d'Hygiene Alimentaire. *British Journal of Addiction*, **79**, 221–5.

Chick, J., Lloyd, G., and Crombie, E. (1985). Counselling problem drinkers in medical wards: A controlled study. *British Medical Journal*, **290**, 965–7.

Curran, W. J., Arif, A. E., and Jayasuriya, D. C. (1987). *Guidelines for assessing and revising national legislation on treatment of drug and alcohol-dependent persons.* World Health Organization, Geneva.

Den Hartog, G. L. (1982). *A decade of detox: Development of non-hospital approaches to alcohol detoxification—A review of the literature.* Substance Abuse Monograph Series. Division of Alcohol and Drug Abuse, Jefferson City, MO.

Drummond, D. C., Thom, B., Brown, C., Edwards, G., and Mullan, M. J. (1990). Specialist versus general practitioner treatment of problem drinkers. *Lancet*, **336**, 915–18.

Hagen, R. E. (1985). Evaluation of the effectiveness of educational and rehabilitation efforts: Opportunities for research. *Journal of Studies on Alcohol*, **46** (Suppl. 10), 179–83.

Hawks, D. V. (1980). The meaning of treatment services for alcohol-related problems' in developing countries. In *Alcoholism treatment in transition*, (ed. G. Edwards and M. Grant), pp. 199–204. University Park Press, Baltimore.

Hoffmann, N., Ninonueve, F., Mozey, J., and Luxenberg, M. (1987). Comparison of court-referred DWI arrestees with other outpatients in substance abuse treatment. *Journal of Studies on Alcohol*, **48**, 591–4.

Holder, H. and Parker, R. N. (1992). Effect of alcoholism treatment on cirrhosis mortality: a 20-year multivariate time series analysis. *British Journal of Addiction*, **87**, 1263–74.

Holder, H., Longabaugh, T., Miller, W. R., and Rubonis, A. V. (1991). The cost effectiveness of treatment for alcoholism: A first approximation. *Journal of Studies on Alcohol*, **52**, 517–40.

Hunt, G., Klingemann, H., and Takala, J. P. (1992). Introduction. In *Cure, care, or control. Alcoholism treatment in sixteen countries*, (ed. H. Klingemann, J. P. Takala, and G. Hunt), pp. 1–7. State University of New York, Albany, NY.

Ivanets, N. N, Anokhina, I. P., Egorov, V. F., Valentik, Y. V., and Shesterneva, S. B. (1992). *Cure, care or control. Alcoholism treatment in sixteen countries*, (ed. H. Klingemann, J. P. Takala, and G. Hunt), pp. 9–22. State University of New York, Albany, NY.

Institute of Medicine (1979). *Healthy people: The Surgeon General's report on health promotion and disease prevention: Background papers*. Department of Health, Education and Welfare, (Public Health Service) (DHEW (PHS)) Publication No. 79-55071A, Washington, DC.

Institute of Medicine (1990). *Broadening the base of treatment for alcohol problems*. National Academy Press, Washington, DC.

Keller, M. (1986). The old and new in the treatment of alcoholism. In *Alcohol interventions*, (ed. D. L. Strug, S. Priyadarsini, and M. M. Hyman), pp. 23–40. Haworth, New York.

Klingemann, H., Takala, J. P., and Hunt, G. (ed.) (1992). *Cure, care, or control. Alcoholism treatment in sixteen countries*. State University of New York, Albany, NY.

Kreitman, N. (1986). Alcohol consumption and the preventive paradox. *British Journal of Addiction*, **81**, 353–63.

Kristenson, H., Trell, E., and Hood, B. (1982). Serum of glutamyl-transferase in screening and continuous control of heavy drinking in middle-aged men. *American Journal of Epidemiology*, **114**, 862–72.

Kristenson, H., Ohlin, H., Hulten-Nosslin, M., Trell, E., and Hood, B. (1983). Identification and intervention of heavy drinkers in middle-aged men: Results and follow-up of 24–60 months of long-term study with randomized controls. *Alcoholism: Clinical and Experimental Research*, **7**, 203–9.

Larsson, G. (1983). Prevention of fetal alcohol effects: An antenatal program for early detection of pregnancies at risk. *Acta Obstetrica et Gynaecologica Scandinavica*, **62**, 171–8.

LeGo, P. M. (1968). Le depistage précoce de l'ethylisme. *Presse Médicale*, **76**, 579–80.

LeGo, P. M. (1977). *Le depistage précoce et systématique du buveur excessif.* Riom Laboratoires, France.

Ludwig, A. M. (1988). *Understanding the alcoholic's mind: The nature of craving and how to control it*. Oxford University Press, New York.

Mäkelä, K., Room, R., Single, R., Sulkunen, P., and Walsh, B. (1981). *Alcohol, society and the state*, Vol. 1. Addiction Research Foundation, Toronto.

Mäkelä, K. (1991). Social and cultural preconditions of Alcoholics Anonymous (AA) and factors associated with the strength of AA. *British Journal of Addiction*, **86**, 1405–13.

Mann, R. E., Smart, R., Anglin, L., and Rush, B. (1988). Are decreases in liver cirrhosis rates a result of increased treatment for alcoholism. *British Journal of Addiction*, **83**, 683–8.

Mann, R. E., Smart, R., Anglin, L., and Adlaf, E. (1991). Reductions in cirrhosis deaths in the United States: Associations with per capita consumption and AA membership. *Journal of Studies on Alcohol*, **52**, 361–5.

McIntosh, I. D. (1982). Alcohol-related disabilities in general hospital patients: A critical assessment of the evidence. *International Journal of the Addictions*, **17**, 609–39.

Miller, W. R. and Hester, R. K. (1986). Matching problem drinkers with optimal treatments. *Treating addictive behaviors: Processes of change*, (ed. W. R. Miller and N. Heather), pp. 175–203. Plenum, New York.

Miller, W. R. and Munoz, R. F. (1976). *How to control your drinking*. Prentice-Hall, Englewood Cliffs, NJ.

Miller, W. R. and Taylor, C. A. (1980). Relative effectiveness of bioliotherapy, individual and group self-control training in the treatment of problem drinkers. *Addictive Behaviors*, **5**, 13–24.

Moore, M. H. and Gerstein, D. R. (ed.) (1981). Panel on alternative policies affecting the prevention of alcohol abuse and alcoholism. *Alcohol and public policy: Beyond the shadow of prohibition*, pp. 16–47. National Academy Press, Washington, DC.

Moser, J. (1974). *Problems and programmes related to alcohol and drug dependence in 33 countries*. WHO Offset Publication No. 6. World Health Organization, Geneva.

Moser, J. (ed.) (1985). *Alcohol policies in national health and development planning*, Report No. 89. World Health Organization, Geneva.

Nichols, J. L., Weinstein, E. B., Ellingstad, V. S., and Struckman-Johnson, D. L. (1978). The specific deterrent effect of ASAP education and rehabilitation programs. *Journal of Safety Research*, **10**, 177–87.

Nilssen, O. (1991). The Tromso Study: Identification of and a controlled intervention on a population of early-stage risk drinkers. *Preventive Medicine*. **20**, 518–28.

Reis, R. E. (1983). The findings of the comprehensive driving under the influence of alcohol offender treatment demonstration project. *Abstracts and Reviews in Alcohol and Driving*, **4**, 10–16.

Roman, P. M. (1981). From employee alcoholism to employee assistance; deemphases on prevention and alcohol problems in work-based programs. *Journal of Studies on Alcohol*, **42**, 244–72.

Roman, P. M. and Gilbert, P. J. (1979). Alcohol abuse in the US and the USSR: Divergence and convergence in policy and ideology. *Social Psychiatry* **14**, 207–16.

Romelsjö, A. (1987). Decline in alcohol-related in-patient care and mortality in Stockholm County. *British Journal of Addiction*, **82**, 653–63.

Rosett, H. L., Weiner, L., and Edelin, K. C. (1983). Treatment experience with pregnant problem drinkers. *Journal of the American Medical Association*, **249**, 2029–33.

Safer, M. A. (1986). A comparison of screening for disease detection and screening for risk factors. *Health Education Research: Theory and Practice*, **1**, 131–8.

Schorling, J. B. (1993). The prevention of prenatal alcohol use: A critical analysis of intervention studies. *Journal of Studies on Alcohol*, **54**, 261–7.

Scott, E. and Anderson, P. (1990). Randomized controlled trial of general practitioner intervention in women with excessive alcohol consumption. *Australian Drug and Alcohol Review*, **10**, 311–22.

Smart, R. and Mann, R. E. (1990). Are increases in treatment levels and Alcoholics Anonymous membership large enough to reduce liver cirrhosis rates? *British Journal of Addiction*, **85**, 1291–8.

Smart, R., Mann, R. E., and Anglin, L. (1989). Decreases in alcohol problems and increased Alcoholics Anonymous membership. *British Journal of Addiction*, **84**, 507–13.

Stoudemire, A., Wallack, L., and Hedemark, N. (1987). Alcohol dependence and abuse. *Closing the gap: The burden of unnecessary illness*, (ed. R. W. Amler and H. B. Dull), pp. 9–18. Oxford University Press.

Swenson, P. R. and Clay, T. R. (1980). Effects of short-term rehabilitation on alcohol consumption and drinking-related behaviors: An eight-month follow-up study of drunken drivers. *International Journal of the Addictions*, **15**, 821–38.

Walker, K. and Shain, M. (1983). Employee assistance programming: In search of effective interventions for the problem-drinking employee. *British Journal of Addiction*, **78**, 291–303.

Wallace, P, Cutler, S., and Haines, A. (1988). Randomised controlled trial of general practitioner intervention in patients with excessive alcohol consumption. *British Medical Journal*, **297**, 663–8.

Weisner, C. (1990). Coercion in alcohol treatment. Institute of Medicine. In *Broadening the base of treatment for alcohol problems*, pp. 579–609. National Academy Press, Washington, DC.

Weisner, C. and Morgan, P. (1992). Rapid growth and bifurcation: Public and private alcohol treatment in the United States. In *Cure, care, or control. Alcoholism treatment in sixteen countries*, (ed. H. Klingemann, J. P. Takala, and G. Hunt), pp. 223–52. State University of New York, Albany, NY.

Wells-Parker, E., Anderson, B. J., Landrum, J. W., and Snow, R. W. (1988). Long-term effectiveness of probation, short-term intervention and LAI administration for reducing DUI recidivism. *British Journal of Addiction*, **83**, 415–21.

Wells-Parker, E., Anderson, B. J., McMillen, D. L., and Landrum, J. W. (1989). Interactions among DUI offender characteristics and traditional intervention modalities: a long-term recidivism follow-up *British Journal of Addiction*, **84**, 381–90.

WHO (World Health Organization Expert Committee) (1980). *Problems related to alcohol consumption*. WHO Technical Report Series 650. World Health Organization, Geneva.

8. Public discourse on alcohol: implications for public policy

Sally Casswell

Introduction

Public discourse concerning alcohol, especially that taking place in the mass media, has become the topic of considerable research attention in the past few decades. Although the mass media have long been channels for public discourse on alcohol, the 1970s and 1980s have seen major changes in its nature and pervasiveness, due in part to developments in the broadcast media. It is probable that communications in the mass media have become a significant influence on the shaping of public consciousness around alcohol issues with consequent implications for the development and implementation of alcohol policies.

This chapter reviews research which has investigated public discourse on alcohol during the past few decades. The questions covered are: What is the nature of public discourse about alcohol policies and drinking and what is the impact of this public discourse particularly in relation to the social climate surrounding alcohol use and the process of policy development?

The nature of public discourse on alcohol and drinking has, for the purposes of this discussion, been broadly categorized into five areas. The first area covered is the portrayal of alcohol in entertainment material; second, advertising of alcohol products by the producers and distributors; third, educational campaigns using the media; fourth, coverage in news media; and fifth, academic discourse. No attempt is made to review all the research which is germane to these five aspects of public discourse. Rather, illustrative examples and reviews are cited.

The key players in this public discourse include the vested interest groups: the media, advertising and sports industries, as well as the producers and distributors of alcohol. It may also include citizen organizations; local, regional, and national governments; national and international alcohol agencies; public health advocates, researchers; and the general public. Each of these groups have particular perspectives and information which they enter into the public debate. There is undoubtedly a complex and interdependent relationship between public discourse and public consciousness about drinking and alcohol policies. This chapter briefly describes the way researchers and commentators in the past few decades have researched and described the relationship.

Changes in the technology and economics of the mass media

The decades of the 1970s and 1980s have seen many dramatic changes in the mass media. The most apparent change has been the growing pervasiveness of television watching. In the United States, the number of homes with television sets doubled from 1954 to 1964, rising from 56 to 92 per cent; by the 1980s a television set was switched on in the average US home for seven hours every day (Gitlin 1983). Similarly in the United Kingdom television occupied between 30 and 40 per cent of most people's available free time and was their major source of information and entertainment (Garnham 1990). An average Australian's use of television, at 29.5 hours per week, has been contrasted with the time spent reading, an average of 19 minutes per week (Saunders 1993). The use of satellites to broadcast television across national boundaries has exposed many parts of the world to foreign-made programmes, particularly those originating from the United States. Even in those developing countries which have not yet established television stations and where television sets are rare, communal viewings of video recordings of television programmes are a regular event.

Technological developments in television have been accompanied by changes in ownership. Industrial consolidation has led to the ownership of television stations (and other media) by industrial conglomerates, as just one of many profit-making opportunities (Gerbner 1990). The objectives of the mass media are not only to entertain, persuade, and inform but also to make a profit (Atkin and Arkin 1990). The increasing reliance on advertising revenue and a reduction in resources for public sector broadcasting (Rowland and Tracey 1988) has encouraged the public health sector and governments to look to the commercial sector to broadcast educational messages and they, in a climate of public concern over alcohol problems, have been willing to do so (DeJong *et al.* 1992). As a consequence, the distinction between commercial advertising of alcohol and public health messages has become somewhat blurred in some countries (Mosher and Jernigan 1989; Comiti 1990).

The reliance on advertising revenue and the consequent need for a mass audience have also contributed to an increased emphasis on entertainment material in the mass media. Entertainment programmes proliferate and television movies have replaced network documentaries in the United States (Montgomery 1990). Entertainment material, particularly on television, has therefore become a significant vehicle for the portrayal of alcohol and a considerable amount of research effort in the 1970s and 1980s has been devoted to its description and analysis.

The nature of the public discourse on alcohol

Portrayal of alcohol in entertainment material

Research analysing the portrayal of alcohol in television has usually (although not exclusively, for example, see Heilbronn 1988) been framed in terms of its potential impact on drinking and alcohol-related problems and has looked at the frequency of portrayals and the consequences of drinking. Other media: film, novels, music, and magazines, have more often been analysed as indicators of cultural beliefs (for example, Beckley and Chalfant 1979; Paakkanen 1982; Falk and Sulkunen 1983; Heiskala 1988).

US television entertainment programmes have received most research attention, and content analyses carried out in the 1980s provide a consistent picture of frequent use of alcohol in positive social contexts. Refusals to drink were few and far between. The portrayal of intoxication or other negative consequences of drinking was rare. Regular characters suffered the consequences of heavy drinking less often than non-regulars, and stars seemed to be given near immunity (Partanen and Montonen 1988). Alcohol beverages were shown being consumed far more often than non-alcohol beverages, a pattern which is the reverse of daily life (Signorielli 1990). British television also portrays alcohol use very frequently with very little portrayal of negative consequences of drinking (Hansen 1988). In both the United States and United Kingdom television programmes, drinking tends to be an incidental, background feature whereas in Finnish television alcohol tends to be in the foreground and negative consequences of drinking are often shown (Montonen 1989). Swedish television was similar to US programmes in the frequent portrayal of drinking with relatively few negative consequences but was nevertheless described as more negative in tone than US programming (Nowak 1986, cited in Partanen and Montonen 1988).

The frequency of drinking scenes on US television increased dramatically through the 1970s until the mid 1980s (Signorielli 1987; Wallack *et al.* 1990). However, in both the United States and the United Kingdom there has been a decline in the frequency of portrayal of alcohol use after 1984 (Wallack *et al.* 1990; Pendleton, *et al.* 1991). But although Wallack *et al.* (1990) found that the portrayal of drinking on prime time television had gone down in the mid to late 1980s there was little substantive change in the nature of its portrayal: 'when problems do occur, they are treated at the individual level, factors external to the individual that are important to the prevention and treatment of alcohol problems are seldom addressed, and the community aspects of alcohol issues are rarely explored'.

Concern in the United States over the possible cumulative effects of the portrayal of alcohol in entertainment material has led researchers and public health advocates to engage in collaborative efforts with media personnel to influence the portrayal of alcohol in entertainment material (Breed and De Foe 1982; DeJong and Winsten 1990).

Alcohol advertising

Advertising is a significant aspect of communication about alcohol. World-wide expenditure on advertising rose sixfold from the mid 1960s to the mid 1980s and alcohol, one of the world's largest advertising categories, reached US$3 billion world-wide (Clark 1988).

Advertising for all products in the 1970s and 1980s became less product-oriented and more directed towards people's desires and dreams. Alcohol was no exception; it has been described as the 'supreme image product' (Clark 1988). In the words of a consultant psychologist to the alcohol industry writing in the 1980s:

> More and more it seems the liquor industry has awakened to the truth. It isn't selling bottles or glasses or even liquor. It's selling fantasies. Lifestyle approaches have come into favour as the most effective way for the liquor industry to promote its wares. Psychologically, for consumers to be attracted to these ads, they need to be attracted to the people in them, to identify with the fantasies they create (Nathanson-Moog 1984).

There has been considerable research analysis and description of the themes of alcohol advertising. Relatively large-scale content analyses of US alcohol advertisements in magazines and on television have been carried out (Atkin and Block 1981; Breed and De Foe 1979; De Foe and Breed 1979; Finn and Strickland 1982). Partanen and Montonen (1988), in their review of advertising messages, describe the most dominant theme as an indirect appeal associating the drink in question with a desired outcome, frequently a life style suggesting wealth, prestige, success, or social approval. Drinking is depicted as a normal and desirable part of life. The brand becomes symbolically invested with the positive attributes of the life style itself.

Advertising gains much of its power from the culture's shared myths. For example, in cultures like the United States, Australia, and New Zealand, where the myth of the frontier—of physical challenge and risk-taking—is powerful, beer advertising gains by association. Even if the frontier is closed to most men, they may still re-enact this myth and demonstrate their masculinity through the ritual of beer-drinking (Postman *et al.* 1988; Wyllie *et al.* 1989). Content analyses which have ignored the cultural meaning of the messages and focused only on observable measures, such as the presence or absence of under-age people on the screen, have been criticized for their superficial nature (Strate 1991; Thorson in press; Saunders and Yap 1991).

The themes of alcohol advertising are similar to the themes of alcohol portrayal in Anglo-American entertainment material. Indeed, the boundaries between the two have become somewhat blurred through practices such as product sampling in which corporations provide film studios with free products to use as props (Herd 1983). Indirect advertising has also been described on Finnish television (Montonen 1985, cited in Partanen and Montonen 1988). Placing goods, including alcohol products, in television programmes and movies began as an organized business in the United States in the late 1970s. By the mid 1980s there were about 30 companies operating in Hollywood (Clark 1988). Not only the product's presence on screen but the way in which it was presented was controlled: 'the beer being promoted will be drunk by the hero; the villain will drink another brand' (Clark 1988).

One of advertising's functions in large marketplaces is to differentiate brands (which in reality are often virtually identical in terms of taste, colour, and alcohol content so as to appeal to different sectors of the market). Research carried out on behalf of the beer industry has identified different personality types, including problematic alcohol users, to whom different brands appealed (Ackoff and Emshoff 1975) and content analyses have identified advertising apparently targeted at heavy users, women, youth, and ethnic minorities (Jacobsen *et al.* 1983; Clark 1988).

While most of the research describing and analysing alcohol advertising has come from industrialized countries it has been observed that in many developing countries alcohol products are advertised using whatever media are available. In countries without well-developed communication systems sponsorship of sporting and cultural events is a frequent form of advertising (for example, Sinclair 1983; Casswell 1986).

Sponsorship by the alcohol industry is a form of advertising also widely employed in industrialized countries, sometimes as a way of circumventing restrictions on alcohol advertising (for example, Casswell *et al.* 1989). Even when direct advertising of alcohol brands is possible, sponsorship has the added advantage of improving the corporate image of the industry.

Many countries have restrictions on alcohol advertising. Several countries, particularly those with governmental-monopoly retail sales of alcohol, have partial bans on alcohol advertising. For example, Sweden prohibits advertising of medium- and high-alcohol beer and there is a voluntary ban in the United States on distilled spirits advertising on television.

Media education campaigns

Educational messages using mass and local media have a long history in the prevention of alcohol-related problems. The temperance movement made extensive use of newspapers and posters to communicate a message of moderation (Wallack 1981).

Developments in the broadcast mass media provided attractive channels for campaigns aiming to educate the public about alcohol use and these contributed to the public discourse on alcohol in many countries in the 1970s and 1980s. They have been a major focus of efforts to prevent alcohol-related problems. Their popularity has been rivalled only by school-based education; both strategies are popular in part because of their easily accessed audience.

Whereas, early mass media campaigns often relied on brief, unco-ordinated efforts utilizing single media channels, the 1980s saw a greater emphasis on 'an integrated series of communication activities, using multiple operations and channels, aimed at populations and target audiences, usually of long duration with a clear purpose' (Flay and Burton 1990). A further defining characteristic of an educational campaign is the predominantly one-way nature of the communication: 'A public information campaign seems to represent someone's intention to influence someone else's beliefs or behaviour using communicated appeals' (Paisley 1981).

Many of the mass media campaigns which have been described in the alcohol problem prevention literature in the 1970s and 1980s have had a moderation theme. Moderation tends to be left ill-defined but generally connotes limits on the quantity of alcohol consumed in a drinking session and less clearly limits on the frequency of drinking occasions (but some contexts are seen as inappropriate). Moderation generally implies normalized drinking of alcohol in social situations, without adverse consequences. Development of the moderation theme was in keeping with the sociocultural model of alcohol problem prevention popular in the 1960s and 1970s which looked for reduction of harm associated with alcohol use by an integration of alcohol into everyday life, accompanied by more education about what were appropriate ways of drinking (Room 1989). Also supporting moderation education, the latter part of the 1970s and 1980s has seen a popularization of the concept of a healthy life style to prevent ill health (Lalonde 1974; USDHEW 1979) and alcohol use along with tobacco, exercise, and diet has been a focus of general healthy life style education and health-promotion efforts.

Prevention messages in the mass media have included: strategies for reducing intake, such as switching to non-alcoholic beverages; portrayal of the negative effects of intoxication or chronic heavy use; portrayal of the positive consequences of moderate use; and recommendations about appropriate levels of alcohol intake (for example, Leathar 1979; Blane and Hewitt 1980; Wallack and Barrows 1983; Comiti 1990).

Although there has been widespread acceptance of most of these strategies, the provision of specific guidelines for appropriate, sensible, or safe levels of use has been more controversial. Recommendations about the amount it is 'safe' to drink have been promulgated in small media format in a number of countries, especially by medical agencies. They have been broadcast in the mass media less often. In the north-east of England, a 1981 campaign asked 'Five pints of beer every day is too much for your own good. True or false?' and recommended 'two or three pints, two or three times a week' and in Western Australia the 1988 Drinksafe campaign used a number of mass media channels to publicize the Health Department's recommended daily limits for consumption (Clark and Knowles 1990). In the Netherlands, by contrast, the Ministry of Welfare, Public Health, and Cultural Affairs decided not to promulgate guidelines for safe levels citing the fact that most safe limits focus exclusively on physical harm; safe weekly amounts overlook binge drinking; safe drinking advice offers heavy drinkers a 'good story'; and safe limits do not apply to unhealthy people and high-risk groups (Kolstad 1992).

A recent innovation in small media alcohol education in the United States has been the introduction of health warning labels on alcohol beverage containers. These were mandated by the US federal government in 1989 and warn of the risk of birth defects and impairment of ability to drive a car or operate machinery. Prior to the US' move, Colombia (in 1974) and Mexico (in 1985) had introduced a general warning about harm to health on container labels.

Another very common topic of mass media campaigns throughout the 1970s and 1980s has been drinking and driving (Hewitt and Blane 1984). By the mid 1980s anti-drinking and driving messages had become the most prevalent of the US government public service television advertisements (Atkin 1989) and were also a common theme for alcohol industry funded moderation advertising.

In the United States, analysis of such industry-originated moderation advertising has suggested that the themes and images used in much of this advertising are consistent with the beer companies' regular brand promotions, which works to the detriment of providing a clear, unambiguous public health message. During the late 1980s and early 1990s US industry-originated moderation advertising has moved from commercials that resembled public service educational messages to introduce pro-drinking themes and imagery typical of brand promotion advertising (DeJong *et al.* 1992).

News coverage of alcohol issues

The news media disseminate information and stimulate discussion about public policies; they legitimize policy options in the eyes of policy-makers and the public (Milio 1986). However, the coverage of alcohol issues in news and information programming, while clearly an important part of the public discourse on alcohol, has received relatively little research attention in the past two decades, particularly when compared with the focus on alcohol in entertainment programmes, advertising, and mass media education campaigns.

In North America in the 1970s, coverage of alcohol issues was found to be low compared with coverage of illicit drug use (Smart and Krakowski 1973) and with coverage of other social issues (issues which were, however, judged less important than alcohol by the public) (Hubbard *et al.* 1975). This was at a time when the emphasis in public and bureaucratic thinking about alcohol-related problems remained on providing an institutional system to treat alcohol problems once they occured, rather than the development of public policies to minimize their occurrence (Room 1984). The then pervasive ideology of Alcoholics Anonymous also defined alcohol problems as a private individual matter (Beauchamp 1988). A shift towards recognition of the role of public policies in the prevention of alcohol-related problems occurred in the research and policy arena in the late 1970s (see below). No US research appears to have looked for a reflection of this academic discourse in news programming. In the Finnish press, however, a liberal stance was found to be replaced by more control-oriented thinking around 1974 (Piispa 1981, cited in Partanen and Montonen 1988).

Drinking and driving issues have been the topic of news coverage in which there has been the most increase during the 1980s. There was little coverage of alcohol's role in car crashes in US newspapers in the late 1970s, according to an analysis by Breed and De Foe (1978), but the early 1980s saw a dramatic increase in coverage of drinking and driving issues in the news media, reflecting in part the activity of citizen advocacy groups in this area (Luckey *et al.* 1984, cited in Atkin 1989; McCarthy and Harvey 1989).

An analysis of newspaper coverage in New Zealand in the early 1980s similarly showed that concern over drinking and driving issues received considerable coverage (Stewart and Casswell 1993). However, there was little coverage of public policies on alcohol. More space was filled with material which reflected alcohol as a business commodity. Product information, especially about wine, has been a noticeable part of news coverage in countries in which wine consumption has been on the increase (for example, Stewart and Casswell 1993; Qwerin 1989).

In the late 1980s and early 1990s a new factor has entered the news coverage on alcohol issues in the form of widespread reporting of research suggesting a beneficial effect of drinking on prevention of premature mortality from coronary heart disease. This has been linked implicitly, if not explicitly, with public policy issues in that the beneficial effects of moderate alcohol consumption are used to argue against the application of public policies which affect the total population (Casswell 1993).

Academic discourse

The academic discourse on alcohol is confined to a much smaller audience: primarily researchers, tertiary teachers, bureaucrats, and policy-makers, compared with the mass audiences for advertising, entertainment, and news material. However, it is likely to be influential beyond its more immediate audience in terms of changing conceptualizations of alcohol issues and in the subsequent negotiation of public policies on alcohol.

A report written by an international group of researchers under the leadership of the Finnish researcher Kettil Bruun, published in 1975, *Alcohol control policies in public health perspective*, was 'widely noted' among the international research and policy communities (Room 1984). This report came after some decades of emphasis on the individual alcoholic and the need to provide treatment services, an emphasis which had excluded discussions of policies affecting the availability of alcohol. Providing a clear contrast the report concluded: 'Changes in the overall consumption of alcoholic beverages have a bearing on the health of the people in any society. Alcohol control measures can be used to limit consumption: thus, control of alcohol availability becomes a public health issue' (Bruun *et al.* 1975, p. 90).

The US National Academy of Sciences report, *Alcohol and public policy: Beyond the shadow of prohibition*, published three years later (Moore and Gerstein 1981) was described as 'having become a common discussion item, a touchstone that people can use to certify the legitimacy and complementarity of a broad band of possible preventive measures. It has become part of discussion about what a problem is and what can be reasonably done about it' (Gerstein 1984, p. 8).

The increased recognition of the alcohol environment as an important contributor to alcohol-related problems and of public policies as effective prevention strategies fitted well with the public health model (Mosher and Jernigan 1989). The Annual Review of Public Health carried major articles on alcohol policy in 1984 (Room), 1988 (Ashley and Rankin), and 1989 (Mosher and Jernigan). Similarly the framework of health promotion, as promulgated by the WHO Regional Office for Europe during the 1980s, with its emphasis on the development of healthy public policy, also provided a sympathetic context for discussion of alcohol policies (Bennett *et al.* 1992).

The impact of the public discourse on alcohol

Research investigating the impact of aspects of public discourse have varied in the theoretical perspectives assumed. Two important dimensions have been: (1) the length of time over which effects are expected to occur (short- versus long-term effects), and (2) the extent to which the media effects were presumed to impact directly on the individual's behaviour, rather than to interact with personal characteristics, with interpersonal experiences or (an even less direct mechanism) impact on the social climate and public policy rather than directly on the individual's behaviour.

The evaluation research which has aimed to measure the impact of purposive interventions, such as alcohol advertising or mass media education campaigns, has most commonly looked for relatively short-term effects at the level of individual beliefs, attitudes, and behaviour. Many of the educational efforts to prevent alcohol-related problems, and their evaluations, were based on an assumption that increasing knowledge about the potentially adverse effects of alcohol would influence that individual's attitude toward alcohol and subsequently his or her behaviour. Mass media campaigns were initially directed toward a relatively undifferentiated mass audience and, in keeping with the knowledge-attitude-behaviour model, the underlying assumption was of direct influence of media messages on the individual's beliefs, attitudes, and behaviour (Wallack 1981; Dorn and South 1983). Although the extensive literature evaluating the impact of mass media campaigns of weeks or months duration has found some evidence of increased knowledge and, less consistently, change in attitudes, there has been no support for an impact of mass media campaigns directly on drinking behaviour (Moskowitz 1989). Similarly, the experimental research investigating the impact of alcohol advertising on drinking also assumed a direct, even shorter-term effect (Atkin in press). The experimental studies of alcohol advertising have looked for short-term direct effects on observed alcohol consumption and, somewhat inconsistently, these have been reported (Kohn and Smart 1984, 1987; Wilks *et al.* 1992).

News media coverage, in contrast with the portrayal of alcohol in entertainment, advertising, and educational campaigns, has not been expected to have direct effects on drinking, but rather to influence the climate of opinion surrounding alcohol issues and to serve a gate-keeping function, influencing which issues enter the political agenda and in what form (Partanen and Montonen 1988).

However, television coverage of the possible reduced risk of coronary heart disease from alcohol may also have had a short-term direct effect on behaviour suggesting the importance of the novelty and acceptability of a media message. Following a televised discussion by scientists and doctors of the merits of drinking wine, especially red wine, to protect against heart disease, a burst of wine-buying was recorded by sales tracking data from supermarkets in the United States. Eight months after transmission of the programme, sales of red wine had jumped by 45 per cent and sales of white wine by 10 per cent (The wine industry: withering or heartening 1992). A recent example of a direct short-term effect on behaviour in the opposite direction, also from Texas in the United States, were small sharp decreases in injury from motor vehicle collisions; these followed extensive mass media publicity of two successful lawsuits against licensed premises which had served alcohol to people who subsequently caused the death of others (Wagenaar and Holder 1991). In both of these cases, the media coverage provided new information which was of considerable relevance to the recipients and appeared to have direct effects on the behaviour of, in the one case, operators of licensed premises and, in the other, people who perceived themselves to be potential coronary heart disease victims or found this to be a useful justification. Decreases in fatal traffic crashes in the first part of the 1980s have also been partially attributed to the dramatic increase in news media coverage of drinking and driving issues in the United States (Hingson *et al.* 1988).

Other theoretical perspectives which have been influential in public discourse research areas have assumed a more gradual and contributory effect of the messages being disseminated. Social learning theory describes the influence of modelled behaviour and its consequences on the observer. In this model, expectancies may be learned but not acted upon immediately if factors in the environment militate against it (Bandura 1977, 1986). Similarly, cultivation theory (Gerbner *et al.* 1986) stresses the cumulative absorption of media content, rather than an immediate impact. Very small influences may accumulate given the considerable exposure experienced, particularly to television. In the United States, the heaviest watching children's group are children aged 2 to 5 who watch 25 hours weekly (Clark 1988). Television watching has been described by Gerbner (1990) as more like a ritual than the use of any other popular medium; most viewers watch by the clock rather than by the programme. Between the ages of 2 and 65 an average of nine years of television are watched in the United States. The media draw on the surrounding reality to produce their own symbolic reality, which then enters into the collective experience and provides the audience with values and behavioural models for their everyday life (Gerbner *et al.* 1986). There is some evidence that television portrayal of alcohol use may have its greatest impact when viewers are unable to check back to personal experiences (Hansen 1986). It is possible, therefore, that the impact of the portrayal of alcohol in United States entertainment programmes or in commercial advertising may be stronger in developing countries which have less widespread experience of commercial alcohol use.

While such theoretical perspectives have largely informed analysis of entertainment material on television, similar ways of framing the effects of mass media education campaigns have also become current in the 1980s: 'more attention is given to the intermediate or indirect effects of communication that may cumulatively contribute to the sorts of major attitude changes or overt behaviour changes that earlier campaigns sought . . .' (Rogers and Storey 1987).

In the light of theoretical perspectives which emphasize a cumulative absorption of mass media messages, Atkin (1989) described correlational surveys of longer-term exposure to alcohol advertising and self-reported drinking and beliefs about drinking as providing the most externally valid data on the advertising–consumption relationship. Such investigations of alcohol advertising effects have looked for a relationship between self-reports of exposure to advertising and other relevant variables, including self-reported behaviour, attitudes, and beliefs. These studies have found small but significant relationships between exposure to alcohol advertising and higher levels of self-reported consumption, and relevant attitudes (Strickland 1982, 1983; Atkin *et al.* 1984; Atkin and Block 1984). A recent study of children in the United States aged from 10 to 14 years used non-recursive modelling with latent variables to assess the relationship between children's awareness of alcohol advertising and beliefs about drinking and intentions to drink (Grube and Wallack 1994). Children who could correctly identify more beer advertisements held more favourable beliefs about drinking and indicated that they intended to drink more frequently as adults. These effects were maintained even when the reciprocal effects of knowledge and beliefs on awareness of advertising were controlled. A recent longitudinal study carried out in New Zealand has also shown a relationship between recall of alcohol advertising at age 15 and adolescent alcohol consumption (Connolly *et al.* 1994).

A similar correlational approach to the evaluation of mass media education campaigns is possible but has not yet been undertaken. The relatively low levels of exposure to educational campaigns may reduce the chances of finding such a relationship. In the New Zealand longitudinal study no relationship was found between recall of moderation advertising and alcohol consumption in contrast to the effect of alcohol advertising. The inability of educational messages to monopolize the issue in the mass media, due to alcohol's extensive and uncritical portrayal in advertising and entertainment material, has been proffered as an important reason to expect that few if any changes can be achieved by mass media educational campaigns in isolation (Wallack 1980, 1990).

The recipient of the communication has been more clearly acknowledged as an active player in theoretical perspectives which have shaped recent research. Individuals selectively use media channels and messages to satisfy their needs for information (Rubin 1986) and process messages in terms of their prior beliefs and experiences (Ajzen and Fishbein 1975; Petty and Cacioppo 1981). The individual's uses of the media act as intervening variables influencing the ultimate effect of a media message. This perspective has resulted in an increased emphasis in the 1980s on formative evaluation techniques to design campaigns which resonate with identified sectors of the audience (Flay and Burton 1990) and less expectation of undifferentiated effects across a mass audience. The selective use of messages is also relevant to policy development in that information which substantiates a preferred policy position, for example from research, is selectively attended to and used to justify the policy stand (Moskalewicz 1993).

A further relevant theoretical perspective on the media, particularly the news media, is its role of agenda setting; that is, keeping alcohol issues to the forefront of public attention, especially the attention of policy-makers (McCombs and Shaw 1972). Milio (1986) has described the role of words as part of an information strategy to define the issues and range of acceptable policy options. 'When the strategy can be extended to the media, the persuasive force is multiplied because, among other things, the issues and solutions so defined are legitimised for debate, if not for acceptance, in the eyes of policymakers, the public and other interest groups' (Milio 1986). For example, the epidemiological evidence suggesting reduced risk of coronary heart disease among those drinking alcohol has been seen as contributing to the alcohol policy debate in New Zealand (Casswell 1993).

Also relevant to public discourse on alcohol are the theoretical perspectives that deal with what governs the nature of the messages which are communicated via the mass media. These include issues of ownership, funding, and control of the media (Garnham 1990; Gerbner 1990) and also analysis of the role of key players in the field as sources of information for the media (Schlesinger 1990). Access to the mass media to debate and legitimate policy options is often fiercely contested and selectively applied by media personnel. The trends in the past decades towards greater reliance on advertising revenue in the broadcast media have impacted on public health advocates' access (Atkin and Arkin 1990). The importance accorded the struggle for access to the news media suggest the participants' belief in the importance of media coverage of policy options as part of the process of policy adoption. This is supported by the limited amount of analysis available, primarily in the drinking and driving area. It is clearly a symbiotic relationship with media debate probably increasing the likelihood of policy development, and policy development (particularly legislation) providing material for media coverage.

Media advocacy has developed as a response to the recognition of the importance of access to the mass media to debate policy issues. It has been defined as the strategic use of the mass media to advance a social or public policy objective (Wallack 1990). Case studies of media advocacy in the alcohol area have suggested an impact in shifting the terms of the debate around alcohol policies. A campaign on alcohol advertising in Switzerland in the early 1980s, for example, did not succeed in introducing restrictions but meant that, in the years following the campaign, discussion of alcohol-related problems was very likely to include reference to the issue of alcohol advertising (Muster 1985).

In a case where the campaign was unsuccessful in achieving its immediate objective there appeared to have been shifts in the social climate surrounding the issue. Following the tax initiative in California, which took place in 1990, the extensive media advocacy campaign appeared to have contributed to a lasting shift in public opinion despite the failure of the initiative itself. Six months after the election, public support for tax increases was higher than before the campaign and the authors of the case study suggested: 'The issue's new visibility and obvious strong public support were likely among the key factors in the legislature's enactment of a 1992 budget that included an increase in alcohol excise taxes for the first time in twenty years' (Advocacy Institute 1992).

Another area in which the impact of widespread media coverage may have impacted on the social climate is that of drinking and driving casualties. The media debates preceding and surrounding the introduction of legislation have influenced the social climate surrounding drinking and driving. This can be measured in terms of cumulative changes in the public's attitudes to drinking and driving, as measured in repeated random sample surveys (for example, Hingson *et al.* 1987; Perkins 1990) and also the passing of legislation with increased punitive penalties and sometimes a preventive aim. Content analysis showed dramatic increase in media coverage of the drinking and driving issue in the first part of the 1980s during which US state legislators enacted hundreds of new drinking and driving laws (McCarthy and Harvey 1989; Snortum and Berger 1989; Hingson *et al.* 1988). This has been attributed to the impact of citizen advocacy groups (Zimring 1988; Wolfson 1989).

Where legislation with a general deterrence aim (such as random breath-testing in Australia) has been passed and supported by ongoing media coverage it has resulted in long-term behaviour changes (Homel 1988). Although it is not possible to separate the effects of the 'social stew' of public policy change and media messages it is likely that both contribute to changes in the social climate (Snortum and Berger 1989; Homel 1993).

The possible impact of other aspects of the public discourse on alcohol, such as commercial advertising and educational campaigns, on the conceptualization of alcohol-related problems and appropriate ways of dealing with them have also been recognized (Partanen and Montonen 1988). For example, while some direct effects of alcohol advertising has been documented, it is possible that the more significant effects of alcohol advertising are on the social climate surrounding alcohol. It has been suggested that alcohol advertising communicates a meta-message of society's approval of alcohol (Postman *et al.* 1988) and in turn reduces the likelihood of other public policies being implemented (van Iwaarden 1983; Farrell 1985).

Even the apparent direct impact of advertising bans in reducing alcohol consumption and alcohol-related problems, as measured by Saffer (1991), may reflect the public debate surrounding the introduction of such restrictions and the fact that the social climate had reached a stage at which such bans were possible, as much as a direct effect at the individual level. It is likely that such a social climate was also encouraging of other policy changes which impact on behaviour.

Mass media educational campaigns aimed at influencing individual behaviour may also have an effect on the social climate surrounding alcohol use. Perhaps the meta-message communicated by the broadcast of campaigns on the highly visible and symbolically powerful electronic mass media is one of societal concern and disapproval. In support of this hypothesis are the findings from an evaluation of a mass media campaign aimed at reinforcing moderate drinking among young New Zealand men. Exposure to this campaign influenced general population support for alcohol policies on price, availability, and advertising (Casswell *et al.* 1989).

The mass media campaign may have influenced the social climate in part because it served as an agenda setting function for the local news media; in the cities receiving the mass media campaign more local news coverage of policy and educational issues occurred, relative to cities without the campaign (Stewart and Casswell 1993). It may also be of relevance to the impact on social climate that moderation campaigns such as this one (which used sexual attraction and mateship to promote reducing consumption) had not been broadcast in New Zealand before. Nor were there competing alcohol industry advertisements on the broadcast media at that stage. The impact on the social climate of similar campaigns might be less in a culture such as in California where the frequency of television beer advertising was such that it was difficult in the 1980s to create moderation advertisements that were clearly discriminated as such by the audience (Wallack and Barrows 1983).

A further example of measured changes in beliefs, beyond the specific goals of a mass media educational campaign has been documented. The introduction of policy governing the use of alcohol in recreational facilities in Ontario, Canada, was publicized using a number of mass media channels and the evaluation showed that this increased not only intention to comply with the specific policies targeted but support for public policies on alcohol more generally (Glicksman *et al.* 1990).

Further discussion of the impact of mass media educational campaigns on the social climate regarding alcohol use has focused on the anti-drinking and driving campaigns of the 1980s. It has been suggested that the dominance of the anti-drinking and driving message has communicated an unintentional meta-message to young drinkers: that sensible or safe drinking is that which is not followed by driving, regardless of the amounts consumed and level of intoxication reached (Divers and Zipursky 1993; Wagenaar 1992). Similar concerns have been expressed over industry advertising such as the Seagram's campaign: 'Seagrams goes with everything but driving' (Mosher and Jernigan 1989).

Conclusion

Documentations of the public discourse on alcohol in research literature illustrate that the portrayal of drinking and alcohol issues differs markedly depending on the origin and purpose of the communication. The most dominant portrayal in many cultures is that found in entertainment and advertising, which tends to normalize and sanitize alcohol use, and neither the experiences of alcohol-related problems nor the research-based knowledge on alcohol policies contribute as much to the public discourse. The range of material provides opportunity for the active recipient of the media material to pay selective attention to the messages which best fit their individual needs. The concerned parent will notice more of the arguments in favour of increasing the minimum drinking age while the daughter may be more familiar with Bacardi's latest advertising campaign.

However, despite this selective attention, it is possible that the different portrayals of alcohol all contribute in some way to the overall social climate. For example, even if the active recipient of the advertising message is not directly influenced, his or her perception of the acceptability of drinking in the situation portrayed may change. Research effort has tended to deal with different aspects of the public discourse separately but, analysis of the whole, their relative weight, and their inter-textual relationships may be relevant for an understanding of the impact of public discourse on the process of policy development.

During the 1980s, the theoretical perspectives about the way in which the media impacts on people's lives appear to have become less prone to overestimate the media's direct effects. At the same time, however, the results from studies of sudden changes in exposure to media messages (related to advertising bans) and of brief exposure to advertising messages encouraging drinking have shown some measurable effects on aggregate and individual level alcohol consumption. Similarly, studies of the cumulative effects of exposure to commercial mass media messages have also suggested some impact on beliefs about alcohol and drinking on consumption.

For a clearer understanding of the likely impact of mass media messages, research will also need to look for beverage- and brand-specific effects in relation to specific groups of the population and to take into account the active role message recipients take in attending to and interpreting portrayals of alcohol (Hansen 1988; Partanen 1988).

Purposive mass media communications, which aim to have direct effects on consumption, may also be usefully conceptualized as influencing a shared societal perception of drinking and of the appropriate way to handle alcohol at the policy level. So alcohol advertising gives a meta-message of acceptance and approval; education campaigns, particularly when clearly distinguishable from advertising material, may signal that there are legitimate concerns over alcohol-related problems. These media representations are part of the social and political context in which decisions are taken about the development and implementation of public policies, many of which may then have direct impacts on drinking behaviour.

News and commentary are also important aspects of the public discourse and help shape the social climate in which policy decisions are taken.

The media provide a forum for the public expression of different 'convictions, attitudes, and political stances . . . concerning the definition of alcohol-related problems, their causes and appropriate ways of dealing with them' (Partanen and Montonen 1988). The decades of the 1970s and 1980s have seen a recognition by researchers and public health advocates of the significance of the mass media to the public discourse on alcohol. This has resulted in a body of empirical research on media portrayal of alcohol and greater utilization of the media to disseminate research and information—the concept of media advocacy.

The portrayal of alcohol in the public discourse, in the mass media, and also in the newer information technologies (Milio 1992) will undoubtedly remain an important research topic in a future which has been described as the age of participatory democracy (Hancock 1992). The impact of this public discourse on the social climate and the process of public policy development deserves further research.

Acknowledgements

Preparation of this chapter was made possible by core programme funding from the Health Research Council and the Alcohol Advisory Council of New Zealand. I am grateful to Allan Wyllie for comments on an earlier draft.

References

Ackoff, R. L. and Emshoff, J. R. (1975). Advertising research at Anheuser-Busch, Inc. (1963–68). *Sloan Management Review*, **16**, 1–15.

Advocacy Institute (1992). *Taking initiative: the 1990 citizen's movement to raise California excise taxes to save lives*. The Advocacy Institute, Washington, DC.

Ajzen, I. and Fishbein, M. (1975). *Belief, attitude, intention, and behaviour: An introduction to theory and research*. Addison-Wesley, Reading, MA.

Ashley, M. J. and Rankin, J. G. (1988). A public health approach to the prevention of alcohol-related health problems. *Annual Review of Public Health*, **9**, 233–71.

Atkin, C. K. (1989). Mass communication effects on drinking and driving. In *Surgeon General's workshop on drunk driving: Background papers*, pp. 15–34. US Department of Health and Human Services, Rockville, MD.

Atkin, C. K. (in press). Survey and experimental research on alcohol advertising effects. *The Effects of the mass media on the use and abuse of alcohol*. National Institute on Alcohol Abuse and Alcoholism (NIAAA), Washington, DC.

Atkin, C. K. and Arkin, E. B. (1990). Issues and initiatives in communicating health information. In *Mass communication and public health: Complexities and conflicts*, (eds C. Atkin and L. Wallack), pp. 13–40. Sage, Newbury Park.

Atkin, C. K. and Block, M. (1981). *Content and effects of alcohol advertising. Report 1. Overview and summary*. National Technical Information Service, Springfield, VT.

Atkin, C. K. and Block, M. (1984). The effects of alcohol advertising. In *Advances in consumer research*, (ed. T. C. Kinnear), pp. 688–93. Association for Consumer Research, Provo, UT.

Atkin, C. K., Hocking, J., and Block, M. (1984). Teenage drinking: Does advertising make a difference? *Journal of Communication*, **34**, 157–67.

Bandura, A. (1977). *Social learning theory*. Prentice-Hall, Englewoods Cliffs, NJ.

Bandura, A. (1986). *Social foundations of thought and action: A social cognitive theory*. Prentice-Hall, Englewood Cliffs, NJ.

Beauchamp, D. E. (1988). *The health of the republic: Epidemics, medicine, and moralism as challenges to democracy*. Temple University Press, Philadelphia.

Beckley, R. E. and Chalfant, H. P. (1979). Contrasting images of alcohol and drug use in country and rock music. *Journal of Alcohol and Drug Education*, **25**, 44–51.

Bennett, P., Murphy, S., and Bunton, R. (1992). Preventing alcohol problems using healthy public policy. *Health Promotion International*, **7**, 297–306.

Blane, H. T. and Hewitt, L. E. (1980). Alcohol, public education and mass media: an overview. *Alcohol, Health and Research World*, **5**, 2–16.

Breed, W. and DeFoe, J. R. (1978). Bringing alcohol into the open, *Columbia Journalism Review*, **18**, 18–19.

Breed, W. and DeFoe, J. R. (1979). Themes in mass alcohol advertisements: A critique. *Journal of Drug Issues*, **9**, 511–22.

Breed, W. and DeFoe, J. R. (1982). Effecting media change: the role of cooperative consultation on alcohol topics. *Journal of Communication*, **32**, 88–89.

Bruun, K., *et al.* (1975). *Alcohol control policies in public health perspective*, Vol. 25. Finnish Foundation for Alcohol Studies, Helsinki.

Casswell, S. (1986). *Alcohol in Oceania*. Alcohol Research Unit, Auckland.

Casswell, S. (1993). Public discourse on the benefits of moderation: implications for alcohol policy development. *Addiction*, **88**, 459–65.

Casswell, S., Gilmore, L., Maguire, V., and Ransom, R. (1989). Changes in public support for alcohol policies following a community-based campaign. *British Journal of Addictions*, **84**, 515–22.

Clark, E. (1988). *The want makers: Lifting the lid off the world advertising industry: How they make you buy*. Hodder and Stoughton, London.

Clark, K. and Knowles, S. (1990). *The drinksafe campaign, 1988–1990: A review of campaign survey data*. Health Department of Western Australia, Perth.

Comiti, V. P. (1990). The advertising of alcohol in France. *World Health Forum*, **11**, 242–5.

Connolly, G., Casswell, S., Zhang, J. F. and Silva, P. (1994). Alcohol in the mass media and drinking by adolescents: a longitudinal study. *Addiction*, **89**, 1255–63.

DeFoe, W. and Breed, J. R. (1979). Themes in magazine alcohol advertisements: A critique. *Journal of Drug Issues*, **9**, 511–22.

DeJong, W. and Winsten, J. A. (1990). The use of mass media in substance abuse prevention. *Health Affairs*, Summer, 30–46.

DeJong, W., Atkin, C. K., and Wallack, L. (1992). A critical analysis of 'moderation' advertising sponsored by the beer industry: Are 'responsible drinking' commercials done responsibly? *The Millbank Quarterly*, **70**, 661–78.

Divers, P. P. and Zipursky, B. M. (1993). The intended and unintended consequences of promoting 'don't drink and drive' messages. In *Experiences with community action projects: New research in the prevention of alcohol and other drug problems*, (ed. T. K. Greenfield and R. Zimmerman), pp. 59–70. Center for Substance Abuse Prevention (CSAP) Prevention Monograph No. 14. US Department of Health and Human Services, Rockville, MD.

Dorn, N. and South, N. (1983). *Message in a bottle: Theoretical overview and annotated bibliography on the mass media and alcohol*. Gower, Aldershot, UK.

Falk, P. and Sulkunen, P. (1983). Drinking on the screen. An analysis of a mythical male fantasy in Finnish films. *Social Science Information*, **22**, 387–410.

Farrell, S. (1985). *Review of national policy measures to prevent alcohol-related problems*, (unpublished document PAD 85.14). World Health Organization, Geneva.

Finn, T. A. and Strickland, D. E. (1982). A content analysis of beverage alcohol advertising. II. Television advertising. *Journal of Studies on Alcohol*, **43**, 964–89.

Flay, B. R. and Burton, D. (1990). Effective mass communication strategies for health campaigns. In *Mass communication and public health: Complexities and conflicts*, (ed. C. Atkin and L. Wallack), pp. 129–46. Sage, Newbury Park.

Garnham, N. (1990). *Capitalism and communication: Global culture and the economics of information*. Sage, London.

Gerbner, G. (1990). Stories that hurt: tobacco, alcohol, and other drugs in the mass media. In *Youth and drugs: Society's mixed messages*, (ed. H. Resnick), pp. 53–127. Center for Substance Abuse Prevention (CSAP) Prevention Monograph No. 6. US Department of Health and Human Services, Rockville, MD.

Gerbner, G., Gross, L., and Morgan, M. (1986). Living with television: The dynamics of the cultivation process. In *Perspectives on media effects*, (ed. J. Bryant and D. Zillman), pp. 17–40. Lawrence Erlbaum, Hillsdale, NJ.

Gerstein, D. R. (ed.) (1984). *Toward the prevention of alcohol problems: Government, business, and community action*. National Academy Press, Washington, DC.

Gitlin, T. (1983). *Inside primetime*. Pantheon, New York.

Gliksman, L., Douglas, R. R., Thomson, M., Moffatt, K., Smythe, C., and Caverson, R. (1990). Promoting municipal alcohol policies: an evaluation of a campaign. *Contemporary Drug Problems*, **17**, 391–420.

Grube, J. W. and Wallack, L. (1994). Television beer advertising and drinking knowledge, beliefs, and intentions among schoolchildren. *American Journal of Public Health*, **84**, 254–9.

Hancock, T. (1992). Promoting health environmentally. In *Supportive environments for health* (ed. K. Dean and T. Hancock), pp. 3–21. World Health Organization Regional Office for Europe, Copenhagen.

Hansen, A. (1986). The portrayal of alcohol on television. *Health Education Journal*, **45**, 127–31.

Hansen, A. (1988). The content and effects of television images of alcohol: towards a framework of analysis. *Contemporary Drug Problems*, **15**, 249–79.

Heilbronn, L. M. (1988). What does alcohol mean? Alcohol's use as a symbolic code. *Contemporary Drug Problems*, **15**, 229–48.

Heiskala, R. (1988). An exclusively male matter? Alcohol, gender and family in Finnish general magazines and women's magazines in 1955 and 1985. *14th Annual Alcohol Epidemiology Symposium*, California, 5–11 June.

Herd, D. (1983). Images of drinking: distortion or re-creation? In *Alcohol: The prevention debate*, (ed. M. Grant and B. Ritson), pp. 97–104. Croom Helm, London.

Hewitt, L. E. and Blane, H. T. (1984). Prevention through mass media communication. In *Prevention of alcohol abuse*, (ed. P. M. Miller and T. D. Nirenberg), pp. 281–323. Plenum, New York.

Hingson, R. W., Heeran, T., Kovenack, D., Mangione, T., Lederman, R., and Scotch, N. (1987). Effects of Maine's 1981 and Massachusetts' 1982 driving under the influence legislation. *American Journal of Public Health*, **77**, 593–7.

Hingson, R. W., Howland, J., and Levenson, S. (1988). Effects of legislative reform to reduce drunken driving and alcohol-related traffic fatalities. *Public Health Reports*, **103**, 659–67.

Homel, R. (1988). Random breath testing in Australia: A complex deterrent. *Australia Drug and Alcohol Review*, **7**, 231–41.

Homel, R. (1993). Random breath testing in Australia: getting it to work according to specifications. *Addiction*, **88** (Suppl.), 27S–33S.

Hubbard, J. C., DeFleur, M. L., and DeFleur, L. B. (1975). Mass media influences on public conceptions of social problems. *Social Problems*, **23**, 22–34.

Jacobson, M., Hacker, G., and Atkins, R. (1983). *The booze merchants: The inebriating of America*. Center for Science in the Public Interest, Washington, DC.

Kohn, P. M. and Smart, R. G. (1984). The impact of television advertising on alcohol consumption: an experiment. *Journal of Studies on Alcohol*, **45**, 295–301.

Kohn, P. M. and Smart, R. G. (1987). Wine, women, suspiciousness and advertising. *Journal of Studies on Alcohol*, **48**, 161–6.

Kolstad, H. (1992). President's view. *36th International Congress on Alcohol and Dependence*, Glasgow, 16–21 August 1992. *The Globe*, pp. 12–13.

Lalonde, M. (1974). *A new perspective on the health of Canadians*. Government of Canada, Ottawa.

Leathar, D. S. (1979). Communicating through cartoons. *Community Education*, Autumn, 16–22.

McCarthy, J. D. and Harvey, D. S. (1989). Independent citizen advocacy: The past and the prospects. In *Surgeon General's workshop on drunk driving: Background papers*, pp. 247–60. US Department of Health and Human Services, Washington, DC.

McCombs, M. E. and Shaw, D. L. (1972). The agenda-setting function of the mass media. *Public Opinion Quarterly*, **36**, 176–87.

Milio, N. (1986). Health and the media in Australia: An uneasy relationship. *Community Health Studies*, **10**, 419–22.

Milio, N. (1992). New tools for community involvement in health. *Health Promotion International*, **7**, 209–17.

Montgomery, K. C. (1990). Promoting health through entertainment television. In *Mass communication and public health: Complexities and conflicts*, (ed. C. Atkin and L. Wallack), pp. 114–28. Sage, Newbury Park.

Montonen, M. (1989). Alcohol in Finnish television drama: perceptions by viewers. *34th International Institute on the Prevention and Treatment of Alcoholism*, Pontault-Combault, 31 May–9 June.

Moore, M. and Gerstein, D. R. (ed.) (1981). *Alcohol and public policy: Beyond the shadow of prohibition*. National Academy Press, Washington, DC.

Mosher, J. F. and Jernigan, D. H. (1989). New directions in alcohol policy. *Annual Review of Public Health*, **10**, 245–79.

Moskalewicz, J. (1993). Lessons to be learnt from Poland's attempt at moderating its consumption of alcohol. *Addiction*, **88** (Suppl.), 135S–42S.

Moskowitz, J. M. (1989). The primary prevention of alcohol problems: A critical review of the research literature. *Journal of Studies on Alcohol*, **50**, 54–88.

Muster, E. (1985). Work with the media: the popular vote on drug advertising. In *Extending alcohol education*, (ed. M. Grant and R. Waahlbert), pp. 52–61. International Council on Alcohol and Addictions, Lausanne.

Nathanson-Moog, C. (1984). Brand personalities undergo psychoanalysis. *Advertising Age*, 26 July, p. 18.

Paakkanen, P. (1982). *Cultural continuity in Finnish drinking: Alcohol in Finnish literature in 1911–1912 and 1972*, (Report No. 164). Social Research Institute of Alcohol Studies, Helsinki.

Paisley, W. J. (1981). Public communication campaigns: The American experience. In *Public communication campaigns*, (ed. R. E. Rice and W. J. Paisley), pp. 15–40. Sage, Newbury Park.

Partanen, J. (1988). Communicating about alcohol in the mass media. *Contemporary Drug Problems*, **15**, 281–319.

Partanen, J. and Montonen, M. (1988). *Alcohol and the mass media*, (Euro Reports and Studies 108). World Health Organization, Regional Office for Europe, Copenhagen.

Pendleton, L. J., Smith, C., and Roberts, J. L. (1991). Drinking on television: A content analysis of recent alcohol portrayal. *British Journal of Addiction*, **86**, 769–74.

Perkins, W. A. (1990). *Public attitudes towards alcohol-impaired driving and speed*, (Traffic Research Report No. 42). Traffic Research and Statistics Section, Ministry of Transport, Wellington.

Petty, R. and Cacioppo, J. (1981). *Attitudes and persuasion: Classic and contemporary approaches*. Brown, Dubuque, IA.

Postman, N., Nystrom, C., Strate, L., and Weingartner, C. (1988). *Myths, men, and beer: An analysis of beer commercials on broadcast television, 1987*. AAA Foundation for Traffic Safety, Falls Church, VA.

Qwerin, G. (1989). Rules and practices of alcohol advertising. *34th International Institute on the Prevention and Treatment of Alcoholism*, Pontault-Combault, 31 May–9 June.

Rogers, E. M. and Storey, J. D. (1987). Communication campaigns. In *Handbook of communication science*, (ed. C. R. Berger and S. H. Chaffee), pp. 817–46. Sage, Newbury Park.

Room, R. (1984). Alcohol control and public health. *Annual Review of Public Health*, **5**, 293–317.

Room, R. (1989). Alcoholism and Alcoholics Anonymous in US films, 1945–1962: The party ends for the 'Wet Generations'. *Journal of Studies on Alcohol*, **50**, 368–83.

Rowland, W. and Tracey, M. (1988). The breakdown of public service broadcasting. *Intermedia*, **16**, 32–42.

Rubin, A. (1986). Uses, gratifications, and media effects. In *Perspectives on media effects* (ed. J. Bryant and D. Zillman), pp. 1–16. Lawrence Erlbaum, Hillsdale, NJ.

Saffer, H. (1991). Alcohol advertising bans and alcohol abuse: An international perspective. *Journal of Health Economics*, **10**, 65–79.

Saunders, B. (1993). Guarding the guardians: influencing the regulation of alcohol promotions in Australia. *Addiction*, **88** (Suppl.), 43S–51S.

Saunders, B. and Yap, E. (1991). Do our guardians need guarding? An examination of the Australian system of self-regulation of alcohol advertising. *Drug and Alcohol Review*, **10**, 15–27.

Schlesinger, P. (1990). Rethinking the sociology of journalism: Source strategies and the limits of media-centrism. In *Public communication: The new imperatives: Future directions for media research*, (ed. M. Ferguson). Sage, Newbury Park.

Signorielli, N. (1987). Drinking, sex, and violence on television: The cultural indicators perspective. *Journal of Drug Education*, **17**, 245–60.

Signorielli, N. (1990). Television and health: images and impact. In *Mass communication and public health: Complexities and conflicts*, (ed. C. Atkin and L. Wallack), pp. 96–113. Sage, Newbury Park.

Sinclair, J. (1983). *South Pacific Brewery: The first 30 years*. Robert Brown, Australia.

Smart, R. G. and Krakowski, M. (1973). The nature and frequency of drug contents in magazines and on television. *Journal of Alcohol Education*, **18**, 16–23.

Snortum, J. R. and Berger, D. E. (1989). Drinking-driving compliance in the United States: Perceptions and behaviour in 1983 and 1986. *Journal of Studies on Alcohol*, **50**, 306–19.

Stewart, L. and Casswell, S. (1993). Media advocacy for alcohol policy support: results from the New Zealand Community Action Project. *Health Promotion International*, **8**, 167–75.

Strate, L. (1991). The cultural meaning of beer commercials. *Advances in Consumer Research*, **18**, 115–19.

Strickland, D. E. (1982). Alcohol advertising: orientations and influence. *International Journal of Advertising*, **1**, 307–19.

Strickland, D. E. (1983). Advertising exposure, alcohol consumption and misuse of alcohol. In *Economics and alcohol: consumption and controls*, (ed. M. Grant, M. Plant, and A. Williams), pp. 201–22. Gardner Press, New York.

Thorson, E. (in press). Effects of alcohol advertising. *The effects of the mass media on the use and abuse of alcohol*. National Institute on Alcohol Abuse and Alcoholism Monograph, Washington, DC.

USDHEW (US Department of Health, Education and Welfare) (1979). *Healthy people: The Surgeon General's report on health promotion and disease prevention*. US Department of Health, Education and Welfare, Washington, DC.

van Iwaarden, M. K. (1983). Advertising, alcohol consumption and policy alternatives. In *Economics and alcohol: Consumption and controls*, (ed. M. Grant and A. Williams), pp. 223–37. Croom Helm, London.

Wagenaar, A. C. (1992). Designated driver programmes: a commentary on the DeJong and Wallack article. *Health Education Quarterly*, **19**, 443–5.

Wagenaar, A. C. and Holder, H. D. (1991). Effects of alcoholic beverage server liability on traffic crash injuries. *Alcoholism: Clinical and Experimental Research*, **15**, 942–7.

Wallack, L. M. (1980). Assessing the effect of mass media campaigns: an alternative perspective. *Alcohol, Health and Research World*, **5**, 17–29.

Wallack, L. (1981). Mass media campaigns: the odds against finding behaviour change. *Health Education Quarterly*, **8**, 209–60.

Wallack, L. (1990). Improving health promotion: media advocacy and social marketing approaches. In *Mass communication and public health: complexities and conflicts* (ed. C. Atkin and L. Wallack), Sage, Newbury Park.

Wallack, L. and Barrows, D. C. (1983). Evaluating primary prevention in the California 'winners' alcohol program. *International Quarterly of Community Health Education*, **3**, 307–36.

Wallack, L., Grube, J. W., Madden, P. A., and Breed, W. (1990). Portrayals of alcohol on prime-time television. *Journal of Studies on Alcohol*, **51**, 428–37.

Wilks, J., Vardanega, A. T., and Callan, V. J. (1992). Effect of television advertising of alcohol on alcohol consumption and intentions to drive. *Drug and Alcohol Review*, **11**, 15–21.

The wine industry: withering or heartening (1992). *The Economist*, **324:7774**, 26.

Wolfson, M. (1989). The citizen's movement against drunken driving and the prevention of risky driving: a preliminary assessment. *Alcohol, Drugs and Driving*, **5**, 73–84.

Wyllie, A., Casswell, S., and Stewart, J. (1989). The response of New Zealand boys to corporate and sponsorship alcohol advertising on television. *British Journal of Addiction*, **84**, 639–46.

Zimring, F. E. (1988). Law, society, and the drinking driver: some concluding reflections. In *Social Control of the Drinking Driver*, (ed. M. D. Snortum, J. R. Snortum, and F. E. Zimring), pp. 371–84. University of Chicago Press, Chicago, IL.

Part III

Public policy and difficult choices

9. Moderate drinking and public health

Roberta G. Ferrence

Introduction

A large body of evidence implicates consumption of alcohol in a range of diseases, conditions, and damaging behaviours (USHHS 1990). Yet, a growing literature suggests that moderate drinking may provide benefits when compared to abstention. Prospective studies of healthy subjects, case control studies of morbidity and mortality, and ecological studies of drinking patterns and rates of disease and death show repeated, but not consistent, evidence for a protective effect of moderate drinking on coronary heart disease (CHD) and, in some cases, overall mortality. Most studies have used CHD as an outcome measure; some have looked at both CHD and total mortality; others have included cardiovascular disease; few have systematically examined a range of specific causes of death. Other research has related the consumption of alcohol to particular non-CHD causes of death and morbidity, notably breast, oral, and laryngeal cancer.

Early studies showing a lower rate of CHD among moderate drinkers compared to both abstainers and heavy drinkers (the U-shaped curve) lead many to suspect that moderate drinking might be protective. Subsequent research has shown a fairly consistent relationship between levels of drinking averaging about one or two drinks each day and reduced mortality from CHD. Results of this research have been used for developing recommendations about appropriate levels of drinking by government and health agencies (Johns Hopkins University 1992). Media attention has been substantial—particularly following the release of each new study. Industry-associated publications have encouraged moderate drinking as beneficial for the heart (Ford 1988).

Those concerned with public health have been cautious about making recommendations on the basis of this research. First, there is not complete agreement that evidence for a protective effect is conclusive or applies to all populations and subpopulations. Secondly, research on the distribution of consumption of alcohol suggests that increasing total consumption in order to increase moderate drinking would result in disproportionate increases in heavy drinking and attendant problems (Bruun *et al.* 1975). Thirdly, a number of diseases and conditions exhibit a dose-response, rather than a U-shaped relationship with drinking, which could lead to a negative net effect if consumption increased. And finally, a number of alternative methods for reducing CHD and other causes of morbidity and mortality may be more appropriate and have fewer or no negative consequences.

In the light of these issues, an appropriate public health response to the question of moderate drinking must include an examination of all health outcomes associated with drinking, a consideration of methodological issues related to this research, and an analysis of the net effects of changing existing levels of drinking (cf. Casswell 1993). In this chapter, I discuss the first two; other chapters address the third.

Effects of drinking on health

In reviews of the relationship between alcohol and coronary heart disease (Ashley 1982, 1984; Baum-Baicker 1985*a*; Ferrence *et al.* 1986; Klatsky 1990; Beaglehole and Jackson 1992), the large literature on the topic is systematically described and evaluated. Several studies included in these reviews also provide data on alcohol consumption and total mortality (Blackwelder *et al.* 1980; Dyer *et al.* 1980; Kozarevich *et al.* 1980; Klatsky *et al.* 1981; Marmot *et al.* 1981; Cullen *et al.* 1982). The reviews conclude that there is considerable evidence for a protective effect on CHD, but that this evidence is not entirely consistent, that some confounds have not been ruled out, and that there are methodological problems with many studies. Since the task of this chapter is to assess the total effect of moderate drinking on health, it will focus on those studies that include total mortality, total morbidity, or a variety of causes of death or disease. As many recent studies have attempted to deal with criticisms of methods common to these investigations, and have not yet been reviewed, the latest research is emphasized.

Research on drinking and overall mortality and morbidity

A number of prospective, case-control, and ecological studies examine overall mortality and, in some cases, mortality from CHD among middle-aged or older men drinking at levels ranging from life-long abstention to several drinks per day. A few recent studies have compared risk of morbidity and mortality for a range of diseases among younger men (Andreasson *et al.* 1991) and among women (Stampfer *et al.* 1988). In this section, a summary will be given of findings from recent reports that at a minimum examine total mortality (Table 9.1).

The Framingham Study Drinking and subsequent mortality were examined

Table 9.1 Prospective studies of drinking and mortality and morbidity

Study	Year	Follow-up period	*N*	Sex	Age	Drinking measure	Results	Source
Framingham, MA, USA	1950	22 yrs	5209	M/F	40–50	No. of drinkers per month	M: light drinkers lowest; dose-response: cancer, cirrhosis F: no effect	Gordon and Kannel (1984)
Japanese Physicians, Japan	1965	19 yrs	5135	M	–	Past, current, amount	RR[a] occasional and daily/non-drinkers: 0.86, 0.91	Kono *et al.* (1986)
British Regional Heart	1978–80	7.5 yrs	7735	M	40–59	Weekly intake	Lower RR for smokers, manual workers	Shaper *et al.* (1988)
Swedish Conscripts	1969–70	20 yrs	49 464	M	18–21	Weekly intake	Abstainers, light drinkers lowest; RR 2.5+ per day = 2.82	Andreasson *et al.* (1988, 1991)
Nurses' Health, USA	1976	6 yrs	121 700	F	Married	Usual intake past year	1+/day: RR breast cancer 0.6, CHD[b] 0.6	Colditz (1990); Stampfer (1988)
American Cancer Society, USA	1959	12 yrs	250 000	M	40–59	Usual intake 1959	RR occasional, 1, 2/day vs. abstainers = 0.88, 0.84, 0.93	Boffetta and Garfinkel (1990)
Alameda County, CA, USA	1965	19 yrs 15 yrs	4070 4590	M/F	35+	Weekly quantity frequency	Abstainers vs. drinkers higher but not significant	Lazarus *et al.* (1991); Camacho *et al.* (1987)
Normative Aging, USA	1973	12 yrs	1823	M	Mean age 49.5	Drinking previous day at baseline	Mortality slightly higher for non-drinkers. No diff. for CHD non-drinkers vs. mod. drinkers <65 yrs	De Labry *et al.* (1992)
7 countries, Italian rural	1965	15 yrs	1536	M	45–64	Glasses per day	U-shaped, not significant; lowest 30–60 g/day	Farchi *et al.* (1992)
Busselton, W. Australia	1966	23 yrs	2171	M/F	>40	Non/ex-drinker, mild, moderate, heavy drinker	RR Mod/non-drinkers 0.76 total mortality, 0.68 CVD[c] mortality	Cullen *et al.* (1993)

[a] RR, relative risk. [b] CHD, coronary heart disease. [c] CVD, cardiovascular disease.

in 5209 men and women from Massachusetts after a 22-year follow-up, beginning in the early 1950s (Gordon and Kannel 1984). Consumption habits were measured in terms of number of drinks per month. Additional information on drinking was obtained at the seventh biennial exam. Light-drinking males experienced the lowest overall mortality, but differences for non-drinking males were not statistically significant. Total mortality among men varied only slightly by drinking level, with no apparent increase in risk at 90 ounces per month (2520 g—2 to 3 drinks per day). Deaths from cancer among males rose with increasing consumption, and deaths from liver cirrhosis also increased with consumption, with half occurring among those drinking less than 60 ounces (1680 g) per month. CHD mortality decreased with increasing consumption. Drinking by women was unrelated to mortality.

The Japanese Physicians Study Kono *et al.* (1986) investigated the relationship between drinking habit and cause-specific mortality in 5135 Japanese male physicians followed-up over 19 years, beginning in 1965. Self-report data on overall drinking pattern in the past 20 years, current pattern, and amount consumed were obtained for 51 per cent of eligible physicians in western Japan. The relative risk of overall mortality compared to non-drinkers (adjusted for age and smoking status) was significantly higher for ex-drinkers (RR = 1.38) and those drinking 3.2 or more drinks per day (RR = 1.28). Relative risks for occasional and daily drinkers (< 3.2 drinks/day) were slightly, but not significantly, lower (RR = 0.86; 0.91). For specific causes of death, occasional drinkers had significantly lower rates of lung cancer, acute myocardial infarction, and 'other causes' than non-drinkers. Moderate daily drinkers did not experience significantly lower rates of any cancers, CVD, CHD, stroke or other causes than non-drinkers. Heavy drinkers were more likely to die of liver cancer, and non-haemorrhagic stroke. Ex-drinkers had higher rates of CVD, other CHD, and non-haemorrhagic stroke. The investigators suggest that the U-shaped relationship between alcohol and total mortality reported in studies of Western populations may not hold for Japanese populations where the incidence of stroke, which is positively related to consumption, is far higher.

The British Regional Heart Study Shaper *et al.* (1988) report on 7735 British men aged 40–59, selected from general practices throughout the United Kingdom, in 1978–80 and followed for 7.5 years. Self-reported weekly alcohol intake was related to subsequent mortality from all causes, and for CVD separately, with controls for age, smoking habits, and social class. The investigators report a U-shaped relationship with total mortality and CVD, but only among men who were previously diagnosed with cardiovascular disorders. Separate analyses by smoking status and social class indicated that only ex-smokers and manual workers experienced lower mortality at light or moderate drinking levels.

The Swedish Conscripts Study This study involved a 20-year follow-up of 49 464 Swedish male conscripts aged 18–21 (Andreasson *et al.* 1988, 1991). As 97–98 per cent of Swedish men are conscripted, and since the age at recruitment in the study was low, the problem of eliminating those with pre-existing disease was largely eliminated. Mortality at follow-up increased with amount of alcohol consumed. Abstainers had the lowest mortality for both violent and non-violent mortality, which was not significantly different from moderate drinkers (1–100 g per week or less than 1 drink per day). Relative risk of mortality for those drinking more than 250 g per week was 2.82. Main causes of death were suicide and traffic accidents, with a small proportion attributable to alcohol-related disease. Continued follow-up will provide a unique opportunity to examine premature disease-related mortality in this cohort.

The Nurses' Health Study Colditz (1990) assessed the relationship between moderate drinking and the incidence of major chronic diseases over a six-year period among 121 700 married women enrolled in the Nurses' Health Study in 1976. Alcohol consumption was measured in 1980 as usual frequency of intake over the preceding year. The incidence of breast cancer was higher at 0.5 drinks per day (RR = 1.3) and even higher at more than one drink per day (RR = 1.6). The relative risk of CHD declined at the same point to 0.6 and continued to fall with increasing consumption to 0.4. The risk of ischaemic stroke declined in much the same way, while the risk of subarachnoid haemorrhage increased substantially, but not significantly, to 2.4 with any use of alcohol. Hypertension increased significantly at about two drinks per day. Non-significant decreases in risk of gallstones (RR = 0.7) and diabetes (RR = 0.6) also occurred at light drinking levels. The exact number of cases by drinking level is not given, but some idea of the magnitude can be seen by looking at the total number of cases. For those conditions reporting an increase with drinking level, the number of cases for each condition was as follows: breast cancer, 200, subarachnoid haemorrhage, 28, and hypertension, 3275. For conditions in which drinking did not increase morbidity or where drinking appeared to have a protective effect, the numbers were CHD, 200; ischaemic stroke, 66; gallstones, 612; and diabetes, 526. Both gallstones and diabetes were associated with increased body weight. For the same cohort, Stampfer *et al.* (1988) report that moderate drinking was associated with lower mortality from CHD and thrombotic stroke, but increased risk of haemorrhagic stroke.

The American Cancer Society Study Boffetta and Garfinkel (1990) report on a 12-year follow-up of more than 250 000 US men, aged 40–59, enrolled in 1959. Drinking was measured as usual consumption at time of entry. Overall mortality was slightly lower for those drinking occasionally or from 1 to 2 drinks per day compared to non-drinkers (RR = 0.88, 0.84, 0.93). Deaths from cancer increased at 2 drinks per day, accidents at 3 drinks per day, and suicide and liver cirrhosis, with any drinking. Deaths from CHD were slightly lower for drinkers than non-drinkers, but no significant difference was reported across the range from occasional to 6 plus per day. Occasional and irregular drinkers were sometimes classified as non-drinkers and sometimes as occasional or irregular. Smoking history was not controlled in this study, apparently because the investigators believed that giving up smoking for up to 10 years would have no beneficial effect on mortality.

The Alameda County Study Lazarus *et al.* (1991) followed-up a large representative sample of 4070 California residents aged 35 and over recruited in 1965. They examined changes in alcohol consumption from 1965 to 1974 and mortality from all causes and from ischaemic heart disease (IHD) for 1974–84. Respondents were asked about weekly quantity and frequency of alcohol consumption by beverage type.

Among men, long-term abstainers experienced higher risk of death from all causes and from IHD than drinkers, but differences were not statistically significant. No increased risk was seen among men who stopped drinking recently, but women who gave up recently were at higher risk of all causes of death and IHD.

An earlier report on the same study (Camacho *et al.* 1987) involved 4590 subjects aged 35 and older who were followed up for 15 years. Analyses of potential confounders showed a strong negative effect of age, low income, never smoked, low education, and depression. U-shaped relationships were found for disability, fair or poor health, and not being married. With adjustment for age only, they found a slightly U-shaped relationship between drinking level and mortality and IHD. Differences between abstainers, light, and moderate levels were not significant. When the 13 covariates were included in the analysis, the results were unchanged (RR total mortality and IHD mortality were the same for male abstainers = 1.2; female abstainers = 1.1). The investigators tested for a curvilinear association and report a significant alcohol/mortality association only for male all-cause mortality. However, the results are inconclusive since the linear term does not differ significantly from zero. They also found no significant differences between stable abstainers and ex-drinkers after nine years of follow-up.

The Normative Aging Study De Labry *et al.* (1992) followed up 1823 male subjects (mean age 49.5 years), who had been prescreened for serious or chronic disease for 12 years beginning in 1973. Self-reports of drinking the previous day at baseline (none, 1, 2, 3 plus drinks) as well as previous problems with drinking were related to overall mortality and specific cause of death. Overall mortality was slightly higher for non-drinkers than moderate drinkers in three age groups examined; however CHD mortality was no different among non-drinkers and moderate drinkers under the age of 65.

Proportional hazards models controlling for age, cholesterol, systolic blood pressure, and smoking status showed lower CHD mortality among moderate drinkers, but differences were not statistically significant. Surprisingly, men reporting drinking problems were at no greater risk of CHD than other drinkers. The authors attribute the lack of an association with CHD to the smaller number of CHD deaths and to the initial prescreening for hypertension which eliminated men with this risk factor.

The Seven Countries Study: Italian Rural Cohorts Farchi *et al.* (1992) examined total and CHD mortality in 1536 men aged 45–64 followed-up for 15 years (1965–80). Alcohol consumption was measured in terms of glasses of wine or spirits and verified using other sources. Mean consumption of absolute alcohol was 84 g per day, far higher than levels reported in other studies. Because non-drinkers were rare (2 per cent), they were included with 'low-level drinkers'.

Total mortality was lowest in the modal drinking category (30–60 g per day). CVD deaths were significantly higher for the lowest quintile drinkers (0–30 g), whereas deaths from cancer and liver cirrhosis were not. When those with pre-existing CVD were excluded from the analysis, the differences were not statistically significant. CHD deaths showed a similar U-shaped curve, but differences between the first and second quintile were significant only when those with pre-existing disease were excluded.

Proportional hazards models for mortality, with and without those with pre-existing disease excluded, showed U-shaped curves for total, cancer, CVD, and CHD mortality, although none of the relative risks were significantly different from the lowest category. Relative risks for all major diseases only rose above 1.0 for the highest drinking category (mean of 164.7 g per day).

The Busselton, Western Australia Study A 23-year follow-up of the Busselton cohort reports reduced risk of total mortality and cardiovascular mortality for moderate drinkers compared to non-drinkers (Cullen *et al.* 1993). While the relationship of baseline drinking status to total and CVD mortality was not significant when only age and sex were controlled, the addition of nine other variables to the regression model showed relative risks (moderate drinker to non-drinker) of 0.76 and 0.68, respectively. Moderate drinkers comprised 31 per cent of males and only 9 per cent of females. 'Mild' drinkers did not experience significantly lower mortality than non-drinkers.

Problems with the measurement of drinking status in this study may qualify these conclusions. A follow-up in 1975 showed major changes in classification of drinkers after only nine years. Almost half (42 per cent) of those reporting that they were non-drinkers (presumably life-long abstainers) in 1975 had classified themselves as drinkers or ex-drinkers in 1966. Thirteen per cent of non-drinkers in 1966 reported that they had become drinkers in 1975—

Table 9.2 Increased risk of medical conditions associated with moderate consumption of alcohol

Condition	Threshold of risk (g alcohol/day)
Cardiovascular disease	>40
Cerebrovascular disorder	>0
Hepatic cirrhosis	>20 (F)
	>40 (M)
Pancreatitis	>0
Oesophageal cancer	>40
Breast cancer	>35
Spontaneous abortion	>11
Fetal alcohol effects	>20 (60 g on occasion)
Alcohol dependence syndrome	>50

Source: Babor *et al.* (1987).

unusual in a population aged 40 and over—and only 24 per cent of ex-drinkers remained in that category after nine years, with half of the remainder becoming drinkers again and half reporting they were non-drinkers (Cullen *et al.* 1993). The extent to which these differences are due to mis-classification or to real changes in drinking habits is unknown.

Studies of drinking and specific diseases and conditions

While few studies examine the relationship between drinking and health outcomes for the same study population, there are substantial bodies of research that link moderate drinking with various diseases and conditions. Colsher and Wallace (1989) have reviewed this literature for evidence of a biphasic relationship. They conclude that risk of burn injury, falls, and motor vehicle collisions increases with increasing blood alcohol level at the time of the event. Babor *et al.* (1987) have summarized the medical conditions associated with moderate levels of drinking (Table 9.2).

Early studies of motor vehicle accidents by Borkenstein *et al.* and Perrine *et al.* (cf. Babor *et al.* 1987) show substantially increased impairment and risk of collision at blood alcohol concentrations of 50 mg/100 ml. Infrequent drinkers with lower tolerance to alcohol have greater risk of accidents at a given blood alcohol level.

Regular consumption of alcohol interferes with the metabolism of most vitamins and some minerals and stimulates excretion of calcium and magnesium, which may increase risk of osteoporosis (USHHS 1990). The incidence of head and neck cancers increases monotonically with alcohol consumption and synergistically with concurrent cigarette-smoking (USHHS 1990).

Conditions specific to women occur at fairly low levels of consumption. Adverse outcomes of pregnancy are associated with increasing levels of usual drinking. Windham *et al.* (1992) report a relative risk of 1.9 for spontaneous abortion in women drinking seven or more drinks per week. A number of studies report elevated risk of fetal alcohol effects in offspring of women who drank moderate amounts during pregnancy (USHHS 1990: 141–144). Breast cancer is also associated with increased alcohol consumption in many studies. Willett *et al.* (1987) report a 50 per cent increase in risk of breast cancer among women drinking at least one drink per day. Gapstur *et al.* (1992) report increased risk in postmenopausal women who had used non-contraceptive oestrogens and were drinking an average of 5 g of alcohol per day. The strong association of breast cancer with a high-fat diet and with high socio-economic status (which is also related to drinking) may also contribute to this relationship.

Alcohol-related liver cirrhosis may occur in women drinking as little as 20 g per day and men drinking 40–80 g per day (Péquignot *et al.* 1971). Klatsky and Armstrong (1992) report a relative risk of mortality of 7.8 for those drinking 1–2 drinks per day compared to those who drink less or none at all or were ex-drinkers. Pancreatitis increases with any consumption of alcohol (USHHS 1990).

Most studies report a linear relationship between alcohol consumption and hypertension, with no threshold effect (Friedman 1990; Lands and Zakhari 1990). Ueshima *et al.* (1993) report that untreated, mildly hypertensive, moderate drinkers (daily intake =/> 28 ml) who reduce their drinking by half experience significant reductions in blood pressure.

The effect of moderate drinking on stroke varies by type of stroke. While haemorrhagic stroke increases in linear fashion with consumption, there is a threshold effect for ischaemic stroke. Stampfer *et al.* (1988) report an increased risk of subarachnoid haemorrhage in women who drink three to nine drinks per week. Interestingly, a U-shaped relationship was found for ischaemic stroke in Americans, but no such dip occurred in a Japanese population. In the United States, ischaemic stroke accounts for about 70 per cent of all stroke; haemorrhagic stroke occurs more frequently among the Japanese (Lands and Zakhari 1990).

Evidence of benefits of moderate drinking

Baum-Baicker's (1985*a*,*b*) two reviews of the benefits of moderate drinking summarize most of the other evidence. Alcoholic beverages contain small amount of vitamins as well as trace metals and minerals. Alcohol also supplies energy on the basis of 7 calories per gram. Baum-Baicker reviews the psychological effects of drinking, including the reduction of tension, self-consciousness, stress, fear, pain, and depression, and the increase in affective expression and good feelings. Small doses of alcohol are associated with improvements in mood and decreases in depression and tension in several studies. Effects on intellectual functioning are mixed, with some studies reporting small improvements and others small decrements. Expectancies about the effects of alcohol and the social context of drinking may explain some of these relationships. Several studies report benefits of moderate drinking by the elderly, such as increased social interaction, decreased use of psychotropic medication, reduced insomnia, and improved cognitive performance. Alcohol can interact negatively with medications, however, and reports of benefits may be partly or wholly due to other changes associated with the introduction of drinking, such as social events or greater attention from staff in institutions, or to expectancy effects on drinkers.

Methodological issues

Pre-existing disease

Shaper's (1990) review of prospective studies of alcohol and mortality examines the possibility that pre-existing disease accounts for the greater mortality found among abstainers. He argues that the relationship is selective rather than causal, that most non-drinkers (70 per cent) are ex-drinkers who stop drinking as they begin to experience ill-health, and that this group already has symptoms and diseases at the time of screening. Others have argued against this, most usefully by attempting to control for pre-existing conditions by not counting mortality or morbidity early in the follow-up period (De Labry *et al.* 1992). The difficulty remains that the first symptoms of coronary heart disease and cancer, the main causes of death, tend to occur late in the disease process. Screening for disease is rarely intensive enough to identify premorbid conditions. Furthermore, the higher prevalence of many diseases among non-drinkers may make them unsuitable as a baseline group (Shaper 1993).

Inadequate measures of variables

Drinking The measurement of drinking in studies linking alcohol with mortality is often inadequate (Ferrence *et al.* 1986, Knupfer 1987; Colsher and Wallace 1989). Major prospective studies which began many years ago often rely on one to three-day dietary recall information, or fail to collect subsequent information on changes in drinking levels. Since most of these studies were not originally designed to examine the effect of moderate drinking, information on patterns of drinking and drinking history is rarely obtained.

Drinking levels are usually daily averages calculated on the basis of weekly or monthly frequency. Drinkers who abstain during the week and drink heavily on weekends, a typical pattern for many drinkers, are grouped with those who regularly drink small amounts—a relatively rare pattern (Knupfer 1987).

Studies of self-reporting of alcohol consumption suggest that drinkers underestimate their drinking and tend to ignore periods when they drank more heavily (Poikolainen 1985). Former heavy drinkers, for example, might be misclassified as life-long abstainers or former light drinkers if they deny earlier heavy drinking. Based on what we know about underestimates of drinking, the 'optimum' levels reported in many studies (generally one to two drinks per day, but often three, four, or five) could be considerably higher.

Lazarus *et al.* (1991) examined changes in drinking patterns between 1965 and 1974 among women and men in the Alameda County Study. Of those who were non-drinkers in 1965, 22 per cent of women and 32 per cent of men moved to light and moderate drinking categories within nine years. Among moderate drinkers, 37 per cent of women and 39 per cent of men moved to light or non-drinking categories over the same period. This substantial movement between drinking categories suggests that categorizing subjects according to drinking level may be far more complex than it appears, and that regular monitoring of subjects in long-term follow-up studies may be necessary to make any valid inferences about the effect of drinking level on health. Similar movement among drinking categories occurs in the Busselton study (Cullen *et al.* 1993).

These findings raise the issue of the meaning of moderate drinking. If we had full drinking histories, how would we classify someone who drank heavily as a youth, moderately as a younger adult, lightly after age 50, and stopped altogether at age 70? Such patterns may be typical of a substantial part of the population, yet the respondent would be classified differently depending on age of recruitment.

Reports linking moderate drinking to reductions in mortality and CHD provide a range of drinking levels that get called 'moderate drinking'. In fact, the groups with the lowest mortality are usually referred to as moderate drinkers, whether they actually drink occasionally or heavily each day. In the Italian rural cohort (Farchi *et al.* 1992), for example, the high-risk category of light drinkers would be classified as moderate in some studies. In most studies, the moderate category is far above the average consumption of the general population. By contrast, social researchers tend to define moderate drinking in terms that imply low frequency, rarely drinking to intoxication, and not damaging to health or other aspects of life (cf. Babor *et al.* 1987).

Smoking Most studies report that they control for smoking status, but the strong relationship between drinking and smoking makes that difficult. Heavy drinkers who have never smoked are rare as are heavy smokers who are lifelong abstainers. Gordon and Kannel (1984) remark on the close association between drinking and smoking and express concern that they may not have been able to disentangle the effects. Kozlowski and Ferrence (1990) re-analysed data from some of the major alcohol and mortality studies (Marmot *et al.* 1981; Klatsky *et al.* 1981; Friedman and Kimball 1986). They report that the U-shaped curve is most pronounced for very heavy smokers and flattens with amount smoked. Among never smokers, mortality is similar for abstainers and for those drinking two or fewer drinks per day. Dyer *et al.* (1977) did differentiate between former and never drinkers. Analysis of their data clearly showed that former drinkers accounted for almost all the excess mortality among non-drinkers (Kozlowski and Ferrence 1990). Shaper *et al.* (1988) report similar findings, with only ex-smokers showing lower mortality among non-drinkers.

A recent report extends these findings to coronary heart disease. Nyboe *et al.* (1991) report similar results for the risk of first acute myocardial infarction in the Copenhagen City Heart Study. Daily drinking was reported to be 'protective' for very heavy smokers, although the rate of acute myocardial infarction was double that of non-smoking non-drinkers. The most likely explanation for the high relative risk (RR = 6.7) among non-drinking heavy smokers is not that drinking is protective, but that former heavy drinkers are over-represented in this group (Kozlowski and Ferrence 1990). The importance of being able to differentiate heavy from moderate and light smokers is clear from the Danish study, since the effect was not strong below 30 g (about 30 cigarettes) per day.

Smoking history is also important, particularly when total mortality is the outcome measure. Former smokers are more likely to have higher socio-economic status (SES) than never smokers. In younger populations, current smokers are more likely to be lower in SES, so that future studies will find that former smokers are more likely to be lower in SES (Ferrence 1990). This is important because mortality is inversely related to social status, whereas drinking is positively related to social status. Thus, male moderate drinkers are most likely to be higher SES and former smokers. Male heavy drinkers and former drinkers are more likely than moderate drinkers to be lower SES and to be current smokers. Controlling for education does not necessarily eliminate this bias since comprehensive measures of SES are not normally used in such studies.

Age This is always included in studies of drinking and mortality, but age categories, rather than exact age, are generally used. Since non-drinkers are on average older than drinkers, and since mortality rates approximately double in successive five-year age categories (Walker *et al.* 1987), small differences in the age distribution within categories could produce sizeable differences in mortality in older samples. In Boffetta and Garfinkel's (1990) study of alcohol consumption and mortality, for example, age is treated as a categorical variable in most of the analysis. When entered as a continuous variable, however, no significant differences in mortality were found between occasional and daily drinkers (Ferrence and Kozlowski 1991).

The 'healthy subject' effect

The age at which subjects are selected and the method of selection may produce misleading findings in studies of the effect of drinking levels on health. The best designed studies of the effects of drinking level are prospective cohort studies. In most cases, a group of healthy subjects is followed up for several years. The outcome is the presence of diagnosed disease or death. Exposure to alcohol is measured at baseline and, in some studies, at various follow-up points. The ideal design would be a lifetime follow-up of subjects recruited as young adolescents, before they begin their drinking careers or at least by age 20. In most studies, however, subjects are selected at older ages when they may already have developed alcohol-related diseases. De Labry *et al.* (1992), for example, excluded subjects who had diagnosed heart disease, cancer, diabetes, and hypertension. The age of subjects ranged from 20 to 79. If moderate and heavy drinkers are more likely than abstainers to be excluded at this point, and this seems likely, since drinkers more often smoke and have hypertension and other conditions related to drinking, the remaining drinkers would be healthier and probably more resistant to alcohol-related diseases than the abstainers.

Since subjects for prospective studies are usually selected through medical or insurance systems, as volunteers, or through professional associations, individuals who are in hospitals or other institutions or are in poor health, are generally excluded. In studies that use medical insurance plans for recruitment, unemployed or uninsured individuals are excluded. All of these considerations lead to the selection of subjects who are not only healthier than average, but may be more likely to be healthy if they are drinkers.

Support for this hypothesis comes from Walker *et al.* (1987). who studied non-participants in a prospective study of cardiovascular disease in British middle-aged men. Non-participants were younger, more often unmarried, and of lower SES. They had higher overall mortality and were probably, on the basis of these demographic characteristics, more likely to be drinkers and smokers.

In many cases, it is inappropriate to factor out pre-existing disease because some conditions are causally related to both drinking and mortality (Ferrence and Bondy 1994). Rothman (1986) and Weinberg (1993) caution that 'confounders' must not function as intervening variables in the causal path between exposure and disease. Conditions, such as hypertension and breast cancer, may be causally related to moderate drinking and are certainly associated with increased risk of mortality. Thus, they should not be screened out or controlled for in the analysis. The only clear way around the dual problem of inappropriate confounders and controlling for pre-existing disease is to start with young cohorts or to use more intensive methods of examining and analysing the data. The typical practice of entering a dozen or more variables into a regression does not always provide a clear picture of the interrelationships among variables.

Characteristics of abstainers

Life-long abstainers are reported to be older, lower in socio-economic status, to live in rural areas, to be religious, to have relatives with alcohol-related problems (Hughes *et al.* 1985; Wannamethee and Shaper 1988), to have higher depression scores, and to experience more depressive symptoms following life events than light or moderate users (Bell *et al.* 1977; Neff and Husaini 1982). While the higher rate of depression has been attributed to the lack of alcohol as a stress reducer (Baum-Baicker 1985*b*), a more plausible hypothesis is that depressed people socialize less. The amount of alcohol consumed by light or occasional drinkers seems hardly sufficient to prevent depressive symptoms if one is prone to them.

Camacho *et al.* (1987) examined characteristics of subjects by drinking level in the Alameda County Study. While abstainers clearly were very different from drinkers (older, more often female, black, disabled, non-smokers, low income, in poor health, not married, inactive, low education, depressed, and with no organization memberships), adjusting for these covariates in logistic regression had no effect on risk of mortality. The possibility that such major differences may not be fully amenable to statistical control needs to be considered (Kozlowski and Ferrence 1990).

Dietary confounders

Diet is an important factor in many diseases, and may be responsible for one-third of all cases of CHD and cancer in the West (USHHS 1988). Diet is also implicated in hypertension, stroke, diabetes, obesity, and dental disease. Most studies do not control for diet, although data are often collected; furthermore, the narrow range of dietary habits within most study populations may make controls ineffectual. Cross-cultural comparisons, such as in the Seven Countries Study, would provide the best means of controlling for diet, but other differences could make this impractical.

Dietary fat. Since a high intake of dietary fat, particularly saturated fat, is a risk factor for heart disease, cancer, and possibly other diseases, differences in fat intake between moderate drinkers and abstainers could affect their risk of disease (Keys *et al.* 1986).

Fish. Regular intake of fish may be protective for heart disease, due to the effect of omega-3 fatty acids (Fehily *et al.* 1982; Kromhout *et al.* 1985; Phillipson *et al.* 1985).

Milk products. Popham *et al.* (1983) report that the consumption of milk proteins accounts for most of the relationship between drinking and ischaemic heart disease mortality. They hypothesized that a component of lactose found in unfermented milk products might be atherogenic.

Other possible confounders

Another concern is that moderate drinkers included in recent investigations may be using acetylsalicylic acid (ASA) for prevention of coronary heart disease (S. Zakhari personal communication). ASA is often used to counteract the effects of drinking and is known to potentiate the effects of drinking if used beforehand (Roine *et al.* 1990). New therapies, such as ASA, are also most likely to be adopted first by high-status males who are more likely than lower-status males to be moderate drinkers and in good health. Surveys with adequate data on ASA consumption and drinking patterns could be analysed to determine patterns of use by sex, age, social class, and drinking level.

Length of follow-up

Most prospective studies follow-up healthy middle-aged men for a period of from 2 to 20 years. What this provides is an investigation of a select population of healthy individuals over a relatively short period when only a few of them will die. While short-term follow-up results may coincide with those obtained in longer periods, confidence intervals tend to be large, and patterns may change over time. The Swedish Conscripts Study (Andreasson *et al.* 1991), for example, found a slightly elevated mortality among abstainers compared to light drinkers after 15 years which had reversed by 20 years.

Differences in the study 'window', that is, the period in a subject's life from selection to follow-up, can greatly affect findings. The purpose of research on drinking and mortality is to look at premature, rather than ultimate mortality, since everyone dies at some point. What most of these studies lack are measures of attributable risk (AR) and potential years of life lost (PYLL) for a range of diseases and conditions for entire birth cohorts of men and women recruited early in life. There comes a point where low-risk groups experience mortality similar to that of high-risk groups, because more of the latter group have died off. Studies in which subjects are selected at older ages when significant mortality has already occurred, may produce distorted results (for example, De Labry *et al.* 1992).

U-shaped curves

The relationship between drinking and coronary heart disease (CHD) is not the only U-shaped or biphasic one described in scientific literature (Colsher and Wallace 1989). Several studies report higher mortality at both the lowest and highest levels of body weight (USHHS 1988). Other research indicates higher mortality at both low and high levels of cholesterol (Frank *et al.* 1992). It might be useful to study all such U-shaped relationships in the same population in an effort to discover whether some common factor might at least partially explain them. Likely confounders include pre-existing disease, diet, tobacco use, age, and social class. While these factors are at least roughly controlled for in most studies, coarse measurement of several confounding factors could have a substantial effect.

The possibility that those who deviate most from the social norms of their society, may be at increased risk of health problems needs to be considered (Ferrence *et al.* 1986). Lifelong abstainers form a very small proportion of the population in Western countries and probably even less of most study populations. Comparisons with societies in which abstinence is the norm and 'moderate drinking' unusual may shed some light on this issue. Certainly, it seems unlikely that the low cholesterol levels associated with increased mortality in Western societies would show the same relationship in Far Eastern countries where average cholesterol levels are much lower.

Mortality for the Italian rural cohorts of the Seven Countries Study (Farchi *et al.* 1992) showed a similar U-shaped pattern, even though the consumption levels associated with each category were far higher than those reported in other studies. Although most differences were not statistically significant, mortality was highest among those in the lowest and highest drinking quintiles.

Although some have argued that the protective effect must be real since other diseases do not show a U-shaped relationship with drinking (Marmot and Brunner 1991), it should be recognized that the typical curve for drinking and CHD is not an inverse dose-response curve but really a modified dose-response curve with, typically, only a small rise at the beginning. In most cases, light drinkers are not at significantly higher risk of CHD mortality than moderate drinkers. In the majority of studies, only lifelong abstainers, a very small proportion of most Western populations, show higher mortality.

The balance sheet for alcohol

In summary, the literature reviewed here presents an inconclusive picture of the effect of moderate drinking on total mortality. The author concurs with the assessment of Colsher and Wallace (1989, p. 213) who conclude:

> The general absence of a bidirectional dose-response relationship for most of the conditions reviewed and for general measures of morbidity offers little support for an overall health-promoting effect of low to moderate alcohol intake.

Much of the research has been carried out on white middle-class males in western countries. Evidence for a protective effect for women and non-

Western populations is not as strong. Regular light or moderate drinking appears to have at least a small beneficial effect on CHD morbidity and mortality. However, in many populations, this is balanced by the increased incidence of hypertension, liver cirrhosis, and possibly breast cancer, and other diseases that increase in a dose-response manner with consumption. None of the studies reviewed actually present data in the form of disease-specific attributable risks or potential years of life lost so that meaningful comparisons can be made across drinking levels. With the exception of the Swedish Conscripts Study, adverse effects of accidents and violence associated with alcohol, which occur primarily in younger populations, are not included in measuring the total impact of drinking. Only lifelong prospective studies can present a full picture.

The search for a mechanism to explain a protective effect on CHD and some types of cardiovascular disease (CVD) has focused on lipid levels and platelet aggregation. Previous research suggests that an inverse relationship between high-density lipoprotein cholesterol (HDL-C) level and CHD (Gordon *et al.* 1989) may explain the protective effect of drinking on CHD. However, a recent study of the effect of different drinking levels on lipid values (Seppä *et al.* 1992) found no significant difference between abstainers and moderate drinkers.

The current interest in the apparent protective effect of red wine in French drinkers, who apparently eat large amounts of cheese yet experience lower rates of CHD mortality than North Americans, has led to some research on the topic. While at least part of the difference can be explained by historically lower fat intake among the French who only recently began eating a higher fat diet (Nestle 1992), Frankel *et al.* (1993) report that the non-alcoholic phenolic substances in red wine are potent inhibitors of oxidation of low-density lipoprotein and may reduce risk of heart disease.

Much of the evidence suggests that any protective effect may be highly specified. There is some evidence that only heavy smokers are protected. Few heavy smokers are light or abstinent drinkers, unless they are former heavy drinkers (Kozlowski and Ferrence 1990). Many studies have excluded women and populations whose life style is very different from that of Western countries. It is worth noting that CHD is a life style disease and is rare in populations with low-fat diets and low rates of smoking. It may be that alcohol is beneficial only for those with high-fat intake or high-saturated fat intake. Whatever the size of the effect, diet explains far more of the variance in CHD mortality than moderate drinking. Rates of CHD in Crete and Japan, for example are only a small fraction of those in Western countries (Keys *et al.* 1986). A recent report on older Danish men found alcohol protective only for the 10 per cent of men with the Lewis phenotype Le(a-b-), who are genetically at higher risk of ischaemic heart disease (Hein *et al.* 1993).

Recommendations for two or fewer drinks a day appear to be based on studies which report reduced CHD mortality among light and moderate drinkers compared to non-drinkers. These recommendations generally ignore the evidence linking moderate alcohol consumption to other diseases and conditions. Current recommendations generally suggest no more than two drinks per day, with less or none for pregnant women, the elderly, those on medication, and those who are ill (USHHS 1988, 1990). However, the US Surgeon General (USHHS 1988) cautions that:

> Since heavy drinking has numerous adverse effects, including several on the cardiovascular system . . . , the use of alcohol, even in moderate quantities, for its possible beneficial effects on CHD is not recommended.

Marmot and Brunner (1991) relate recommendations to the larger issue of general alcohol consumption. They cite results from the Intersalt study which concludes that an increase of one drink per day would lead to a 10 per cent increase in heavy drinking (Rose and Day 1990); they conclude that the balance of harm and benefit precludes recommending drinking to prevent CHD. Artificial attempts to change the relationship between average and heavy consumption would have to involve rationing or medical prescriptions of alcohol for those who might benefit.

When one considers the reality of making recommendations, only lifelong abstainers qualify on the basis of research findings as a potential target group. Yet, it is unlikely that anyone would recommend that members of this group begin drinking. Many dislike alcohol, abstain for religious or health reasons, or feel they are at risk of dependency. Most older males who are at risk of CHD already have conditions, such as hypertension, which may be worsened by moderate drinking.

Exemptions from recommendations to drink moderately are typically treated as an afterthought, but should give us pause. Consumers Union (1993), for example, concludes their article, *Drink to your health?* with these comprehensive criteria for abstention: a history of abstention; a history of dependency on licit or illicit drugs; a family history of alcoholism or depression; a personal history of depression or anxiety; medical conditions such as liver disease, abnormal heart rhythms, an enlarged heart, a previous haemorrhagic stroke, peptic ulcers, gout, pancreatitis, high blood levels of triglycerides; a strong family history of breast cancer; early menstruation; having no children or having a child at a late age; late onset of menopause; chronic insomnia; sleep apnoea; use of tranquillizers, sleeping pills, anticonvulsants, certain painkillers, antihistamines, heart medications, such as nitrates and beta blockers, use of aspirin or non-steroidal anti-inflammatory drugs; and operating vehicles or equipment that require good co-ordination.

A careful analysis of an appropriate data set would be required to determine just how many of us can safely drink. However, it is clear that the proportion of the population who would be exempted from the apparent benefits of moderate drinking would be substantial, and that recommending guidelines for the general population is not a simple task.

The research agenda

Recent studies of drinking and mortality and drinking and CHD have tried to address some of the issues raised by critics of this research. In response to Shaper's (1990) concerns, attempts have been made to eliminate those with pre-existing disease and to separate lifelong abstainers from former heavy drinkers (Jackson *et al.* 1991; Boffetta and Garfinkel 1990; De Labry *et al.* 1992). The extent to which the former effort has been successful is unclear.

Several issues remain:

1. Why is a protective effect found at such high levels of consumption, in some studies as high as four to five drinks daily, when these levels are known to result in adverse health outcomes?
2. What are the characteristics of abstainers in these studies, and are there factors associated with life-long abstention that explain increased level of risk?
3. Are there small differences in age resulting from the use of categorical rather than continuous measures of age in the analysis that bias results?
4. Many of the divergent findings have come from populations with different drinking levels and eating habits (Andreasson *et al.* 1991; Kono *et al.* 1986). To what extent are North American findings replicated in other countries, especially in those with very different life styles?
5. Tobacco use and particularly heavy use appears to be strongly involved in the relationship between drinking and mortality. More research is needed to clarify this interaction.
6. Since diet, particularly saturated fat intake, is a major factor in CHD, cancer, and other causes of death, more detailed information on dietary history and recent changes is needed in follow-up studies.
7. In general, more attention needs to be paid to how well controls are controlling for the factor in question. As well as age, smoking, and diet, other factors, such as socio-economic status, exercise, and social support, need to be carefully controlled. Potential intervening variables need to be built into statistical models rather than adjusted for in the analysis.
8. To what extent are protective effects evident in women, the elderly, and young people? Are there different net effects for these groups?
9. What are current perceptions of possible benefits of moderate drinking on the part of physicians and the public?
10. Have there been changes in personal behaviour and advice-giving on the part of physicians and the public regarding possible benefits of moderate drinking?

11. What would be the effects on drinking levels and resulting problems in different populations if the public were advised that moderate drinking could be beneficial?

12. Since most smokers and illicit drug users are also drinkers, what would be the potential effect on rates of smoking and illicit drug use if average consumption of alcohol were increased?

Acknowledgements

The contributions of Mary Jane Ashley and Lucia Farinon to this project are gratefully recognized.

References

Andreasson, S., Romelsjö, A., and Allebeck, P. (1988). Alcohol and mortality among young men: A longitudinal study of Swedish conscripts. *British Medical Journal*, **83**, 1021–5.

Andreasson, S., Romelsjö, A., and Allebeck, P. (1991). Alcohol, social factors and mortality among young men. *British Journal of Addiction*, **86**, 877–87.

Ashley, M. J. (1982). Alcohol consumption, ischemic heart disease and cerebrovascular disease: an epidemiological perspective. *Journal of Studies on Alcohol*, **43**, 869–87.

Ashley, M. J. (1984). Alcohol consumption and ischemic heart disease: the epidemiologic evidence. In *Research advances in alcohol and drug problems*, (ed. R. G. Smart *et al.*), Vol. 8, pp. 99–147. Plenum, New York.

Babor, T. F., Kranzler, H. R., and Lauerman, R. J. (1987). Social drinking as a health and psychosocial risk factor. In *Recent developments in alcoholism*, (ed. M. Galanter), Vol. 5, pp. 373–402. Plenum, New York.

Baum-Baicker, C. (1985*a*). The health benefits of moderate alcohol consumption: a review of the literature. *Drug and Alcohol Dependence*, **115**, 207–27.

Baum-Baicker, C. (1985*b*). The psychological benefits of moderate alcohol consumption: a review of the literature. *Drug and Alcohol Dependence*, **115**, 305–22.

Bell, R., Keeley, K., and Buhl, J. (1977). Psychopathology and life events among alcohol users and non-users. In *Currents in alcoholism*, (ed. F. Sexias), Vol. III, pp. 103–26. Grune and Stratton, New York.

Blackwelder, W. C., Yano, K., Rhoads, G. G., Kagan, A., Gordon, T., and Palesch, Y. (1980). Alcohol and mortality: the Honolulu heart study. *American Journal of Medicine*, **68**, 164–9.

Boffetta, P. and Garfinkel, L. (1990). Alcohol drinking and mortality among men enrolled in an American Cancer Society prospective study. *Epidemiology*, **1**, 342–8.

Bruun, K., *et al.* (1975). *Alcohol control policies in public health perspective*, Vol. 25. Finnish Foundation for Alcohol Studies, Helsinki.

Camacho, T. C., Kaplan, G. A., and Cohen, R. D. (1987). Alcohol consumption and mortality in Alameda County. *Journal of Chronic Diseases*, **40**, 229–36.

Casswell, S. (1993). Public discourse on the benefits of moderation: implications for alcohol policy development. *Addiction*, **88**, 459–65.

Colditz, G. A. (1990). A prospective assessment of moderate alcohol intake and major chronic diseases. *Annals of Epidemiology*, **1**, 167–77.

Colditz, G. A., *et al.* (1985). Moderate alcohol and decreased cardiovascular mortality in an elderly cohort. *American Heart Journal*, **10**, 886–9.

Colsher, P. L. and Wallace, R. B. (1989). Is modest alcohol consumption better than none at all? An epidemiological assessment. *Annual Review of Public Health*, **10**, 201–19.

Consumers, Union (1993). Drink to your health? *Consumer Reports on Health*, **5**, 21–4.

Cullen, K. J., Stenhouse, N., and Wearne, K. L. (1982). Alcohol and mortality in the Busselton Study. *International Journal of Epidemiology*, **11**, 67–70.

Cullen, K. J., Knuiman, M. W., and Ward, N. J. (1993). Alcohol and mortality in Busselton, Western Australia. *American Journal of Epidemiology*, **137**, 242–8.

De Labry, L. O., Blynn, R. J., Levenson, M. R., Hermos, J. A., Lo Castro, J. S., Vokonas, P. S. (1992). Alcohol consumption and mortality in an American male population: recovering the U-shaped curve-findings from the Normative Aging Study. *Journal of Studies on Alcohol*, **53**, 25–32.

Dyer, A. R., *et al.* (1977). Alcohol consumption, cardiovascular risk factors and mortality in two Chicago epidemiologic studies. *Circulation*, **56**, 1067–74.

Dyer, A. R., *et al.* (1980). Alcohol consumption and 17-year mortality in the Chicago Western Electric Company Study. *Preventive Medicine*, **9**, 78–90.

Farchi, G., Fidanza, F., Mariotti, S., and Menotti, A. (1992). Alcohol and mortality in the Italian rural cohorts of the Seven Countries Study. *International Journal of Epidemiology*, **21**, 74–81.

Fehily, A. M., Millbank, J. E., Yarnell, J. W. G., Hayes, T. M., Kubiki, A. J., and Eastham, R. D. (1982). Dietary determinants of lipoproteins, total cholesterol, viscosity, fibrinogen, and blood pressure. *American Journal of Clinical Nutrition*, **36**, 890–6.

Ferrence, R. G. (1990). *Deadly fashion: The rise and fall of cigarette smoking in North America 1990–1979*. Garland, New York.

Ferrence, R. G. and Bondy, S. (1994). Re: Alcohol and mortality in Busselton, Western Australia [letter]. *American Journal of Epidemiology*, **139**, 544–6.

Ferrence, R. G. and Kozlowski, L. T. (1991). Moderate drinking and coronary health [letter]. *Epidemiology*, **2**, 311–12.

Ferrence, R. G., Truscott, S., and Whitehead, P. C. (1986). Drinking and coronary heart disease: findings, issues, and public health policy. *Journal of Studies on Alcohol*, **47**, 394–408.

Ford, G. (1988). *The benefits of moderate drinking: Alcohol, health and society*. Wine Appreciation Guild, San Francisco.

Frank, J. W., Reed, D. M., Grove, J. S., and Benfante, R. (1992). Will lowering population levels of serum cholesterol affect total mortality? Expectations from the Honolulu Heart Program. *Journal of Clinical Epidemiology*, **45**, 333–46.

Frankel, E. N., Kanner, J., German, J. B., Parks, E., and Kinsella, J. E. (1993). Inhibition of oxidation of human low-density lipoprotein by phenolic substances in red wine. *Lancet*, **341**, 454–7.

Friedman, H. S. (1990). Alcohol and hypertension. *Alcohol Health and Research World*, **14**, 313–19.

Friedman, L. A. and Kimball, A. W. (1986). Coronary heart disease mortality and alcohol consumption in Framingham. *American Journal of Epidemiology*, **124**, 481–9.

Gapstur, S. M., Potter, J. D., Sellers, T. A., and Folsom, A. R. (1992). Increased risk of breast cancer with alcohol consumption in postmenopausal women. *American Journal of Epidemiology*, **136**, 1221–31.

Gordon, D. J., *et al.* (1989). High-density lipoprotein cholesterol and cardiovascular disease: four prospective American studies. *Circulation*, **79**, 8–15.

Gordon, T. and Kannel, W. B. (1984). Drinking and mortality: The Framingham Study. *American Journal of Epidemiology*, **120**, 97–107.

Hein, H. O., Sorensen, H., Suadicani, P., and Gyntelberg, F. (1993). Alcohol consumption, Lewis phenotypes, and risk of ischaemic heart disease. *Lancet*, **341**, 392–6.

Hughes, J., Stewart, M., and Barraclough, B. (1985). Why teetotallers abstain. *British Journal of Psychiatry*, **146**, 204–8.

Jackson, R., Scragg, R., and Beaglehole, R. (1991). Alcohol consumption and risk of coronary heart disease. *British Medical Journal*, **303**, 211–16.

Johns Hopkins University (1992). *Is alcohol good for the heart? Johns Hopkins Medical Letter*, October.

Keys, A., *et al.* (1986). The diet and 15-year death rate in the seven countries study. *American Journal of Epidemiology*, **124**, 903–15.

Klatsky, A. L. (1990). Alcohol and coronary artery disease. *Alcohol Health and Research World*, **14**, 289–300.

Klatsky, A. L. and Armstrong, M. A. (1992). Alcohol, smoking, coffee, and cirrhosis. *American Journal of Epidemiology*, **136**, 1248–57.

Knupfer, G. (1987). Drinking for health: the daily light drinker fiction. *British Journal of addiction*, **82**, 547–55.

Kono, S., Ikeda, M., Tokudome, S., Nishizumi, M., and Kuratsune, M. (1986). Alcohol and mortality: a study of male Japanese physicians. *International Journal of Epidemiology*, **15**, 527–32.

Kozarevic, D. J., McGee, D., Vojvodic, N., Racic, Z., Dawber, T., and Gordon, T. (1980). Frequency of alcohol consumption and morbidity and mortality: The Yugoslavia cardiovascular disease study. *Lancet*, **1**, 613–16.

Kozlowski, L. T. and Ferrence, R. G. (1990). Statistical control in research on alcohol and tobacco: an example from research on alcohol and mortality. *British Journal of Addiction*, **85**, 271–8.

Kromhout, D., Bosschieter, E. B., and Coulander, C. D. L. (1985). The inverse relation between fish consumption and 20-year mortality from coronary heart disease. *New England Journal of Medicine*, **312**, 1205–9.

Lands, W. E. M. and Zakhari, S. (1990). Alcohol and cardiovascular disease. *Alcohol Health and Research World*, **14**, 305–12.

Lazarus, N. B., Kaplan, G. A., Cohen, R. D., and Leu, D.-J. (1991). Changes in alcohol consumption and risk of death from all causes and from ischaemic heart disease. *British Medical Journal*, **303**, 553–6.

Marmot, M. G. and Brunner, E. (1991). Alcohol and cardiovascular disease: the status of the U-shaped curve. *British Medical Journal*, **303**, 565–8.

Marmot, M. G., Rose, G., Shipley, M. J., and Thomas, B. J. (1981). Alcohol and mortality: a U-shaped curve. *Lancet*, **1**, 580–3.

Neff, J. and Husaini, B. (1982). Life events, drinking patterns and depressive symptomatology: The stress-buffering role of alcohol consumption. *Journal of Studies on Alcohol*, **43**, 301.

Nestle, M. (1992). Wine and coronary heart disease [Letter]. *Lancet*, **340**, 314–15.

Nyboe, J., Jensen, G., Appleyard, M., and Schnohr, P. (1991). Smoking and the risk of first acute myocardial infarction. *American Heart Journal*, **122**, 438–47.

Péquignot, G., Chabert, C., and Sydoux, H. (1971). Increased risk of liver cirrhosis with intake of alcohol. *La Revue de L'Alcoolisme*, **20**, 191–202.

Phillipson, B. E., Rothrock, D. W., Connor, W. E., Harris, W. S., and Illingworth, D. R. (1985). Reduction of plasma lipids, lipoproteins, and apoproteins by dietary fish oils in patients with hypertriglyceridemia. *New England Journal of Medicine*, **312**, 1210–16.

Popham, R. E., Schmidt, W., and Israel, Y. (1983). Variation in mortality from ischemic heart disease in relation to alcohol and milk consumption. *Medical Hypotheses*, **12**, 321–9.

Roine, R., Gentry, R. T., Hernandez-Munoz, R., Baraona, E., and Lieber, C. S. (1990). Aspirin increases blood alcohol concentrations in humans after ingestion of ethanol. *Journal of the American Medical Association*, **264**, 2406–8.

Rose, G. and Day, S. (1990). The population mean predicts the number of deviant individuals. *British Medical Journal*, **301**, 1031–4.

Rothman, K. J. (1986). *Modern epidemiology*. Little, Brown & Co, Boston.

Seppä, K., Sillanaukee, P., Pitkäjärvi, T., Nikkilä, M., and Koivula, T. (1992). Moderate and heavy alcohol consumption have no favorable effect on lipid values. *Archives of International Medicine*, **152**, 297–300.

Shaper, A. G. (1990). Alcohol and morality: a review of prospective studies. *British Journal of Addiction*, **85**, 837–47.

Shaper, A. G. (1993). Alcohol, and the heart and health [editorial]. *American Journal of Public Health*, **83**, 799–801.

Shaper, A. G., Wannamethee, G., and Walker, M. (1988). Alcohol and mortality in British men: explaining the U-shaped curve. *Lancet*, **ii**, 1267–73.

Stampfer, M. J., Colditz, G. A., Willet, W. C., Speizer, F. E., and Hennekens, C. H. (1988). A prospective study of moderate alcohol consumption and the risk of coronary disease and stroke in women. *New England Journal of Medicine*, **319**, 267–73.

Ueshima, H., *et al.* (1993). Effect of reduced alcohol consumption on blood pressure in untreated hypertensive men. *Hypertension*, **21**, 248–52.

USHHS (US Department of Health and Human Services) (1988). *The Surgeon General's report on nutrition and health*. Prima, Rocklin, CA.

USHHS (US Department of Health and Human Services) (1990). *Seventh special report to the US Congress on alcohol and health*. National Institute on Alcohol Abuse and Alcoholism (NIAAA), Rockville, MD.

Walker, M., Shaper, A. G., and Cook, D. G. (1987). Non-participation and mortality in a prospective study of cardiovascular disease. *Journal of Epidemiology and Community Health*, **41**, 295–9.

Wannamethee, G. and Shaper, A. G. (1988). Men who do not drink: A report from the British Regional Heart Study. *International Journal of Epidemiology*, **17**, 307–16.

Weinberg, C. R. (1993). Toward a clearer definition of confounding. *American Journal of Epidemiology*, **137**, 108.

Willett, W. C., Stampfer, M. J., Colditz, G. A., Rosner, B. A., Hennekens, C. H., and Speizer, F. E. (1987). Moderate alcohol consumption and the risk of breast cancer. *New England Journal of Medicine*, **316**, 1174–80.

Windham, G. C., Fenster, L., and Swan, S. H. (1992). Moderate maternal and paternal alcohol consumption and the risk of spontaneous abortion. *Epidemiology*, **3**, 364–70.

10. The economic evaluation of alcohol policies

Christine Godfrey and Alan Maynard

Introduction

The consequences of alcohol misuse produce problems in areas such as: mental and physical health; productivity and other employment problems; drink driving and other alcohol-related accidents; crime and public disorder; and social and family issues. These problems affect drinkers, their families, and the rest of society. Recent studies designed to use monetary values to measure some of these effects include: Rice *et al.* (1990) for the United States; Chetwynd and Rayner (1985) and Rayner and Chetwynd (1987) for New Zealand; Collins and Lapsey (1991) for Australia; and Maynard (1992) for England and Wales. The estimates for England and Wales in 1990 prices are given in Table 10.1.

The normal approach in these studies is to estimate direct health care costs associated with alcohol-related conditions and the indirect costs (usually in terms of productivity loss) of both morbidity and premature mortality. Other direct and indirect costs of accidents and criminal activity are also often included. Figures are prevalence based and relate to a particular time period usually one year. This methodology, usually referred to as a cost of illness approach, results in a summary figure which can be used in policy debates to signify the magnitude of alcohol-related problems. The estimates have, however, been subjected to a number of criticisms both by industry lobbies and for methodological reasons (for example, Heien and Pittman 1989; Godfrey and Powell 1987).

Rather than measuring total costs an alternative approach is to consider the factors which influence 'value for money' among the alternative interventions available to tackle alcohol-related problems and misuse. In particular, what incremental benefits can be produced at what additional cost by small changes in policy? As well as the social efficiency of different programmes, an additional criterion is the fairness of different policies; that is, who bears the costs of changes of policies and who gains the benefits.

Unfortunately, few economic evaluations of alternative strategies for

Table 10.1 The social costs of alcohol use: 1990 (£mn)

1. The social cost to industry	
(a) Sickness absence	964.37
(b) Housework services	64.78
(c) Unemployment	222.23
(d) Premature deaths	870.76
2. Social cost to the National Health Service	
(a) Psychiatric hospitals, inpatient costs (alcohol psychosis, alcohol dependence syndrome, non-dependent use of alcohol)	26.51
(b) Non-psychiatric hospitals, inpatient costs (alcoholic dependence syndrome, alcohol cirrhosis and liver disease)	10.64
(c) Other alcohol-related inpatient costs	109.41
(d) General practice costs	2.79
3. Society's response to alcohol-related problems	
(a) Expenditure by national-related problems	0.44
(b) Research	0.80
4. Social cost of material damage	
(a) Road traffic accidents (damage)	138.62
5. Social costs of criminal activities	
(a) Police involvement in traffic offences (excluding road traffic accidents)	6.53
(b) Police involvement in road traffic offences (including judiciary and insurance administration)	19.36
(c) Drink-related court cases	24.18
Total (excluding unemployment and premature death)	1368.43
Total (including unemployment and premature death)	2461.42

controlling alcohol misuse have been undertaken and, therefore, there are few case studies which can be used to aid policy decisions. The purpose of this chapter is to draw together information about the costs and benefits of different types of policy, outline common methodological problems, and provide some guidelines for the collection of data to aid decision-making in particular countries and situations.

Economic criteria and policy choices

Economic evaluations involve the comparison of the costs and benefits of two or more interventions. A checklist of potential costs and benefits associated with any policy are outlined in Table 10.2. The benefits from the policy options are the reductions in alcohol-related problems and improvements in public health. These benefits, both to the individual (private) and to the rest of society (third party or external), will depend on the effectiveness of each intervention.

Table 10.2 Checklist of potential costs and benefits of alcohol policies

1. Benefits and averted costs for individuals and family
   Contribution to quantity and quality of life of:
   - Immediate health benefits and reduced risk of future ill health (including loss of life)
   - Improved employment prospects and earnings
   - Social functioning
   - Reduction in risk of arrest for drunkenness, drinking and driving, violence
   - Other benefits: (a) less worry to families, (b) increased welfare from reduced spending on alcohol
2. Benefits (or averted costs) to third parties
   - Reduced future health care costs
   - Productivity and training gains for employers
   - Reduced criminal activity and criminal justice costs
   - Reduced social care, housing service demands etc.
   - Reduced accidents, fires—resource and third-party harm benefits
3. Direct costs of the policy
   - Administration and implementation costs, e.g., for taxes, liquor licences
   - Resource costs, e.g., media campaigns, provision of services, criminal justice costs
4. Indirect costs
   - Costs to other agencies, e.g., employers costs of workers in treatment, social care demands arising from increased health care treatments
   - Spillover effects on other alcohol-related problems
5. Costs to individuals and families
   - Direct costs of policy, e.g., expenses involved in treatments, travelling costs from availability controls
   - Indirect costs, especially loss of 'benefits' from alcohol consumption

The cost associated with each policy option can also be divided into direct costs of a programme, which include, for example, the costs of treatment or administration of licensing controls, and the indirect costs such as the value of lost productivity to employers from those undergoing treatment. Individuals may also incur direct costs such as expenses or time taken in treatment or extra expenses acquiring alcohol because of licensing restrictions.

The indirect costs include potential personal lost benefits from reduced alcohol consumption. Alcohol consumption is, for a considerable proportion of the population, a pleasurable experience. Economists usually consider the amount consumers are 'willing to pay' as a measure of this private benefit of consuming any good. In an efficient economy consumers will consume up to the point where the extra (marginal) benefit from consuming an additional drink is just equal to the cost, both monetary and the expected health and other problems, associated with that drink. That is, marginal private costs and benefits are equal at this point. While some prevention policies seek to change behaviour by persuasion or information others are 'imposed' across all drinkers. Examples are taxes and restrictions on availability. Such policies can distort the desired consumption pattern and thus consumers can suffer a loss in benefit or welfare. These calculations, however, assume alcohol is a normal good and that consumers are the best judges of their own welfare.

Two circumstances can alter these calculations and imply that the normal economic measures of the private benefits of alcohol consumption may be overstated. The first factor is the level of population awareness of the problems associated with inappropriate or excessive drinking. If drinkers are fully informed and rational in the economic sense, that is, they are the best judges of their own well-being, the potential costs will be taken into account when making decisions about how much and where to drink. However, if consumers are not fully informed, their assessment of private costs may be below the 'true' level and hence they will drink more than if fully informed. In these circumstances prevention policies by reducing consumption may improve the balance between costs and benefits and bring 'economic' welfare improvement. In these circumstances, including the full loss of 'benefit' from reductions in alcohol consumption in an assessment of a prevention policy would bias the evaluation of the coercive policy compared to an alternative without this characteristic.

Dealing with dependence is more complex. One definition of addiction is that addicted individuals gain no benefit at all from drinking. Therefore, a change in consumption patterns to other goods will produce benefits, in addition to health gains and reductions in other problems, not costs (Pogue and Sgontz 1989). More sophisticated 'rational' addiction models suggest a more dynamic approach is needed to understand these issues (Becker and Murphy 1988). These models, by allowing for tolerance, reinforcement, and withdrawal costs, can be used to describe many aspects of dependent behaviour. With such factors, drinkers demanding restrictive policies, such as taxes, can be shown to be rational in that for an individual they could improve the ratio of private costs to private benefits (Crain *et al.* 1987).

The benefits from alcohol vary across the different type of drinkers in a population. The more informed and less dependent the drinker the more likely he/she is to suffer a 'loss' if coercive prevention policies are imposed to set against any gain in benefits to both private and third parties from the reduction in alcohol-related problems. This mixture of drinkers will vary across time and countries.

In choosing the policy strategy towards alcohol misuse it is necessary to consider how the pattern of these different costs and benefits vary across the different types of interventions. The policy choices available to reduce the public health burden of alcohol problems can be divided into three groups: population-based policies such as tax, advertising, availability controls or health promotion campaigns; problem-directed policies such as specific drink driving initiatives; and direct interventions such as brief interventions, treatments, and rehabilitation programmes.

The first group of policies considered are those used primarily to change overall levels of alcohol consumption among the population. This group of policies may be directed primarily at consumers (demand), for example, tax levels or at producers and distributors (supply), for example, regulations on where and when alcohol can be sold, but they all 'distort' the alcohol market in some way through price, quality of the goods, or conditions of sale. Such strategies may be seen as relatively 'blunt' instruments as rather than being directed at those with problems they affect all drinkers. However, as discussed in other chapters these are generally the policies where effectiveness has been demonstrated.

The second group of policies are those directed at specific alcohol-related problems such as drink driving or alcohol-related offences. These policies are more targeted and hence are less likely to affect the non-problem drinker. However, there is a danger that one problem may be reduced at the risk of leaving others unaffected or even increased. In evaluating these policies it is therefore important to consider all the indirect effects and to have comparative measures on the costs of the problems at which specific programmes are directed.

The third group of policies includes all those interventions directed at individual drinkers. Many 'treatments' are only offered to those drinkers with the most problems or those at the severely dependent stage. Successful interventions have potentially therefore a major impact for improving the individual's quality of life but would have to reach a large proportion of this group to have a noticeable impact on the population level of problems. For some interventions such an expansion may have considerable cost implications.

The checklist of the different types of costs and benefits from Table 10.2 is applied in turn to each of these type of policies. Available research on the size of costs and benefits and the factors which influence them are reviewed. Finally, the distributional impacts of each policy, that is, fairness issues, are considered.

Population-based policies

Four distinct types of population policies are considered: (1) taxation; (2) information and health-promotion policies; (3) advertising; and (4) availability controls.

1. Taxation

Taxation is one of the most direct ways available of reducing alcohol consumption through increasing prices. Prices are one of the major influences on alcohol consumption and the benefits from this policy arise from the reduction in consumption and consequent reduction in problems. Studies have examined the relationship between changes in prices and alcohol consumption and have considered the effect of prices and taxes on alcohol-related problems such as liver cirrhosis and drink related traffic accidents (Saffer and Grossman 1987; Cook and Tauchen 1982). The benefits of tax policy will be enjoyed both by individuals and third parties.

Unlike tobacco, where similar price responsiveness has been found across different countries, price elasticities for alcohol vary across countries (see Österberg, Ch. 6, this volume). Price responsiveness also differs across beverages with the most popular drink in a country usually being the least responsive to price changes. These sort of differences would imply a uniform change in prices would not result in an equal reduction in consumption across the beverages.

The benefits from increased prices will be reduced if income is also increasing. For example, Godfrey and Maynard (1992) suggest that a 5 per cent annual increase in price in the United Kingdom would reduce alcohol consumption by 31 per cent by the year 2000 but this reduction would be reduced to 20 per cent if income grew at 2 per cent per annum and alcohol consumption would be 14 per cent higher if income were to grow at 3 per cent per annum.

A further limit to potential benefits from a taxation policy is the extent to which increases in taxes result in higher prices. This depends on the actions of manufacturers and distributors who may decide to reduce their profits rather than passing on tax increases in full to the consumer. This is a potential problem if the industry decides to oppose a prevention strategy. In practice, however, announcement of a tax change have been used by manufacturers to increase prices by more than the tax change (Cook 1981; Godfrey *et al.* 1992).

Imposing tax increases are usually assumed to result in few additional direct costs. In most countries, the costs of collecting extra tax are small compared to the costs of changing other taxes such as income tax. There is, however, the possibility of indirect costs. Large tax increases may result in increases in smuggling or illegal home-brewing and hence increases in enforcement costs. The change from consuming licit to illicit alcohol can also have additional health consequences. The likelihood of increases in home-brewing or distilling vary from country to country.

Taxation can be a blunt instrument policy with any increases being borne by all drinkers not just those with problems. The distribution of 'lost benefits' will be uneven with the fully informed and non-dependent drinkers, for example, bearing the full amount of lost benefits from, say, an increase in taxation. This compares to alternative policies which may only change the behaviour of those who are ill-informed or dependent.

The importance of distinguishing the costs and benefits for different types of drinkers will depend on the policy question being addressed and the current tax and problem level in any country. For example, Richardson and Crowley (1992) did not make any adjustment for lack of information or dependence on their measure of benefits of alcohol consumption. Their measure was based on consumers' willingness to pay for alcohol as a normal good. The calculated value of the willingness to pay for alcohol was compared to the total social costs of alcohol in Australia, in order to make some recommendations about tax levels. They concluded that because costs were much larger than these estimated benefits from consumption there was evidence to support a substantial rise in alcohol taxes. Hence, in this analysis the potential 'overstatement' of the benefits of alcohol do not alter the conclusions. In other circumstances, the comparison of costs and benefits of different policies may not be clear-cut. To adjust the 'benefit' measure where the proportion unaware of the dangers of consumption or the number who are 'addicted' is not known requires other assumptions (see Godfrey 1991, for further discussion). While this approach would not necessarily give definitive answers it does provide a framework within which policy discussions can take place.

An additional issue when considering the fairness of tax as a prevention strategy is the burden it imposes on lower-income families. Unlike tobacco, however, alcohol is generally highly responsive to income changes. This implies that those on higher incomes consume more and hence bear more of the tax burden for this good.

2. *Information and health-promotion policies*

Population-based information policies include warning labels, direct health campaigns, and media coverage of alcohol-related issues. The common theme is that these activities affect the knowledge consumers have about the harmful effects of alcohol. The prevention policies are designed to give information or reduce misinformation. Well-informed consumers may reduce their consumption and the related problems. Certain information campaigns may be directed at minimizing problems rather than reduction of consumption.

Direct education, especially media campaigns, have the most obvious visible resource costs. The cost-effectiveness of stand alone media campaigns has been frequently questioned (for example, Grant 1989). There may be wider benefits from such activity, however, including the role they play in agenda-setting and generating 'free' media coverage. The UK Department of Transport found the majority who were aware of drink driving campaign messages got their information not from their sponsored TV, newspaper, and poster advertisements but from news coverage on television and in the newspapers about the campaign (Harrison and Tether 1990).

An alternative way of using limited resources is to concentrate information activities on a particular day. Evaluation of national no-smoking days have suggested that these activities are a cost-effective way of reducing smoking (Townsend 1984) but it is unclear whether the more complex messages associated with sensible drinking will have similar results. Media campaigns with more extensive community action may be required (Casswell *et al.* 1990).

Requiring industry to supply information through labelling is a means of shifting some of the direct costs of information policy from the taxpayer to the industry and hence the consumers of alcohol. As well as information on the products there can also be requirements for displaying information at the point of sale. Legislation or voluntary agreements are not costless to introduce. Consultation, lobbying, and enacting legislation imposes costs, although labelling policies may require less enforcing and monitoring than advertising or licensing controls.

A major contrast between information and taxation policies is their effects on lost benefits from changes in alcohol consumption. The changes resulting from information policies are voluntary. Those who, after the receipt of information, still value alcohol consumption more than the cost they expect from that consumption are unlikely to change their behaviour.

3. *Advertising controls*

The effects of advertising on alcohol consumption is a controversial area with considerable dispute between health and trade lobbies about the size of potential benefits of increasing controls of advertising. The effects of misleading advertising on the young is of particular concern. Most studies suggest controls or bans on advertising have small to moderate effects on consumption levels.

Advertising controls involve direct costs in terms of bureaucratic time and enforcement activity. Indirect costs may also occur. Industries will try to subvert regulatory policies, for example, by replacing controlled advertising with activities like sports sponsorship. Such changes in activities may increase consumption and problems or limit their reduction. Alcohol advertising bans may have additional indirect effects. With no advertising, the costs facing firms fall which could be passed on in lower prices. Also, price competition may replace that previously conducted via advertising. Both in the United Kingdom and the United States the spirits industries voluntarily stopped advertising on television as the industries calculated that this 'health' measure was in their collective commercial interest.

One of the major 'costs' highlighted by trade groups is the restraint advertising restrictions have on commercial freedom. This is a rather intangible concept but it could be thought to embrace the belief that restrictions on industries affect competitive structure and hence efficiency. Inefficient firms will waste scarce resources and total welfare in the society will be lower than if all firms were efficient. This inefficiency in industry usually manifests itself as higher prices. This raises a possibility of a health/wealth trade off between different areas of government policy, that is, the same levels of overall social welfare may be possible with different mixtures of alcohol problems and inefficient production. It should be noted, however, that the current structure of the alcohol industry in many countries is far from the economic benchmark model with only a few large companies or even state monopolies. The effect of any change in current policies in terms of additional loss in their efficiency may therefore be small. Existing firms will, however, lobby intensively to retain their present commercial advantages.

Advertising policies may result in some unforeseen costs in terms of reduced 'quality' and variety of good produced. For example, it would be difficult to introduce new products with an advertising ban. This may result in some loss to non-problem drinkers but the consumers' valuation of these effects in relation to alcohol are unknown.

Information and advertising policies are also associated with distributional questions, especially concerning who bears the direct costs of the programmes. Mass media campaigns are usually financed from health budgets or general taxation whereas advertising regulation costs are more likely to fall on the industry initially and hence to the drinker or shareholder. An alternative way of financing health-information programmes is to put a levy on alcohol advertising which shifts the costs back to the industry. This strategy may provide more realistic levels of finance for health education and other prevention policies. Current activities for alcohol health education in the United Kingdom total at most £8mn compared to £160mn on press and TV advertising.

4. Other controls on availability of alcohol

There are a range of other policies which restrict the availability of alcohol. The details of these policies and the acceptability of different options varies across cultures (see the Introduction to this volume). Controls on availability have, however, been found to reduce alcohol consumption and hence problems. Adjustments to regulations or help in enforcing regulations, for example, by server-training can improve the effectiveness and hence benefits from these types of policies.

The 'costs' of different types of regulation on the sale and production of alcohol are similar to those discussed for advertising, particularly the potential for trade-off between wealth or industrial efficiency policies and health. The 1980s saw a general shift to deregulate industries in many countries and relaxations in regulation to increase the availability of alcohol were part of this trend. This may reflect a change in the 'value' given to gains from competition rather than a lowering of the perceived costs of alcohol misuse.

Problem-directed policies

An alternative approach to reducing consumption is to attempt to influence directly the rate of problems. There have, for example, been a range of specific drink driving policies introduced in most countries. Such policies may have additional benefits on other alcohol problems by reducing consumption. Other more direct harm minimization strategies (for example, those directed to reducing intoxication), may leave consumption unchanged or even lead to increases. Some policies may be directed at reducing costs to third parties (for example, reducing public order problems) rather than aiding individual drinkers. This raises the possibility that targeted policies may reduce problems in one area but increase those in others, especially long-term health problems.

Crime, accidents, and reduced productivity were considered in earlier alcohol cost studies, and prevention policies specific to these problems could be devised. In most countries, however, drink driving has received the greatest attention and a wide range of alternative policies have been adopted. Drinking and driving enforcement can involve considerable resource costs but the potential benefits in terms of the value of the reduced fatalities and injuries are also high. Policies may be differentially effective according to how they affect individual perceptions of risks of apprehension and the size of punishment. Random breath-testing (RBT) as carried out in parts of Australia and Finland, for example, are designed to yield a high probability of being stopped across the whole population. The increase in effectiveness and hence benefits is thought to be greater than the increased enforcement costs. If population behaviour changes (for example, population tolerance of drink driving decreases), and the incidence of drink driving incidents which would occur without RBT falls, then the cost-effectiveness calculations also change. In the United Kingdom the government has been reluctant to introduce RBT even though opinion polls suggest a high level of public support. The argument put forward by the government is that such policies impose too high a cost in terms of civil liberties, as another kind of distributional consequence with those not causing problems bearing costs in terms of restrictions on freedom.

Types of crime associated with alcohol range from those which, by definition, are alcohol-related, such as public drunkenness, to others where the role of alcohol is more difficult to quantify, such as crimes of violence or child abuse. The relationship between alcohol and crime is likely to be complex (Ensor and Godfrey 1993). Different crimes have different resource and intangible costs which prevention policies may reduce. Media attention on a particular crime, for example, disorder at sporting events or in city centres, may significantly raise the fear associated with that type of crime.

Any new legislation may restrict civil liberties. For example, concern in the United States about youths' involvement in drink driving fatalities led to increases in minimum drinking ages from 18 to 21. In the United Kingdom concern about football violence and public order offences resulted in banning the sale of alcohol and sports grounds introducing bans on the public consumption of alcohol in certain areas. This contrasts with the attitude of the same UK government to random breath-testing.

For both accidents and crime, therefore, the potential cost-effectiveness of different measures will be affected mainly by 'perceived' valuations about both problem and policy and whether policy-effectiveness results in greater benefits than the resources needed to implement them.

It should also be noted that other general policies may be more cost-effective than alcohol-specific alternatives when considering the outcome in terms of the particular problem. Providing safer environments, such as better cars and safer roads, fitting smoke detectors in private dwellings, etc., may reduce the 'harm' from the misuse of alcohol. Cameron (1979) considered a number of road safety measures and 'combined alcohol safety action countermeasures' was ranked third in terms of potential casualty savings but only 37 when ranked by cost-effectiveness criteria.

Reductions in lost productivity in the workplace may seem to have the highest potential for generating benefits. Current levels of cost do not seem to be reflected in lower wages for those with the highest level of consumption (Cook 1991). These findings would suggest that costs are being mainly borne by workmates, employers, and taxpayers. The costs to individuals may, however, be more complex and Mullahy and Sindelar (1989) suggest that alcohol consumption among the young affects educational attainment and hence occupation and lifetime earnings. Workplace interventions vary especially in the balance between disciplinary and assistance elements. While the setting may vary the type of intervention offered in the assistance-type policies are similar to those offered by health services, and they are reviewed briefly below.

Direct alcohol intervention policies

Increasing alcohol-related services is another alternative means of reducing alcohol-related harm. There are few full economic evaluations of the wide range of 'treatments' offered. Alcohol interventions can be offered for a spectrum of alcohol consumption and problems and in a number of different settings. They have the potential for reducing social as well as health problems and hence reducing third-party as well as individual costs of alcohol misuse.

Two areas of research illustrate the potential for services to achieve benefits in terms of adverted costs. In the United States, a number of studies have examined the effect of a specific alcohol treatment on all other health costs and their results suggest that the costs of treatment may be offset by reductions in other health care expenditures (Holder 1987; Holder and Blose 1992). These studies have not generally included any allowance for potential reductions in other social costs. A second set of studies have examined the relationship between levels of treatment and a number of alcohol problems (Smart and Mann, 1990; Holder and Parker 1992). Increases in the level of treatment have been shown to lead to a fall in certain problems in these studies.

More specific reviews of the potential for cost-effectiveness of different types of interventions have been undertaken (Holder *et al.* 1991; Godfrey 1992). The conclusions that can be drawn from available evidence are that low-cost interventions may be as effective as more expensive treatments for many problem drinkers. Brief interventions may also bring net benefits to a wide range of drinkers but adopting this strategy is not without considerable resource consequences. Other groups will remain in need of more intensive interventions. Matching services to clients may improve outcomes and result in interventions being cost-beneficial to society as a whole.

Summary of available evidence on policy choice

A summary of evidence about the costs and benefits associated with different types of policy is given in Table 10.3. These estimates could be refined for more specific policies and for some countries where more data are available. However, in general there are many unknowns or broadly similar magnitudes of costs and benefits within the different categories.

There are only a limited number of studies which have attempted to compare the benefits from different policies. Saffer and Grossman (1987), for example, suggest that increasing taxes in the United States may be more effective in reducing alcohol-related traffic fatalities than raising the minimum drinking ages. Other non-alcohol-related policies, such as improving cars and roads, can be even more cost-effective when the outcomes are measured in terms of the problem.

Improving estimates: methodological issues and data requirements

The summary evidence suggests that if economic evaluations are to aid policy choice more detailed studies are required. In this section, some of the methodological issues that arise in undertaking such evaluations and the consequent data requirements are discussed.

1. Policy questions and choice of techniques

There are three main types of economic evaluation techniques: cost–benefit analysis; cost effectiveness; and cost utility. The main difference between the techniques, illustrated in Table 10.4, is the method used to evaluate benefits. In cost–benefit analysis all benefits are measured in monetary terms and this technique is useful when the benefits from different policies are mixed. Cost–effectiveness analysis is useful when the policy alternatives being evaluated have effects on the same and easily measured outcome, for example, two alternative ways of saving years of life from alcohol-related causes. This technique may be of only limited use for alcohol policies because the effects of

Table 10.3 Summary of evidence on costs and benefits of alternative policies

Policy	Benefits		Costs		Lost 'benefit' from alcohol consumption	Other individual costs
	Individual	Third party	Direct	Indirect		
Population-based						
Tax	Moderate to high	Moderate to high	Low	Variable	Moderate/High	Low
Information	Unproven	Unproven	High (for media) to moderate	Low	None/Low	Low
Advertising	Low to moderate	Low to moderate	Moderate	Moderate	Low	Low
Availability	Moderate	Moderate	Moderate	Moderate	Moderate	Moderate
Problem-based	Moderate	Moderate	Variable	Moderate/High if other problems increase	None/Low	Variable
Direct interventions	Variable	Variable	Moderate/ High	Moderate	Low	Low/Moderate

Table 10.4 Types of economic evaluation

Method	Cost measurement	Benefit measurement: What?	Benefit measurement: How value?
Cost–benefit analysis	Monetary terms	All effects produced by the alternative	Monetary terms
Cost-effective analysis	Monetary terms	Single common specific variable achieved to varying extents	Common units (e.g., life years) within intervention area
Cost–utility analysis	Monetary terms	Effects of the competing therapies and achieved to differing levels	QALYs or healthy year equivalents (common units across interventions)

alcohol are so wide and there would be a danger in evaluating alternative policies using one outcome measure. Cost–utility analysis has been used most extensively in health care evaluations and outcomes in these studies are measured by indices which take account of changes in both quality and quantity of life of the individuals concerned. These types of measures avoid some of the problems of valuing life which is discussed in more detail below.

Each type of evaluation in Table 10.4 requires slightly different data. However, some items of cost or expected benefits may be the same for each policy alternative, thus reducing data requirements.

2. *Marginal analysis*

Decision-makers frequently have questions about whether to spend an additional US$100 000 on one project or another. To inform these choices requires data about the marginal or incremental attributes of their choices. What additional benefit will investing an additional US$100 000 in intervention *X* produce compared to the additional benefit from investing the increment in resources project *Y*. Data, such as that in Table 10.1 (the total cost of alcohol misuse), are useless for this purpose. These data inform the decision-maker about the total cost of the problem but give no indication which of many policy options will give the biggest bang for the buck. Only studies which show the marginal costs and benefits of intervention options can inform these key choices.

3. *Measuring the value of life*

One of the most serious consequences of alcohol misuse is the premature loss of life. A major benefit from prevention policies is therefore to reduce this burden. Valuing human life, especially in monetary terms, does, however, pose a number of methodological problems.

Pearce and Knight (1989) suggest that the loss of life (or injury and ill-health) has three components:

(1) the individual's own value of life;

(2) the value placed on risks to others. Mooney (1989) suggests this may be an important element in society's valuation of drug problems. This is a wider notion of caring than the intangible pain, grief, and suffering of families and friends of alcohol misusers; and

(3) any other net costs borne by society. This could include productivity losses; that is, the loss of labour resources.

There are three main methods of valuing loss of life: in terms of human capital; willingness to pay; or in natural units. Most of the costing studies, such as reported in Table 10.1, have used the human capital approach. This method consists of considering the loss of earnings over what would have been the expected years of life and discounting this sum to a present value. This is a narrow view of the value of life and does not take into account unemployment and the costs of training. In some social cost estimates, (see Table 10.1), figures are presented excluding an allowance for excess unemployment. The human capital approach remains a discriminatory measure with lower values being placed on those with lower earnings potential. In many studies, values are included for those not currently in productive employment such as the young, home-bound, and the elderly. Adjustments for those not currently employed and 'pain, grief, and suffering' have been included in some studies but this further obscures the bases of the valuation.

An alternative approach is to attempt to measure directly the individual's valuation of life. The methods used, however, yield a wide range of values. Richardson and Crowley (1992), for example, calculate a range between Aus$0.6 million to Aus$4.8 million per life in 1991 values. Generally, this method gives much higher values than the human capital approach. For example, in the United Kingdom, the Department of Transport changed from a human capital to willingness to pay valuation for their calculations of the costs of road traffic fatalities (including those caused by drinking and driving). The human capital value, including an allowance for pain, grief, and suffering which made up 50 per cent of the total, was £283 000. The value chosen using the willingness-to-pay method, based on the minimum value of many experts, was £500 000 (Dalvi 1988). Using these types of estimates will considerably increase the benefits of alcohol prevention policies compared to using a human capital approach. For example, the value of the 30 000 or more alcohol-related deaths which occur annually in England would far exceed the total social cost figure given in Table 10.1.

The willingness-to-pay method is subject to a number of criticisms because of the difficulties of eliciting consistent valuations from individuals and that their valuations are also based on the current distribution of income. This is likely, for example, to give very different values across countries. The coverage of this measure is also not clear, that is, are individuals only including the value of their own lives or are they including an altruistic element? Also, the sums are usually expressed as an average for all lives and hence in their use no distinction is made from saving the life of a 18- or 80-year-old person.

A third approach used frequently in health care evaluations is to use some natural unit, such as life years gained, sometimes quality-adjusted. In using this type of measure it is assumed that from a society perspective it is equitable to value a life year as equal whatever the age, sex, or social class of the recipient. Measures, such as quality-adjusted life years (QALYs) or well-years, have been developed further to include changes in the quality as well as quantity of life and this allows a comparison of life-saving to life-enhancing policies. The disadvantage of this approach is that by presenting the results as net cost per life year or per QALY comparisons are restricted to other 'health'-related areas rather than broader policies which may only include monetary costs and benefits.

Whatever measure is used, some assumption is being made about the relative value of life between individuals and the acceptability of different measures could well vary with political and cultural factors. Hence, in countries with a 'libertarian' tradition, values based on willingness-to-pay methods may seem more acceptable than the equalitarian-based values implicit in most natural unit measures.

4. Should transfer payments be included?

Taxes and other transfers need to be considered to answer questions such as: 'Do drinkers pay their way?' This question relates to 'fairness' (that is, does the tax on alcohol cover the excess expenditure by governments on drinkers?) and not to cost burdens. Tranfer payments include taxes on alcohol and on wages, social security, and state pension payments, and these payments are transfers from drinkers to the government. Such transfers alter the distribution of ownership of resources among individuals in a community.

Another confusion arises from the use of a different type of study which seeks to address the questions about whether drinkers impose third-party costs on society. In these studies the amount of extra tax paid by drinkers (or sometimes those just misusing alcohol) is examined to see if it is sufficient to cover the value of the costs they impose on third parties. If these taxes are not sufficient, that is, there are net external costs from alcohol misuse, this implies that current policies may not be efficient and the total welfare of society could be increased by reducing alcohol problems. In such circumstances, one policy option is to increase tax levels to bring about a behaviour change and it is the behaviour change that would result in increased benefit rather than a change in revenue (which could be negative if consumption was reduced).

Transfers are an important part of two specific types of study. First, the 'fairness' of a policy change may be the issue of primary concern. Secondly, in some studies, the outcome of any change of policy for government finances may be of political importance. However, when considering the balance of total social costs and benefits between different policies, that is, does one policy have a greater gain in welfare than another, transfer payments are neither a cost nor a benefit.

5. Should changes in resources used in the production of alcohol be considered?

From the public health perspective some have claimed that because of the harm associated with alcohol the resources used in production would bring greater welfare if they were used to produce alternative goods. Alternatively, industry lobbies frequently use arguments about the benefits of the alcohol industry in terms of jobs, revenue, and exports, to argue against the imposition of prevention policies (Booth *et al.* 1990). Neither argument can be fully supported by economic theory.

Leu (1983) suggests that the allocation of resources between the production of different goods adapts to consumer preferences in an efficient economy. Benefits or costs of a change of production should not therefore be included in the evaluation of different prevention policies. However, although the economy may be fully adjusting in time, there may be adjustment costs and this creates the 'political' costs to governments which may face a trade-off between health and wealth objectives.

The other extreme position that any resources devoted to alcohol production are wasteful is also difficult to justify. This position could only be upheld for alcohol misusers who were so 'addicted' to alcohol that they received no pleasure or benefit from drinking (Godfrey 1991).

6. Timing and uncertainty

Policies to reduce drinking among young adults are likely to have immediate benefits in terms of fewer alcohol-related accidents but the gain from reducing other health problems may not be realized for 20 to 30 years. Economists usually deal with differential timing by discounting both the costs and benefits to a present value, often using quite a low discount rate (for example, 5 per cent) and subjecting the analysis to only limited-sensitivity analysis. There is, however, some dispute about whether health gains should be discounted in the same way as monetary costs and benefits (Parsonage and Neuberger 1992).

Discounting will give lower weight to future health gains and therefore if applied some prevention strategies will be judged less cost-effective than those with more immediate benefits. Consequently, current research which is revealing high discount rates (perhaps as high as 7–10 per cent) means that investment in health education interventions may be cost-ineffective. For example, many people die every year from alcohol-related accidents. Using the figures for England and Wales and assuming some event/policy resulted in no deaths for one year then a total health gain of 148 500 life years would be achieved over the following 30-year period. However, discounting these benefits by 5 per cent would reduce the present value of these health gains to 85 800 life years, and by 10 per cent the total would only be estimated at 57 000, less than half the undiscounted figure. An accident-based policy, especially one directed at young people, would, in terms of benefits, fall in priority if health benefits are discounted.

Calculating both benefits and costs using an incidence approach requires more information and assumptions about the future than the prevalence estimates. It is necessary to be able to predict how and when changes in alcohol consumption patterns are going to affect different alcohol problems. These types of calculations not only require considerable amount of data but will by necessity involve a degree of uncertainty. Testing the sensitivity of results to changes in assumptions, such as the predicted size and timing of changes in alcohol-related problems, is an important part of developing the use of economic evaluation techniques.

7. Conclusions

The data requirements for the economic evaluations of alcohol policies are considerable. The method requires data on both costs and consequences from the alternative approaches over a number of time periods. Also, it is necessary to have data on the effects of expanding and contracting the scope of each option. Many items are difficult to value. The evaluation techniques are powerful but will not always provide definitive answers. The techniques also require a number of assumptions being made and therefore it is important that checks on any practical evaluation are undertaken. These checks will include questions such as:

1. Have all the relevant policy alternatives been considered in the evaluation study?
2. Is the evidence on which the benefits and costs of the different options robust?
3. Have all the relevant costs and benefits been included and valued appropriately?
4. Have marginal costs and benefits for each option been identified?

5. Have both costs and benefits been discounted?

6. Have all the assumptions been subject to sensitivity analysis?

7. Has the distributional consequences or fairness of the different policies been considered?

Information is limited and it is difficult to enumerate many of the costs and benefits attached to the different individual prevention strategies discussed in this chapter. However, where comparative research has been undertaken there is some evidence that effective population-based approaches may be more cost-effective than problem-based policies. Such tentative findings cannot be generalized too far and the most cost-effective strategy for any country is likely to contain a mixture of population, problem, and direct interventions. A further area considered in this chapter is the effects of different policies on the distribution of costs and benefits between different types of drinkers and this information may also inform policy debates.

Economic evaluations are not value-free and the weights attached to different 'intangible' items will vary between countries, cultures, and over time. Great caution has to be taken, therefore, in giving general conclusions about the cost-effectiveness of different prevention strategies but the techniques allow a more structured discussion about the importance of some of these intangible items.

The balance of total social costs and benefits for each alternative policy is, however, only one potential factor in the decision-making process. It is important to note the perceived 'political' costs of introducing different policies may not be ranked in the same order as they would be using cost-effectiveness (Van Iwaarden 1989). Revenue and employment consequences may not be true economic costs but are factors likely to be taken into account by politicians.

The first requirement for improving estimates of cost-effectiveness of competing policy interventions is establishing the effectiveness of policies on alcohol consumption and problems in properly designed studies, as reviewed in other chapters in this book. There is also considerable scope for methodological improvements in developing frameworks and tackling issues, such as valuing loss of life, and measuring changes in the benefits from alcohol consumption. The use of computer simulations and scenario analysis could also be explored further (Holder and Doria 1990).

The potential for using economic evaluations to further research into the prevention of alcohol problems is considerable. To improve techniques and estimates, however, requires input from a range of disciplines. One purpose of this chapter is to provide one starting point to stimulate these developments, just as earlier social cost estimates stimulated debate about the seriousness of alcohol-related problems.

Acknowledgements

Christine Godfrey gratefully acknowledges the financial support from the Alcohol Education and Research Council London, UK for the project 'Changing the social costs of alcohol misuse'.

References

Becker, G. S. and Murphy, K. M. (1988). A Theory of rational addiction. *Journal of Political Economy*, **96(4)**, 675–700.

Booth, M., Hartley, K., and Powell, M. (1990). Industry: structure, performance and policy. In *Preventing alcohol and tobacco problems*, (ed. A. Maynard and P. Tether), Vol. 1. Avebury, Aldershot, UK.

Cameron, T. (1979). The impact of drinking-driving countermeasures: a review and evaluation. *Contemporary Drug Problems*, **8**, 495–565.

Casswell, S. *et al.* (1990). Evaluation of a mass-media campaign for the primary prevention of alcohol related problems. *Health Promotion International*, **5**, 9–17.

Chetwynd, J. and Rayner, T. (1985). The economic costs to New Zealand of lost production due to alcohol abuse. *New Zealand Medical Journal*, **98**, 694–7.

Collins, D. J. and Lapsley, H. (1991). *Estimating the economic costs of drug abuse in Australia*. Report prepared for the Department of Community Service and Health for use in association with the National Campaign Against Drug Abuse.

Cook, P. J. (1981). The effect of liquor taxes on drinking, cirrhosis, and auto fatalities. *Alcohol and public policy: Beyond the shadow of prohibition*, (ed. M. Moore and D. Gerstein), pp. 255–85. National Academy of Sciences, Washington, DC.

Cook, P. J. (1991). The social costs of drinking. In *The negative social consequences of alcohol use*. Norwegian Ministry of Health and Social Affairs, Oslo.

Cook, P. J. and Tauchen, G. (1982). The effect of liquor taxes on heavy drinking. *Bell Journal of Economics*, Autumn, 379–90.

Crain, M., Deaton, T., Holcombe, R., and Tollison, R. (1987). Rational choice and the taxation of sin. *Journal of Public Economics*, **8**, 239–45.

Dalvi, M. Q. (1988). *The value of life and safety: a search for a consensus estimate*. Department of Transport, London.

Ensor, T. and Godfrey, C. (1993). Modelling the interactions between alcohol, crime and the criminal justice system. *Addiction*, **88**, 477–87.

Godfrey, C. (1991). The social costs of drinking. In *The negative social consequences of alcohol use*. Norwegian Ministry of Health and Social Affairs, Oslo.

Godfrey, C. (1992). *The cost-effectiveness of alcohol services: Lessons for contracting*. YARTIC Occasional Paper 2, Centre for Health Economics, University of York and Leeds Addiction Unit.

Godfrey, C. and Maynard, A. (1992). *A health strategy for alcohol; Setting targets and choosing policies*, YARTIC Occasional Paper 1, Centre for Health Economics, University of York and Leeds Addiction Unit.

Godfrey, C. and Powell, M. (1987). Making sense of social cost studies of alcohol and tobacco. In *The costs of alcohol, drugs and tobacco to society—papers and abstracts*. Institute of Preventive and Social Psychiatry, Erasmus University, Rotterdam.

Godfrey, C., Hardman, G., and Maynard, A. (1992). *Controlling alcohol and tobacco consumption: Scenarios for the 1992 budget*. Centre for Health Economics, University of York.

Grant, M. (1989). Controlling alcohol abuse. In *Controlling legal addictions*, (ed. D. Robinson, A. Maynard, and R. Chester), pp. 63–83. Macmillan, Basingstoke.

Harrison, L. and Tether, P. (1990). Information and voluntary agreements: the policy networks. In *Preventing alcohol and tobacco problems*, (ed. C. Godfrey and D. Robinson), Vol. 2, pp. 25–43. Avebury, Aldershot, UK.

Heien, D. M. and Pittman, D. J. (1989). The economic costs of alcohol abuse: an assessment of current methods and estimates. *Journal of Studies on Alcohol*, **50**, 567–79.

Holder, H. (1987). Alcoholism treatment and potential health care cost saving. *Medical Care*, **25**, 52–71.

Holder, H. and Blose, J. O. (1992). The reduction in health care costs associated with alcoholism treatment: a 14-year longitudinal study, *Journal of Studies on Alcohol*, **53**, 293–302.

Holder, H. and Doria, J. (1990). Computers in prevention research. *Alcohol Health and Research World*, **14**, 246–51.

Holder, H. and Parker, R. N. (1992). Effects of alcoholism treatment on cirrhosis mortality: a 20 year multivariate time series analysis. *British Journal of Addiction*, **87**, 1263–74.

Holder, H., Longabaugh, R., Miller, W. R., and Rubonis, A. V. (1991). The cost effectiveness of treatment for alcoholism: a first approximation. *Journal of Studies on Alcohol*, **52**, 517–40.

Leu, R. (1983). What can economists contribute? In *Economics and alcohol*, (ed. M. Grant, M. Plant, and A. Williams), pp. 13–33. Croom Helm, London.

Maynard, A. (1992). *YARTIC Newsletter 2*. Centre for Health Economics, University of York and Leeds Addiction Unit.

Maynard, A., Hardman, G., and Whelan, A. (1987). Measuring the social costs of addictive substances. *British Journal of Addiction*, **82**, 701–16.

Mooney, G. (1989). What price the humanitarian considerations? *British Journal of Addiction*, **84**, 470–1.

Mullahy, J. and Sindelar, J. L. (1989). Life cycle effects of alcoholism on education, earnings and occupation. *Inquiry*, **26**, 272–82.

Parsonage, M. and Neuberger, H. (1992). Discounting health benefits. *Health Economics*, **1**, 71–6.

Pearce, D. and Knight, I. (1989). *Valuation of non-fatal road accident casualties. An evaluation of alternative approaches*. Paper presented at a seminar on the valuation of non-fatal casualties. Department of Transport, London.

Pogue, T. F. and Sgontz, L. G. (1989). Taxing to control social costs: the case of alcohol. *The American Economic Review*, **79**, 235–43.

Rayner, T. and Chetwynd, J. (1987). The economic cost of alcohol-related health care in New Zealand. *British Journal of Addiction*, **82**, 59–66.

Rice, D. P., Kelman, S., and Miller, L. S. (1990). *The economic costs of alcohol and drug abuse and mental illness, 1985*. Institute for Health and Aging, San Francisco.

Richardson, J. and Crowley, S. (1992). *Taxation to minimise the social and economic costs of alcohol consumption*, (Working Paper 10). National Centre for Health Program Evaluation, Monash University and the University of Melbourne.

Saffer, H. and Grossman, M. (1987). Drinking age laws and highway mortality rates: cause and effect. *Economic Inquiry*, **25**, 403–17.

Smart, R. G. and Mann, R. T. (1990). Are increases in treatment levels and Alcoholics

Anonymous membership large enough to reduce liver cirrhosis rates? *British Journal of Addiction*, **85**, 1291–8.
Townsend, J. (1984). Cost effectiveness. In *Smoking control: Strategies and evaluation in community and mass media programmes*, (ed. J. Croften and M. Wood). Health Education Council, London.
Van Iwaarden, M. J. (1989). An economist in 'alcohol policy country' *British Journal of Addiction*, **84(10)**, 1205–16.

Subject index

Page numbers in bold denote main entries

Name index

Page numbers in bold denote main entries